Cybercrime

Cybercrime focuses on the growing concern about the use of electronic communication for criminal activities and the appropriateness of the countermeasures that are being adopted by law enforcement agencies, security services and legislators to address such anxieties. Fuelled by sensational media headlines and news coverage which has done much to encourage the belief that technologies like the Internet are likely to lead to a lawless electronic frontier, *Cybercrime* provides a more considered and balanced perspective on what is an important and contested arena for debate. It will provide an understanding of the basic issues relating to cybercrime and its impact on society.

The volume is divided into three parts: the first focuses upon electronic criminal behaviour; the second discusses preservation of privacy and liberty, and challenges the danger of surveillance as a tool to combat cybercrime; and the final section is concerned with attempts to draft legislation in order to protect electronic communication users and to facilitate the policing of illegal activities.

This book will be essential reading for students of criminology, public administration, politics, sociology and social policy.

Douglas Thomas is Assistant Professor at the Annenberg School for Communication, University of Southern California, USA. **Brian D. Loader** is Co-Director of CIRA, University of Teesside, UK, and Editor of the international journal *Information, Communication & Society* (www.infosoc.co.uk).

Cybercrime

Law enforcement, security
and surveillance in the
information age

**Edited by Douglas Thomas
and Brian D. Loader**

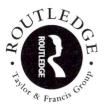

London and New York

First published 2000
by Routledge
11 New Fetter Lane, London EC4P 4EE

Simultaneously published in the USA and Canada
by Routledge
29 West 35th Street, New York, NY 10001

Routledge is an imprint of the Taylor & Francis Group

Typeset in Garamond by Taylor & Francis Books Ltd
Printed and bound in Great Britain by Biddles Ltd, Guildford
and King's Lynn

British Library Cataloguing in Publication Data
A catalogue record for this book is available from the British Library

Library of Congress Cataloging in Publication Data
Cybercrime: Law Enforcement, Security and Surveillance in the
Information Age / edited by Douglas Thomas and Brian D. Loader.
    Includes bibliographical references and index.
    1. Computer crimes – United States – prevention.
    2. Computer crimes – prevention. 3. Privacy, right of.
    I. Douglas, Thomas. II. Loader, Brian, 1958–
    HV6773.3.U5 C93 2000
    364.16'8–dc21   99-049215

ISBN 0–415–21325–8 (hbk)
ISBN 0–415–21326–6 (pbk)

For Kim, William and Christopher

Contents

Illustrations

Figures

Tables

Contributors

Julia D. Babaeva is an associate professor in the Psychology Dept at Moscow State Lomonosov University. Her interests are in the psychology of giftedness and creativity.

William E. Baugh, Jr is vice president, Science Applications International Corporation, and general manager, Advanced Network Technologies and Security Operations. He is former assistant director, Federal Bureau of Investigation. E-mail: William.E.Baugh@Jrcpmx.saic.com

Peter Blume is professor of legal informatics in the Faculty of Law at the University of Copenhagen, Denmark. He is a member of the European Union's Legal Advisory Board, DGXIII and vice-president of the International Federation of Computer Law Associations. He has published a number of books and articles on data protection, legal information retrieval, intellectual copyright and jurisprudence. E-mail: Peter.Blume@jur.ku.dk

Philip H.J. Davies is currently lecturing in sociology at the University of Reading. In 1997 he received his doctorate from Reading on the basis of his dissertation on the structural development of Britain's Secret Intelligence Service (MI6). The author of *The British Secret Services* (Oxford: ABC Clio; Rutgers NJ; Transaction, 1996) and a number of articles in academic and defence publications, Dr Davies is currently engaged in research on changes in the public role of signals intelligence services in the light of the new ICTs and the development of national information infrastructures (NIIs), and information warfare preparedness amongst the newly industrialised countries of Southeast Asia.

Dorothy E. Denning is professor of Computer Science and Communication, Culture, and Technology at Georgetown University. She is author of *Information Warfare and Security* (Addison Wesley, 1999). E-mail: denningcs.georgetown.edu. Web: www.cs.georgetown.edu/ ~denning.

Simone Fischer-Hübner is currently an assistant professor at Hamburg University, Faculty for Informatics. From September 1994 until March 1995 she was a guest professor at the Copenhagen Business School. Institute for Computer and System Sciences. From July 1998 until spring 1999 she was a guest professor at Stockholm University, Department of Computer and System Sciences. Her teaching and research has been focused on IT security and privacy. She is a founding member and secretary of IFIP Working Group 9.6 ('I.T. Misuse and the Law'), secretary of IFIP working group 11.8 ('I.T. Security Education'), member of the National Expert Working Group on I.T. Security Evaluation Criteria and local co-ordinator of the Erasmus/Socrates Program on 'I.T. Security & Safety Education'. E-mail: fischer@informatik.uni-hamburg.de

Margaret Jackson is associate professor in Computer Law at RMIT University in Melbourne, Australia. Her research interests include confidentiality of information in the health sector, the effect of new technology in business, women in management, and computer law issues generally.

Brian D. Loader is co-director of the Community Informatics Research and Applications Unit (CIRA) based at the University of Teesside, UK. He is editor of *The Governance of Cyberspace* (Routledge, 1997), *The Cyberspace Divide* (Routledge, 1998), co-editor with Barry Hague of *Digital Democracy* (Routledge, 1999) and is General Editor of the international journal *Information, Communication & Society* (Routledge).

Gareth Palmer is a senior lecturer in Media Production and Director of the Contemporary Documentary Archive at the University of Salford, UK. His current research focuses on the connections between discourses of social control, the new production contexts of television and the evolving public sphere.

Andrew Rathmell is deputy director of the International Centre for Security Analysis, Department of War Studies, King's College, London, UK. His research interests include Middle East security, intelligence, low-intensity conflict/terrorism and information warfare.

Philip R. Reitinger is a senior counsel for the Computer Crime and

Intellectual Property Section, Criminal Division, Department of Justice, USA.

Olga V. Smyslova is a postgraduate student at the Psychology Department, Moscow State Lomonosov University. Her research is devoted to the psychology of computer hackers.

Paul A. Taylor is a lecturer in the sociology of technology at the University of Salford, UK. His research interests centre around the computer underground and its depiction in cyberpunk fiction. His recent book is entitled *Hackers: Crime in the Digital Sublime* (Routledge 1999).

Douglas Thomas is assistant professor at the Annenberg School for Communication at the University of Southern California. His work focuses on contemporary critical theory and cultural studies of technology. He is author of *Reading Nietzsche Rhetorically* (Guilford, 1998) and *Hacking Culture* (University of Minnesota, forthcoming) and is co-investigator on the Metamorphosis Project at USC, which studies the social, cultural and political impacts of technology and is a member of the Advisory Board for the Center for Cyberculture Studies at the University of Maryland.

Alexander E. Voiskounsky is currently head of the Psychology Department, Moscow State Lomonosov University. His main area of research and teaching is the psychology of information technology usage.

Michael Whine is the administrator of the Community Security Trust and Director of the Defence and Group Relations Division of the Board of Deputies of British Jews. He writes extensively on anti-semitism, political extremism and terrorism.

Preface

This collection of essays is focused upon the growing concern about the use of electronic communication for criminal activities and the appropriateness of the counter measures which are being adopted by law enforcement agencies, security services and legislators to address such anxieties. The contributions from leading international experts in this field of study are drawn primarily from the first special issue of the journal *Information, Communication & Society (ICS)*[1] and subsequently from later issues of the same journal. Fuelled by the sometimes sensational media headlines and news coverage which have done much to encourage the belief that technologies like the Internet are uncontrollable and likely to lead to a lawless electronic frontier, this volume attempts to provide a more considered and balanced perspective to what is an important and contested arena for debate. We thereby hope to provide an understanding of the basic issues relating to cybercrime and its impact on society. By critically assessing the discourse surrounding these issues it is intended to provide a perspective that will both inform and help raise the level of discussion regarding the effects of information and communication technologies (ICTs) on law enforcement, security and privacy.

Such an ambitious task can only seriously be attempted in the company of informed and dedicated scholars. It is our good fortune to have found such figures to share our enterprise and be prepared to offer their thoughts through the pages of this small volume. We are in their debt and thank them for their contributions. The reader may judge for himself or herself whether we have done them equally good service in our choice of structure and editorial support.

The collection commences with an introductory chapter which attempts to provide a clear and succinct exposition of what we mean by *Cybercrime*, the importance of the new challenges it raises and the nature of the responses it evokes from law enforcement agencies, legislators and security analysts. All the contributions are clustered within three separate parts, each beginning with a short editorial overview intended to foreground the main issues and themes and provide overall coherence.

The compilation of this book was greatly assisted by the enthusiastic support we received from Rob Tarling, Imogen Exton and especially Heather Gibson and Fiona Bailey, all of Routledge. We are also grateful to June Ions for giving the manuscript a consistency of appearance which is beyond our capability to master. Our respective employing establishments, the University of Southern California and the University of Teesside, are due a further debt of recognition for providing a working environment conducive to critical reflection. In particular we would like to thank colleagues at the Annenberg School for Communication and the Community Informatics Research and Applications Unit (CIRA) for their stimulating and enjoyable company.

Doug Thomas, Los Angeles
Brian D. Loader, Swainby

Note

1   *Information, Communication & Society* 1.4.1998. For more information about *iCS* you can access the journal website at www.infosoc.co.uk.

1 Introduction

Cybercrime: law enforcement, security and surveillance in the information age

Douglas Thomas and Brian D. Loader

A deep-seated social anxiety can be recognized as a close companion to the recent impressive advances in Internet and web-based information and communications technologies (ICTs). Its popular manifestation through the media of newspapers, magazines, radio and TV broadcasts has often focused upon speculation about the detrimental effects of ICTs upon various aspects of law enforcement, security and social order. The Internet, for example, is frequently depicted as a kind of dark virtual domain inhabited by a mixture of dissenting computer hackers, organized criminals, extremist political groups and purveyors of pornographic images. Interactive ICTs are consequently seen as a means for facilitating anti-social criminal activities which undermine national security and law enforcement and thereby threaten the very social fabric of democratic capitalist societies. Scarce wonder then that we may witness public alarm about the new media as a consequence of such sensational reporting.

But do these highly publicized and sensational selections of the use of ICTs for criminal undertakings provide us with an accurate picture of the perceived threat to our social and economic order? What is the extent of felony on the Internet? Is there not a danger that this publicity may contribute towards a 'moral panic' and a backlash against free expression? Moreover, what are the safeguards to privacy and anonymity in the face of demands for such technologies to be used for surveillance and detection? The challenges facing legal systems, critical national infrastructures and security agencies as a consequence of the use of the new ICTs by criminal activists are certainly nothing short of momentous. The validity and effectiveness of the actions and policies adopted to tackle them however require more considered deliberation than are presently to be found in the hysterical verbiage emanating from most of the popular media.

This short introductory chapter attempts to provide the reader first with a clearer idea of the defining characteristics of *cybercrime* with a brief exploration of some of its most common manifestations before considering a number of themes and issues that arise from attempts to frame legislation enabling secure electronic commerce, the protection of intellectual property rights, data protection for citizens and the safeguard of freedom of expression in a global information age. The intention is thereby to move beyond polemic and emphasize the need for consideration of checks and balances between a number of competing interests, such as, national security and cryptography, individual liberty and effective law enforcement, enhanced protection from the development of transnational policing and concern over democratic accountability.

What do we mean by cybercrime?

One might easily be forgiven for thinking that 'cybercrime' is a rather pretentious expression to refer simply to the use of computers by criminals; merely the latest variant of the ubiquitous prefix *cyber* in a book title to boost sales. There is, after all, nothing very new in the adoption by criminals of new technologies. Cases of bank robbers using portable radios to intercept police transmissions and more recently the utilization of mobile cellular phones for evading police detection provide obvious examples. So too technologies have been an increasingly important aspect of crime detection throughout the twentieth century, including most famously the use of a wireless signal to aid the arrest of Dr Crippen. So what, if anything, is different about cybercrime?

To understand cybercrime as a significantly new phenomenon, with potentially profound consequences, it is necessary it recognize it as a constituent aspect of the wider political, social and economic restructuring currently affecting countries worldwide. In particular, the processes of economic globalization, which are being facilitated by the new ICTs, not only provide the opportunities for the profitable development of international informational markets (Castells 1996) but also simultaneously raise the spectre of new criminal activities arising to exploit them. The very technologies which enable multinational corporations to do business more easily and challenge the individual controls and regulations of nation states also offer the prospect of globally organized criminal networks (Castells 1998). Moreover, the free flow of uncensored information on electronic networks and websites is as attractive to insurgents and extremist groups as it is to dissidents proclaiming their human rights.

Cybercrime can be regarded as computer-mediated activities which are either illegal or considered illicit by certain parties and which can be conducted through global electronic networks. Its distinctiveness is derived from the versatile capabilities provided by the new ICTs. The global connectivity of the Internet, for example, makes it much easier for criminals to act beyond national boundaries to conduct their illegal affairs. It also makes it possible for existing organized crime to use more sophisticated techniques to support and develop networks for drugs trafficking, money laundering, illegal arms trafficking, smuggling and the like. For hackers with the requisite computer skills, a large market exists for security and trade secrets which can be accessed and transmitted electronically. Furthermore, the many-to-many communication which is an essential feature of the Internet enables the production and worldwide dissemination of information and knowledge which could be potentially harmful, threatening or liable to incite violence.

The nascent threat of cybercrime to affect national and international economies, security and social and political relations provides a serious challenge to the future roles and practices of law enforcement agencies and security services. A flexible communications system designed to withstand attack by means of rerouteing messages has also proved difficult for governments to control (Loader 1997). Sources of illegal activity often require advanced computer skills to be detected as a consequence of their anonymous character. More recently however many national and regional law enforcement and security agencies have established dedicated squads to tackle the threat posed by cybercrime. Such a trend has not surprisingly fuelled the imagery in the popular media of the arrival of the sheriff to tame the electronic frontier.

Of even greater significance perhaps is the blurring of the distinction between internal and external security. The transforming qualities of ICTs make it increasingly difficult to distinguish between warfare, terrorism and criminal activities. Extremist political groups, for example, may engage in all three. The trial of Timothy McVeigh for his part in the Oklahoma City bombing provides perhaps the most dramatic illustration to date. Also, national security is vitally dependent upon economic security. A country in the post Cold War period may be more under threat from economic espionage than nuclear assault. The use of ICTs by non-government organizations and international criminal organizations will therefore clearly have an increasingly important impact upon the functioning of law enforcement and security agencies in the information age.

The magnitude of the task was rudely brought home to the British secret intelligence service, MI6, on 12 May 1999 following the publication of over one hundred names of its agents on the Internet. One of its former agents, Richard Tomlinson, was said to be responsible for the disclosure due to his bitterness at the manner of his dismissal from and later treatment by the intelligence service. It began with an introduction stating that:

> This attached list identifies the unprincipled and unscrupulous individuals involved with MI6 worldwide. The list was produced by an honest man who has since left MI6 because he felt that the behaviour of that organisation was unacceptable in a civilised society.
> They are accountable to nobody for their law breaking activities. They are subordinated to the elite people of this country, for example the royal household and the establishment.
>
> (*The Guardian* 15 May 1999)

Whilst many of the names included retired personnel and foreign office diplomats there were enough active agents, often operating in sensitive regions of the world, to place MI6 in a state of alarm. The British Foreign Secretary Robin Cook stated that 'the release of any such list, however inaccurate it may be, is a deeply irresponsible and dangerous act' (*The Guardian* 14 May 1999). A frenzied attempt was made by foreign office lawyers to contain the damage by having the list removed from websites. Within hours however the information had spread throughout the Internet, available on several websites worldwide, and the source of discussion on many chat groups.

This was not the first time that the names of secret agents had been made publicly available. Indeed during the Cold War period each side are believed to have had a pretty clear idea of their respective agents usually operating as diplomats. Yet it does represent a radical departure from the time when the British, or any other government could effectively control the publication of what it considered to be damaging information. As Stephen Dorril remarked of the affair 'The gung-ho world of James Bond, if it ever existed, is receding. The modern spy is a glorified archivist who must depend on his ability to make sense of a blizzard of information in the public domain and whose triumphs will be analytical rather than amatory' (S. Dorril 1999).

Finally, countermeasures to cybercrime also raise fundamental questions for the study of criminology, the law and policing policies. A number of writers and civil rights campaign organizations have been vociferous in their opposition to the technological means adopted to tackle such criminal behaviour which they claim is in danger of being used to increase surveillance and threaten our personal privacy (Davies 1996; Lyon 1994). Unsolicited digital data capture and matching are said to represent a fundamental challenge to our freedom from interference. The very measures instigated for our defence are said to be undermining our rights to free speech and privacy.

Crimes on the Net

A statement by Neil Gallagher, a Deputy Assistant Director for the FBI, to the US Congressional Joint Economic Committee suggested that 'the World Wide Web has allowed for an endless barrage of frauds, scams, intrusions and piracy' (Gallagher 1998). The kinds of crimes instigated on the Net are indeed many and varied. Some of the most common would include the following: *computer network break-ins* – Typically these involve hackers breaking into computer systems and networks to steal data or undertake acts of sabotage such as planting viruses or trojan horses. Some of the most significant threats to commercial enterprise come from *industrial espionage* which concerns the time-honoured tradition of spying upon one's competitors. The arrival of ICTs provides new opportunities for hacking into and obtaining information for sale about product development, marketing strategies and other trade 'secrets'. The expanding value of the technologies themselves also offers significant bounties for those able to capture intelligence as a result of *software piracy*.

With electronic commerce rapidly becoming a major factor in national economies it offers rich pickings for criminals prepared to undertake fraudulent activities. According to Gallagher, in the USA 'the ten most frequent fraud reports involve undelivered Internet and online services; damaged, defective, misrepresented or undelivered merchandise; auction sales; pyramid schemes and multilevel market-ing; misrepresented cyberspace business opportunities and franchises; work-at-home schemes; prizes and sweepstakes; credit card offers; books and other self-help guides; and magazine subscriptions' (ibid.). Something like half a billion US dollars may be lost annually by consumers through *credit card fraud* alone.

Perhaps the source of most public concern over the use of the Internet is to be derived from its potential as a site for *child pornogra-phy*. The very flexibility of the network seems to provide a veritable Pandora's box for controlling the illegal activities of paedophiles intent upon accessing images of children in indecent poses.

Computer systems are also susceptible to attack through the use of *mail bombings*, a process whereby software is designed to instruct a computer to repeatedly send e-mail to a specified electronic address. The effect of such a bombardment can be to flood the recipient's personal account and thereby threaten to shut down the whole system. Furthermore other software programs known as *password sniffers* can undermine the security safeguards of whole computer networks. The identity and password of network users can be monitored and recorded to enable impersonators to access restricted files and documents. A related activity known as *spoofing* also enables illicit access by electronically disguising a computer to resemble another.

Who are the cybercriminals?

Understanding who the new cybercriminals are is not simply a matter of thinking about old crimes in new ways. Cybercriminals, like cybercrime itself, are marked by a fundamental transformation in the way we think about the issue of crime and criminality. Acts considered criminal that merely happen to involve ICTs are of less concern than those which are made possible solely by the use of ICTs. For example, the use of a computer to defraud someone is no different than the use of a telephone or a face-to-face conversation to defraud someone. What makes such crimes cybercrime is when the use of ICTs adds a significant element to the crime which would have been impossible without them. For example, using e-mail or the WWW to defraud hundreds of thousands of people, the use of the Net to spread information inexpensively, anonymously, or in great numbers all change the fundamental nature of the crime being committed, not merely the means by which it is done.

Just as crimes have changed with the growth of ICTs, so too have the categories of criminals who engage in such crimes. There are three basic categories in which we can categorize cybercriminals: hackers and phreaks, information merchants and mercenaries, and terrorists, extremists and deviants.

Hackers and phreaks

Computer hackers and phreaks (telephone hackers) use ICTs to illegally enter computer systems, for the purposes of exploration, information or curiosity. Their crimes, while illegal, are generally not intended to cause damage to data or to reap financial reward. Often hackers and phreaks will engage in pranks, such as rerouteing phone calls or rearranging web pages. While their actions may have financial consequences for individuals, corporations or industry, their primary goal is not to profit from their crimes. In many cases, hackers are out to find bugs or holes in systems, to gain a reputation for daring hacking exploits, or to embarrass industry figures or people in positions of power. A small subset of these hackers, referred to as 'malicious hackers' cause damage, delete or erase files, or make confidential information public. This group may also include hackers who use computer or telephone technology for minor fraud (using stolen credit card information to make purchases, referred to as 'carding'), those who write computer viruses, or those who shut down Internet websites or Internet service providers (known as 'denial of service' attacks).

For the most part, these hackers are driven by a sense of curiosity and most of the damage done by this group is either unintended or incidental. Typical crimes include low-level fraud (usually related to attempts to gain access to computer systems by attaining password information), unauthorized access to computer systems and possession of unauthorized access devices such as passwords or access codes.

Information merchants and mercenaries

In contrast to hackers, information merchants and mercenaries trade in the commercial sale of information, engaging in crimes such as corporate espionage and sabotage, sale and theft of identity information, computer and network break-ins, and large-scale software piracy. While they may use similar tools and techniques as hackers, information merchants and mercenaries are primarily driven by profit. Those involved in attaining and selling information often are hired by competing corporations or are, themselves, former employees for the companies or agencies from which they gather information.

This group refers to anyone using ICTs primarily for the purposes of illegally reaping financial gain. This may involve illegal discovery or access to information, illegal transfer of funds, identity theft, or the buying or selling of illegally obtained information. Also falling into this category are those who use ICTs, such as cryptography, to hide or disguise illegal activity as well as those who exploit ICTs for illegal financial gain.

Terrorists, extremists and deviants

A third group of cybercriminals are those who use ICTs for illegal political or social activity. In distinction to the first two categories, these cybercriminals may use ICTs to engage in terrorism, electronic or otherwise, to promote hate or illegal activities, or to engage in illegal social behaviours such as the transmission of child pornography or engaging in paedophilia online. These groups and individuals often walk the fine line between freedom of expression and illegal activity.

What constitutes this group as cybercriminals is their primary reliance on ICTs to engage in illegal activity. This group includes those engaging in information warfare as well as those who use ICTs to organize illegal political activity or terrorism.

Who's guarding the electronic guards?

All democratic societies require safeguards to ensure the legitimate use of policing methods and the occurrence of transparent deliberation over their future development. Effective law enforcement inevitably requires a balance to be struck between the appropriate intrusion into the everyday dealings and relations between citizens and the rights of the individual to privacy. As with other areas of social and economic life the framework within which such equilibrium may be maintained is being challenged by the emergence of the new ICTs. The primary concern arising from this process of restructuring is that the potentially exaggerated threat from cybercrime may give rise to an equally overblown reaction from the forces of law and security. In a period of 'moral panic' where the much-trumpeted innovative nature of the new media makes the future appear insecure and unpredictable there may well be a tendency for unnecessarily authoritative surveillance to be supported by public acquiescence.

The scope of surveillance technologies to categorize, document and monitor the behaviour of individuals in almost every aspect of their lives is considerable. Indeed, many of the mundane activities we undertake such as using a cash dispensing machine, using a telephone, driving a car, undertaking foreign travel, receiving state benefits, getting junk mail, taking out library books or using a credit card, all require us to transfer personal data to an electronic computer system. Such data can be stored, updated, checked and matched against other personal electronic information such as financial, health, leisure, political or legal records. Each time we undertake an electronic transaction we leave a trace of our behaviour which acts to build up an electronic data profile. We share our world with a hidden electronic persona the existence of which is not known by many citizens but which forms the basis for law enforcement in the information age.

Moreover, the technologies of surveillance available to law enforcement agencies can come from an increasingly wide range of options. CCTV cameras are becoming commonplace in the cities and towns of most countries around the world. Workplace electronic surveillance is also an expanding area of business and technologies of more direct control such as electronic tagging are also on the rise. Of particular interest is the growing demand from some quarters for personal data from separate sources such as insurance and health records to be made available for matching with police and security files. The justification for such data-matching often appears as a rational request for greater organizational efficiency designed to provide a better service to the public. Its opponents maintain that it can lead to a surveillance society where the privacy and freedom of the individual are severely diminished (Davies 1996).

It is clear to us therefore that these debates concerning the threat of surveillance and the right of privacy are central to any discourse concerned with developing an appropriate and effective response to the emergence of cybercrime.

Advancing the debate

The collection opens with Douglas Thomas's chapter which focuses upon the relationship between law and law enforcement and the representation of hackers. It provides an insightful discussion of how the US public has come to understand hackers and hacking in terms of their own fears and displacements of anxiety. In doing so, Thomas traces out the role that representations of the body, both in legal and popular discourse, have played in the construction and prosecution of hackers in the United States. The chapter documents the manner in which the law is unable to adequately cope with 'bodiless' or 'non-corporeal' crimes. In this way the discourse about hackers and hacking, Thomas argues, can be read as symptomatic of a large discourse concerning anxiety over technology and specific fears about loss of control of the body expressed through the theme of addiction.

Paul Taylor's contribution takes as its central theme the ambivalent status of hackers as being perceived, on the one hand, as a group capable of resisting technological authoritarianism, whilst on the other arguably being a classic example of a group dominated by technology. A condition mirrored in both fictional and non-fictional accounts of hacking where such representations reflect our concerns about the best way to control technological ingenuity in a hi-tech age. William Gibson's *Neuromancer* and Douglas Coupland's *Microserfs* are used as the main examples of fictional portrayals of hacking and Taylor argues that the imaginative licence exhibited by their authors ultimately draws upon contemporary concerns over the role technology plays in modern life.

The fourth chapter takes a specific look at Russian hackers, who are often regarded in their own country as having a reputation of being smart and competent. Preliminary results are presented by Alexander E. Voiskounsky, Julia D. Babaeva and Olga V. Smyslova of an ongoing research project being undertaken which is aimed at providing a psychological understanding of Russian computer hackers. Drawing upon data collected from different sources such as face-to-face and computer-mediated (distant) interviews with the hackers themselves, anonymous computer experts and ordinary users, the chapter discloses the perceptions of different groups of the population towards hackers.

Gareth Palmer, in the next chapter, considers the technological and economic transformation of television communications technologies and its consequences for the construction of public perceptions of law and order. Through a close textual analysis of British and American programmes such as *Cops*, *LAPD*, *Crimewatch UK* and *Crimebeat*, Palmer contends that public service broadcasting continues to paternalistically shape the audience as social subjects and as citizens whilst assimilating advanced ICTs. What is of primary importance is the way in which the law is presented as a force working through a watching community and given technical expression through surveillance technology.

The use of surveillance technology, contends Palmer, cannot be dismissed as mere reality-TV. These programmes are officially sanctioned messages which tell us a great deal about the relationship between the broadcaster and the state. Through an analysis of the combination of the mode of address adopted, the presentation of crime and the use of technology Palmer asserts that we can detect the creation of a new definition of citizenship which is very much allied to the operations of the state.

Part II of the volume commences with a thorough investigation into the use of the Internet by criminals and its effect upon law enforcement by two of the world's leading experts in cryptography, Dorothy Denning and William Baugh, Jr. The need to adopt encryption technologies for the development of commercial markets raises the corresponding necessity to police such activities. Denning and Baugh, Jr. point to the costs of detecting criminal behaviour which require decryption. Their extensive interviews with criminal investigators act to alert us to the threat which such technologies pose for effective law enforcement and foregrounds the challenge to policy-makers who also need to consider issues of privacy, human rights and consumer protection.

The threat posed by cybercrime is underlined by the chapter from Philip Reitinger who takes issue with libertarians intent upon defending anonymity on the Net without reference to the difficulties it produces for law enforcement. Reitenger argues that the debate needs to be balanced between the desire for personal privacy and the need for a secure space for electronic commerce to develop. Organizations or individuals who wish to restrict access to their business information and keep it confidential have had limited legal means to achieve their aim. Margaret Jackson's chapter impressively identifies and analyses how international developments may lead to changes to the traditional ways in which business information has been able to be protected by the law, examines what these changes may be and considers the implication for organizations. The effects of three international instruments are explored – the 1992 OECD Guidelines for the Security of Information Systems, the 1994 Trade-Related Aspects of Intellectual Property Rights (TRIPs), a part of the General Agreement on Tariffs and Trade (GATT) and the 1997 OECD Guidelines for Cryptography Policy.

The threat to individual privacy provided by the very existence of global communications systems capable of processing increasingly large amounts of personal data is the subject of the next two chapters by Simone Fischer-Hübner and Peter Blume. They both provide comparative analyses of the approaches taken to personal data protection and the respective dilemmas that they raise. Fischer-Hübner provides a clear and valuable discussion of privacy and security risks in the global information society. International examples of the EU, United States, Singapore, Japan and Canada further enable a critical evaluation of the approaches to privacy protection adopted for different information infrastructure programmes. Such cultural diversity suggests how difficult it is to develop a common harmonized approach to privacy protection. The chapter concludes with a consideration of the possibilities for designing information infrastructures which are adequate for both social and privacy requirements.

Peter Blume's contribution is focused upon the extent to which legal regulations designed to protect citizens either can or should also be used to protect citizens who break the law. In particular Blume is concerned to elucidate the central dilemma between data protection on the one hand and the pursuit of crime prevention on the other. This fundamental conflict between individual privacy and public protection is explored through a consideration of Danish legislation, the Council of Europe police data recommendation and directive 95/46 EC and the rules of the Schengen and Europol Convention. Blume concludes his chapter by suggesting that whilst the privacy of criminals may be threatened by current legislation it may still be possible to construct sound data protection which enables necessary crime prevention.

The final part of the book begins with an examination by Andrew Rathmell of a particularly pernicious form of potentially subversive behaviour commonly known as information warfare (IW): the deliberate targeting of an organization's information activities in order to disrupt or destroy that organization. It is increasingly regarded as a threat by armed forces, governments and corporations alike. There is a perception that sub-state groups, or empowered small agents (ESA), pose a particular problem because they may find it easier than formally organized opponents such as states to exploit ICTs to leverage limited resources into disproportionate political, economic or military damage on target organizations. A key reason why ESAs are thought likely to be effective prosecutors of IW is that they seem to embody network forms of organization and such forms of organization are supposed to enhance effectiveness in information-age conflict.

Rathmell however contends that current assumptions derived either from grand theoretical approaches, from a straight transference of experiences in the high-technology commercial sector, or from anecdotal evidence of particular groups that have adopted infrastructure targeting and have effectively exploited ICTs, are limited in their explanatory value. By a critical examination of these assumptions Rathmell seeks to build a more systematic model for assessing the IW capabilities of sub-state groups. In particular he focuses upon organizational structure and organizational culture as the locus of capability for IW, rather than on the indicators of tangible technical IW capabilities that populate most existing assessment mechanisms.

An expansive analysis of one group of political extremists, the far right, who are using the new media for subversive activities, is provided by Michael Whine. Since the mid-1980s German neo-Nazis have been using the Internet to organize racist violence, and in the early 1990s US militias, and then white supremacists, began to use it to network and build their movements. All have realized the potential the Internet offers for anonymity, bridging distances and publishing material which would otherwise not be published because of its illegal or offensive nature. These are new benefits which previously were unavailable to them. Public concern however is now impelling international bodies to consider the harmful effects of illegal material on the Internet and legislation is being enacted to force states to act. Government spokesmen in the UK have stated that the medium by which hate material is published is immaterial and that it will be prosecuted, provided it falls within the UK's jurisdiction. The police and prosecuting authorities have been rather more cautious but there now appears to be a clear intent, in UK and elsewhere, to prosecute.

The final chapter by Philip Davies considers the potential impact of the new ICTs upon the security policies of nation states and its reforming qualities upon security organization and practices. Consideration is given to the consequences of the new media for *intelligence* activities. Davies identifies two competing approaches to the development of information intelligence which have so far emerged. The first takes its tenor from the Gibsonian depiction of wired hackers penetrating a global electronic communications web, which anticipates the continuance of highly sophisticated technical security responses (TECHINT). The second alternative scenario suggests that the threat to security is more likely to come from the more low-tech and pervasive activities of transnational organized crime and terrorism, producing a requirement for new forms of human intelligence (HUMINT). After providing a clear critical appraisal of these alternatives Davies maintains that intelligence policy-makers will need to develop strategies which are based upon an understanding of the interdependency between both the human and technical approaches to intelligence.

Concluding comments

The following chapters we hope provide a critical and informative contribution to the debate about the challenges posed by the new technologies to law enforcement and the need to safeguard privacy and security in the information age. The effectiveness of policy-making in this area will be dependent upon the quality of debate generated and we sincerely hope that this small contribution adds something to the deliberations of what we consider to be a significant challenge to the civil order. Opinions to the contrary can only add to such an important debate and the authors welcome contributions from those who wish to make them.

Part I

Perceptions of cybercriminals

Hackers, insurgents and extremist groups

Themes and issues identified

The idea of cybercrime has, in many ways, become synonymous with hackers and hacking. Films, TV and science fiction novels have portrayed hackers as everything from 'data cowboys' on the electronic frontier to digital vigilantes for hire in cyberspace. This part raises a number of issues related to hackers and hacking, exploring both the myths and realities of hacker culture and criminality.

Hackers are perhaps the most easily identified group of cybercriminals and as a result they have come to represent, in the media, in entertainment and in the popular imagination, the risks and dangers of new ICTs. Often, these risks and dangers are more imagined that real, but they do serve to reveal a great deal about public perceptions of the relationships between new media technology and crime. Specifically, hackers are often markers of the fragility of new ICTs, representatives of the risks of new information technologies and the potential for danger. They also personify a new breed of outlaw, constantly challenging accepted definitions and ideas about technology, security and privacy.

Hackers, as pioneers on the 'digital frontier', find themselves at the limits of the law, in a space where commonly accepted notions of law and order become complex and uncertain. The most basic example, that of trespass, is utterly confounded by notions of virtual space. How can a hacker be accused of trespassing on someone else's property when his or her physical presence is located hundreds or even thousands of miles away? It is a problem that ICTs introduce into the law which hackers exploit to full advantage.

As the notion of crime changes, so does the object of crime. The law itself is forced to wrestle with the ambiguous nature of information as property, a theme continually explored throughout this volume. With physical objects it is easy to understand the crime of theft, of depriving someone of the possession and use of physical property. With information, the issue is more complex. When a hacker copies a piece of information or even views it without permission, is he or she guilty of theft? Hackers, by exploring and exploiting issues of secrecy, question precisely what it is that gives information its value. In doing so, they pose fundamental challenges to the structure of the law and the value and definition of property.

Often seen as 'computer geniuses' or experts, hackers are also positioned in the popular imagination in relation to questions of technological domination. Hackers express, in the most extreme terms, contemporary society's relationship to ICTs themselves. In doing so, they explore for us issues of technological domination and control. From news stories to the literature of science fiction, hackers are often made to stand in for our concerns, anxieties, hopes and dreams of a future dominated by ICTs.

The essays in this part explore the role of hackers and insurgents in terms of broad social implications, examining their relationship to crime, criminality, technological domination and social, cultural and national identity. In each case, as these essays demonstrate, hackers tell us a great deal about both how ICTs function in contemporary society and how public perceptions of technological control and mastery influence the creation, construction and application of cybercrime both in the law and in the public imagination.

2 Criminality on the electronic frontier

Corporality and the judicial construction of the hacker

Douglas Thomas

The image of the hacker in the popular imagination is primarily the result of mass media reporting (particularly of high-profile hacker cases) and popular culture representations. Those representations often portray hackers as criminals, playing on cultural stereotypes and rampant fears that over-reliance on technology makes us vulnerable. There is, however, a second, more important, characterization of hackers that serves to relocate them within a very particular set of discursive constructs. Specifically, in the discourse of law enforcement (and media reports stemming from law enforcement), hackers are often described in terms that relate to physical presence, particularly physical presence which focuses on their bodies.

Such representations, beginning with law enforcement and even the laws themselves, continually spill over into the mass media and popular culture accounts of hackers and hacking. In one such instance, the film *Hackers* (1995), the chief law enforcement officer for the film, Richard Gill (played by Wendell Pierce), describes hackers as follows: 'Hackers penetrate and ravage delicate private and publicly owned computer systems, infecting them with viruses and stealing sensitive materials for their own ends. These people ... they're terrorists.'[1] The image of secret service agent Richard Gill in the movie is meant to reflect both the hyperbole with which hackers are represented and the shallowness with which hackers are understood. Gill's description of hackers becomes something of a mantra, repeated continually throughout the film, making clear the fact that Gill, like many of the law enforcement officers he represents, has no idea what he is talking about. Instead, he is reciting a canned speech that is both sensationalistic and wildly inaccurate.

For all the hyperbole of Gill's statement, one aspect rings particularly true – law enforcement is obsessed with the corporeal. The highly sexualized metaphors of penetration and ravaging, set against the delicacy of sensitive computers and data, suggests that hackers are rapists. Further, it makes a clear connection to the personification of information and makes it impossible to consider hackers solely in terms of the tools that they use. Technology, even to law enforcement, has become a problem of human relations, not merely a question of the tools that hackers use.

The separation of technology, conceived of as a problem of human relations, from the technical, formulated as a problem of instrumentality and utility, forces us to rethink several key aspects of the concepts of law and punishment. The problem has often been discussed as a technical one, presenting law and disorder on the electronic frontier as a 'blend of high technology and outlaw culture' (Hafner and Markoff 1991: 9). In fact, there is a commonplace insistence, particularly in law enforcement, that there is nothing unusual about computer crime *per se*; what is unusual is the means by which hackers accomplish their tasks. To much of law enforcement, hackers are 'common criminals' using uncommon means. Even defenders of hackers, such as Mitchell Kapor, argue for a distinction to be made. 'Much of what is labeled "computer crime" ', he argues, 'would constitute a crime regardless of the particular means of accomplishment. Theft of a lot of money funds through manipulation of computer accounts is grand theft. Does a computer make it any grander?' (Kapor 1993). The answer would appear to be 'yes' considering the manner in which 'computer crime' is described and detailed in both the media and in books documenting hackers' stories.

There is a second dimension to the notion of computer crime which problematizes this seemingly simple notion of 'computer crime'. Specifically, what is most commonly prosecuted in hacker cases is not the crime itself, what we might think of, for example, as electronic trespassing. Instead, the most common laws used to prosecute hacking cases are written around the possession of technology, characterized as 'unauthorized access devices'. Taken literally, 'computer crime' often means the ownership of a computer or of technology itself. In some cases even the mere possession of it constitutes a criminal offence. Such is the case with Ed Cummings (Bernie S.), who was incarcerated, and held as a 'danger to the community', for being in possession of a 'red box', a small modified Radio Shack speed dialler that was altered to emit tones which would allow him to make free telephone calls from public pay phones. The first count of the indictment charged Cummings with 'custody and control of a telecommunications instrument, that is a speed dialer, that had been modified and altered to obtain unauthorized use of telecommunication services through the use of public telephones'. The second alleged that Cummings had 'custody and control of hardware and software, that is, an IBM "Think Pad" laptop computer and computer disks, used for altering and modifying telecommunications instruments to obtain unauthorized access to telecommunications service.'[2] In essence, Cummings was charged with possession of technology – the computer literally became the crime.

It is important to note the fact that the possession of technology has become equated with and even been made to go beyond the performative act of its use. Here, the performative act that is illegal is *ownership* of the technology itself – not its use. Hacking, then, is constituted as a crime around the notion of the possession of technology. The reasons why are simple. Hacking is an act that threatens a number of institutionally codified, regulated and disciplined social mechanisms, not the least of which is the law. Hacking, as an activity, enters and exposes the foundational contradictions within the very structure of social existence. Two of those primary structures are the relationships between technology, law and the body, and the importance of the notion of secrecy in the operation of culture. In many ways, hacking at once performs and violates these central tenets, exposing them for what they are (often self-interested, violent contradictions), while performing them as a means to subvert social, cultural and political forces.

Hacking and the fear of technology

At the most basic level, the reaction to hacking and hackers can be understood as a broader reaction to the threat of technology. However, it should be noted that within this dynamic, technology itself is not *precisely* what is feared. The tools themselves are in all actuality completely benign. What is threatening and what hackers and hacking expose, is the fact that as a *relational* concept that mediates the connection between and among people, technology is almost *never* benign. In this sense, people fear hackers because they exploit the relational dimensions of technology in a way that makes people question not only their own relationship to technology, but also their relationship to the world. Accordingly, part of the fascination with hacking has to do with what is not understood about it as an activity and that lack of understanding is the source of a genuine sense of fear. As Hafner and Markoff explain it:

> For many in this country, hackers have become the new magicians:
> they have mastered the machines that control modern life. This is
> a time of transition when young people are comfortable with a

new technology that intimidates their elders. It's not surprising that parents, federal investigators, prosecutors and judges often panic when confronted with something they believe is too complicated to understand.

(Hafner and Markoff 1991: 11)

This analysis is correct up to a point. However, to leave this misunderstanding of hacking as a technical problem and to explain it as a response to a 'fear of the new' or as a technophobic response to modern inventions seems insufficient, particularly in terms of law enforcement and the judicial system. Lawyers and jurists confront things they don't understand on a daily basis. When doctors stand up to testify about spinal cord injuries, or lab technicians present DNA evidence, or engineers explain complicated issues in patent disputes, judges, lawyers and prosecutors don't panic. The elements that need to be rethought in this dynamic are twofold. First, we must consider the relationship between cultural notions of technology and punishment. Second, we need to consider the problem of 'computer crime' within several new thematics: anxiety over technology, displacement and the culture of secrecy.

The problem of the relationship between technology and punishment has, in most analysis, primarily been conceived as a technical one. What needs to be examined is a more extended questioning of the problems of technology and punishment, which is to say, a reconceiving of the problem of punishment as a question of technology, as a question of human relations. This presents us with two lines of inquiry: what is the relationship between technology and punishment?; and in what ways and to what ends have various readings of technology, the technical and punishment been deployed in representing, understanding and misunderstanding hacker culture?

Understanding technology and punishment

Foucault sets out four guiding principles for understanding the relationships between technology and punishment. First, he writes:

Do not concentrate the study of punitive mechanisms on their 'repressive' effects alone, on their 'punishment' aspects alone, but situate them in a whole series of their possible positive effects, even if these seem marginal at first sight. As a consequence, regard punishment as a complex social function.

(Foucault 1995: 26–27)

As a methodological precaution, this makes a great deal of sense, particularly in terms of the relationship between technology and punishment. If the goal of law enforcement is to 'protect' us from high tech hoodlums, as is so often claimed, the question remains: what is it that is being 'protected'? And what does it mean to be 'protected'? What are the 'positive effects' of protection? Such a question seems easily answered at first sight, until one realizes that most hackers, and almost all of the high-profile cases which have been prosecuted, do not involve common crimes. Hackers who enter systems and do nothing more than look around, or even copy files, do not profit from their crimes, generally do not do anything harmful or malicious, and do not cause any loss to the companies, organizations or businesses that they intrude upon. Most often what hackers are accused of and prosecuted for is 'trespassing' and 'possession of unauthorized access devices'. That is, they are prosecuted for their presence, virtual though it may be. The judicial system is protecting us not from the actions of hackers, but from the presence, or the possibility of the presence, of hackers.

Here, we can identify one of the primary problems that confronts law enforcement: if presence is to be considered a crime, one needs something to be present. That presence cannot be merely a 'virtual' presence, but instead must be linked in some real manner to the physical world. In short, hacking needs a body. This body, however, cannot just be any body. It must be a body that has a particular call to the exercise of punishment, discipline or regulation, which leads us to Foucault's second methodological premise: 'Analyze punitive methods not simply as consequences of legislation or as indicators of social structures, but as techniques possessing their own specificity in the more general field of other ways of exercising power. Regard punishment as a political tactic' (Foucault 1995: 27). In the case of the hacker, the technology of punishment must also be read as not just a technology of the body, but as a politics of the body as well. We must understand that the virtual presence of the hacker is never enough to constitute crime – what is always needed is a body, a real body, a live body, through which law can institute its well-established exercises of power.

Third, Foucault insists that, instead of 'treating the history of penal law and the history of human sciences as two separate series', we 'make the technology of power the very principle both of the humanization of the penal system and of the knowledge of man' (Foucault 1995: 27). As such, Foucault poses the question as to whether or not there is a 'common matrix' or 'a single process of "epistemologico-juridical" formation' which gives rise to both the questions of law and human relations. If so, then we ought to focus our attention on the commonality found in both the discussion of the law and human relations and particularly the points of intersection between the two. Nowhere in the discourse surrounding hacking is this more clear than in the manner in which hackers are characterized as criminals. Indeed, the question of how exactly one characterizes hackers reveals a great deal about attitudes towards both law and humanity. Hence, the discourse that surrounds the criminal nature of hacking reveals a great deal about broader social understandings of criminality, technology and culture.

Finally, Foucault summarizes, in his fourth methodological statement, the manner in which the 'soul' and the 'scientific' are injected into the discourse of punishment as 'the effect of a transformation of the way in which the body itself is invested by power relations' (Foucault 1995: 27). Broadly speaking, the more metaphysical and the more scientific the discourses of punishment become, the more they reveal themselves as technologies of power directed at the body.

Technology and punishment: the body and memory

Technology has never been a stranger to punishment. It is easy to see how, particularly in the twentieth century, technology had, in fundamental ways, constituted punishment; it is one of the primary means by which power is deployed, networked and regulated.

Technology, like all mechanisms of power, is also a means of resistance. As such, at moments, we are able to redefine and redeploy discourse and events in locally resistant ways. If we maintain that technology is a relational, rather than a technical phenomenon, it becomes even more clear that it functions as one of the more complex networks of power. Relationships with technology infect every aspect of human communication and technology mediates nearly every form of relationship. Even the most basic forms of face-to-face communication can be subject to recording, eavesdropping or some other form of electronic snooping. In that sense, all human communication has at some level become public, insofar as all human relationships are mediated by and through technology that always threatens/promises to make that communication and those relationships public. Technology has become nothing more than the sum of and ordering of human relations that are in some manner mediated.

The connection between technology and punishment is as old as human civil relations. As Nietzsche argued, it is precisely the connection between technology and punishment that allowed human relations to become codified and regulated. One can read Nietzsche's *On the Genealogy of Morals*, perhaps one of the most insightful treatises on the relationship between culture and punishment, in just this light. Nietzsche insists on the separation of origins and utilities of things (particularly punishment), arguing that 'the cause of the origin of a thing and its eventual utility, its actual employment and place in a system of purposes, lie worlds apart' (Nietzsche 1997: II, 12). Nowhere is this more clearly established than in his reading of the origins of punishment. Technologies of punishment evolved from the need to 'create a memory in the human animal', and accordingly, the 'answers and methods for solving this primeval problem were not precisely gentle' (ibid.: II, 3). What Nietzsche provides for us is the initial connection between human relations and technology: if one is to live in a civil society, one must follow certain rules, rules which are contrary to nature, and even contrary to human survival. Hence, we find the very possibility of a civil society rooted in the technology of memory.

To call memory a technology is to suggest that it operates through a kind of mechanism that mediates human relations, and, as Nietzsche argues, punishment is precisely the technical mechanism by which we mediate all human relations through memory:

> Man could never do without blood, torture, and sacrifices when he felt the need to create a memory for himself; the most dreadful sacrifices and pledges (sacrifices of the first-born among them), the most repulsive mutilations (castration, for example), the cruelest rites of all religious cults (and all religions are at the deepest level systems of cruelties) – all this has its origin in the instinct that realized that pain is the most powerful aid to mnemonics.
>
> (Nietzsche 1997: II, 3)

This sense of punishment, whatever else one can say about it, has been effective. The body, as we have seen time and time again, *learns* and *remembers*. The origin of punishment is then creating a memory, not in the psychical consciousness, but with and through the body as a physiological solution to the problem of memory.

There is a tendency to confuse the origin of punishment with the purpose of punishment. We tend to seek out a particular use or purpose for punishment (e.g. deterrence, revenge, retribution) and ascribe that as the origin of punishment. In doing so, we mistake the technical utility for the technology itself. Punishment has a technical aspect, a means by which punishment is performed, which has as *its* goal a 'purpose'. But, as we have already seen, the basic technology which informs the understanding of the origin of punishment is the need to create a memory, *mnemotechnics*. While memory serves to define and mediate human relations, the infliction of pain serves only instrumental and therefore technical ends.

Memory as a technology relies on the technical, or physical, aspects of punishment; the technical aspect of punishment can never be divorced from the technology of memory. Punishment is, and always remains, *mnemotechnics* (literally, the combination of memory and technology) – 'If something is to stay in the memory it must be burned in: only that which never ceases to *hurt* stays in the memory' (Nietzsche 1997: II, 3).

Technology's relationship to punishment, however, does not end with this originary moment. Instead, technology has been the force that has propelled punishment, developing increasingly sophisticated ways to monitor, discipline, correct and institutionalize norms, values and ideals. This partnership between technology and punishment has always followed two basic principles: first, that it is the *body* and not the mind which remembers, and, second, that the most powerful form of discipline comes not from an external implementation of coercion, but when the subjects of punishment actually incorporate the system of punishment into their life and begin to regulate themselves.

Hackers understand both these principles. They understand that if the 'crime' cannot be connected to a body, it cannot be punished. Moreover, they realize that, for the most part, the connection between technology and punishment is, at least in one sense, very tenuous. Those who enforce the law have almost no understanding of the technology that is used to break the law. As one hacker, Chris Goggans, describes his visit by federal agents:

> So they continued on in the search of my house and when they found absolutely nothing having to do with computers, they started digging through other stuff. They found a bag of cable and wire and they decided they better take that, because I might be able to hook up my stereo, so they took that.
>
> (Gilboa 1994: 37)

Indeed, law enforcement realizes that information that catches hackers and allows for prosecution is not going to be computers, disks, or stereo cable, but instead the most valuable information will usually come from other hackers. Most hackers who are caught and/or sentenced are caught as a result of being turned in by another hacker. It is a hacker's relationship with other hackers, coupled with the threat of severe penalties for lack of cooperation, that provides information for most arrests. The technology most commonly deployed by law enforcement is a technology that, like hacking itself, is more relational than technical.

One of the ways that law enforcement monitors hackers is by keeping careful watch on the relationships and networks that hackers set up among themselves. Evidence from and of these networks, usually the testimony of other hackers, is the most powerful evidence marshalled in criminal prosecutions of hackers. The most notorious hacker informer is Justin Tanner Peterson ('Agent Steal'), who worked for the FBI in the early 1990s informing on fellow hackers. However, in most cases, the principal evidence comes from 'other hackers' who have usually been bullied into cooperation by the threat of unusually high penalties and the threat of lengthy prison sentences.

There is an additional side to technology's relationship to the body that demands exploration as well. While it is the hacker's body that must be found, identified and ultimately prosecuted, the relationship of hacking to the law has become curiously incorporeal in another sense. The most common legal indictment against a hacker is 'possession of counterfeit, unauthorized and stolen access devices'.[3] Literally, this refers to passwords.[4] Access devices are items that allow one entry to a computer system and can be read as secrets which provide verification of identity. The parameters as to what constitute these access devices are written broadly (counterfeit, unauthorized and stolen passwords would all count), but what is most remarkable about the law is that one never needs to use these access devices to be found guilty, all one needs to do is *possess* them. The constitutive act of possession is thus transformed juridically into the performative act of hacking. Legally, hacking ceases to be an activity, but is reduced to a possession. All that needs to be proven is two things: first, that the hacker had the access devices in their possession and, second, that they are indeed 'counterfeit, unauthorized, or stolen', which is to say that they have the quality of the secret.

Because these issues revolve around questions of identification, what is at stake is the juridical reconstitution of both the hacker and the subject. The premise of this law regarding access devices is that the information or the access device is, at some level, a secret shared between the system (who can authorize its use) and the user, who utilizes that system. That is, it expresses a relationship between them which is characterized by secrecy. But that relationship also produces a sense of identity. The performative act of sharing the secret, which occurs each time the user logs on, also betrays that user's identity. The system 'knows' who is logging on precisely because that person (supposedly) is the only one who shares in the secret.[5] Without the quality of secrecy, each user could be anyone, and therefore, the relationship would not perform any sort of identity at all. By typing in a password, what the system is doing is, in essence, verifying the identity of the person on the other side – making sure they are not counterfeit or unauthorized. But that identity is, in all instances, a virtual identity, one which can be performed independently of the body. Identity, in this space, then, is reduced to a constitutive property – either I have the identity (e.g. possess the secret) or I do not. Identity, in this virtual space, is severed from the body and, in that manner, becomes 'performable' by another simply by knowing the secret. At this moment, the space between the performative and constitutive becomes undecidable – the act (if we can call it an act) of *knowing a secret* is indistinguishable from the act of *performing an identity*.

It is this separation of body and identity that makes the act of hacking possible and it is this separation that is taken up by the law. Nowhere in this law does the hacker have to perform anything. The only quality that the hacker needs to manifest is a constitutive one – proof that the hacker knows a secret that they are not supposed to know. How they got that information and whether or not it is used, which is to say performed, is of no consequence. The law itself affirms a crucial moment of secrecy, where simply knowing someone else's secret constitutes, legally, the performance of their identity.

Hacking the panopticon: reading hacking as resistance

Most hackers understand what is at stake in relation to law enforcement and regard it as something of a game, a game that law enforcement is all too willing to play. It is, in none too simple terms, a game of watching and being watched. But, in all cases, what must be watched is the body, precisely the thing which is absent in the space of the hacking.

Passwords constitute the most basic form of 'unauthorized access devices', but there is a second function that these devices serve in relation to the body and identity. An 'unauthorized access device' can also be considered a device which masks the user's true identity. These devices, then, also create one secret as they mask or obscure another.

One of the more common examples is the use of hacked cellular phones. These phones, which are altered to appear to belong to someone else (making their use both free and untraceable) serve to erect a barrier between hackers and the network that they seek to enter. That barrier shields the hacker's body from the act of hacking. The system can monitor every act that the hacker performs, but they cannot locate the body which is performing the actions. The body, then, becomes the *secret* that the law must uncover and the law against unauthorized access devices is aimed at precisely that secret. As a result, the law is positioned as protecting certain institutional secrets and preventing other 'unauthorized' ones.

Hacking can be read in relation to this notion of a 'culture of secrecy' which figures so prominently in the relationship between hackers and law enforcement. In what we can think of as an 'incitement to discourse', the secret always plays a crucial role. It is the manner by which discourse can both be 'confined to a shadow existence' and be 'spoken of *ad infinitum*' (Foucault 1978: 35). Foucault, for example, maintains that the *illusion* of the secret operates in such a way as to position its object *outside of discourse*, and that only through a 'breaking of a secret' can we 'clear the way leading to it' (ibid.: 34). Put in different terms, access to the object of secrecy *appears* only to be possible through a breaking of the secret. This, however, is always only an illusion – it is the tension between the 'shadow existence' and the 'proliferation of discourse' which marks the force of the secret. As long as the object of secrecy appears *outside of discourse* it can be talked about openly.

This dynamic is steadfastly at work around issues of technology. The discourse around technology has exploded in the past decade, particularly with the growth of the Internet. What is talked about, in terms of hackers at least, is the manner in which hackers themselves exist in a shadowy space of secrecy, possessing near mystical powers that allow control of technology that itself is beyond discourse. The hackers themselves are coded in such a way that they literally become the secret that needs to be broken. And the discourse surrounding hacking reveals little about hackers themselves, but, instead, tells us a great deal about social attitudes toward technology. Again, the discourse about technology reveals to us society's *relationship* to technology, which is marked by the function of the secret.

This secrecy is regulated by a system of panopticism, an all-seeing system of surveillance which serves to instil a sense of always being watched in those who are subjected to it. Panopticism generates its power not by continually monitoring, but by making it impossible to determine if you are being monitored at any given time. As a result, it is *always possible* that you are being watched and it is impossible to determine with certainty if you are not being watched. It is the process by which subjects learn to govern and discipline themselves, internalizing the thought that they are continually under observation. The structure of panopticism exploits the secret in two ways through the dynamic of surveillance. Those who monitor do so by exploiting a secret – which is that one never knows if one is being watched. The secret, then, whether or not there is a guard in the tower, preserves the power of the panoptical gaze. That gaze, however, is aimed precisely at the notion of secrecy itself. Panopticism's goal is the complete removal of the space where secrecy can operate – ideally, in a panoptical space, no one operates in secret because it is always possible that one's actions are being watched. What is watched, and this is of crucial importance, is the body and the space which the body occupies. In terms of hackers, however, that body and that space are rendered 'unwatchable'. One can watch a hacker's actions, even monitor them, online, but this means nothing until they can be attached to a real body and therefore become prosecutable.

The hacker can be read in this respect as a figure who both deploys and disturbs the notion of the secret. In short, hackers' use of the secret is made possible by the space that the broader culture of secrecy opens up. It is the connection of the secret to the hacker's body that the law targets. Simply finding the body is not enough, the law must attach the body to a secret. In one case in March 1990, Chris Goggans was raided by secret service agents in just such a quest. As he recalls the events, Agent Foley approached him after a thorough search of the premises and confronted him with some business cards he had made up which read 'Eric Bloodaxe, Hacker' along with a small US treasury logo. Goggans responded to Foley: 'Well, it doesn't say anywhere on there "Chris Goggans, Special Agent". It says, "Eric Bloodaxe, Hacker". Whoever this Eric Bloodaxe character is. It might be me, it might not. I'm Chris Goggans and that says 'Eric Bloodaxe, Hacker" (Gilboa 1994: 38). The connection would not be enough to convict Goggans of anything. Instead, Foley insists that there must be some secret to be told and he utilizes the threat of the law in an effort to extract that secret. As Goggans explains:

> He says, 'Well if you don't tell us everything that there is to know about your higher ups, we are going to be pressing state, local and federal charges against you.' I said, 'On what grounds?' He goes, 'We want to know everything about your higher ups.' Which I'm

thinking, gosh, I'm going to have to turn in the big man, which is ludicrous, because there is no such thing as a higher up, but apparently they thought we were a part of some big organization.

(Gilboa 1994: 38)

The secret can, in essence, multiply. Failing to connect Goggans to the secret physically, the law enforcement effort was to connect other bodies to Goggans through discourse. Literally, the demand was for Goggans to break the secret – 'tell us what we want to know' – and to connect other bodies to other secrets.

Addiction and technology: rethinking the cyberbody

The body is the locus of criminality and deviance, as well as punishment, justice and correction. It is identifiable, definable and confinable. Taking up the mantle of cyberpunk science fiction, hacking envisions a world without bodies, in which hackers exist, first and foremost, as virtual beings. Such an incorporeal nature is generally thought of as a technical invention, perhaps best described by William Gibson in his envisioning of cyberspace in his 1984 novel, *Neuromancer*.[6] In *Neuromancer*, Gibson tells the story of Case, a computer cowboy, who after stealing from his employer was neurologically damaged so that his body could no longer interface with the computer matrix as kind of punishment or payback. Describing the protagonist's now defunct relationship to the technological, Gibson writes:

> For Case, who'd lived for the bodiless exultation of cyberspace, it was the Fall. In the bars he'd frequented as a cowboy hotshot, the elite stance involved a certain relaxed contempt for the flesh. The body was meat. Case fell into a prison of his own flesh.
>
> (Gibson 1984: 6)

The primary vision of hacking, then, is founded in the hacker's reliance upon, and often addiction to, the technological. The infliction of such punishment is not confined, however, to the world of the future. In the everyday world of hacking and 'computer crime' the elimination of the technological is the greatest threat the hacker faces, and, not unlike Case's employers, judges are fond of prescribing penalties for hackers which include forbidding them to access technology such as telephones, computers or modems.[7] The modern judicial system attempts to legally produce the equivalent of Case's neurological damage.

The 1988 arrest, trial and conviction of Kevin Mitnick, one of the more notorious hackers, provide a striking parallel to Gibson's character Case. During the trial itself, the judge 'sharply restricted his telephone access', allowing Mitnick to only call 'those numbers that had been approved by the court' (Hafner and Markoff 1991: 342). After being found guilty (and serving prison time), Mitnick's relationship to the technological was diagnosed as 'compulsive' and after his release 'the conditions of Kevin's probation prohibited him from so much as touching a computer, but once he demonstrated that he could control his behavior, he was allowed to search for computer work, although he was still prohibited from using a modem' (ibid.: 343). Even more striking are the conditions of probation for Kevin Poulsen, who was given the following 'special conditions' of supervision for probation:

> you shall not obtain or possess any driver's license, social security number, birth certificate, passport or any other form of identification without the prior approval of the probation officer and further, you shall not use for any purpose or in any manner, any name other than your legal true name; you shall not obtain or possess any computer or computer related equipment or programs without the permission and approval of the probation officer; and you shall not seek or maintain employment that allows you access to computer equipment without prior approval of the probation officer.[8]

Poulsen wrote:

> It got even more interesting when I was released. When I reported to my P.O., he explained to me that, not only could I not use any computer, with or without a modem, but that I couldn't be in the same room as a computer. I had to look for a job with an employer that had no computer equipment on the premises. 'Oh, and by the way, don't forget that you have to pay $65,000.00 in restitution in the next three years.'
>
> (Poulsen, 'Many Happy Returns')

Characterizations of compulsive behaviour were not only employed by the courts. The notion of addiction was used by Mitnick's lawyers in an effort to get a reduced sentence. After his arrest in 1988, Mitnick's 'lawyer convinced the judge that Mr Mitnick's problem was similar to a drug or gambling addiction' (Markoff 1994). After his release, Mitnick was sentenced to six months in a halfway house, complete with a twelve-step programme for drug and alcohol offenders.

The notion of addiction, particularly in Mitnick's case, is specifically located in terms of the body. As Hafner and Markoff describe him, Mitnick was 'plump and bespeckled', 'the kind of kid who would be picked last for the school team', and 'his pear-shaped body was so irregular that any pair of blue jeans would be an imperfect fit' (ibid.: 26). In almost all accounts, his body is written as the *cause* of his addiction. Harriet Rossetto, his counsellor from the centre in Los Angeles, where Mitnick underwent his treatment, attributes his addiction to computers as a result of the fact that 'He is an overweight computer nerd, but when he is behind a keyboard he feels omnipotent' (Markoff 1994). Even John Markoff, a staff writer for the *New York Times* who had followed Mitnick's story for a number of years, characterized an almost involuntary reaction relationship between technology and Mitnick's body. 'During the treatment program', Markoff writes, 'Mr Mitnick was prohibited from touching a computer or modem. He began exercising regularly and lost more than 100 pounds' (ibid.). What Markoff and others seem to suggest, is that it is the physical connection to technology itself that perverts and deforms the body. Joshua Quittner, writing for *Time*, reports the connection in precisely the same way. 'As a condition of his release from jail in 1990, he was ordered not to touch a computer or modem. By June of 1992 he was working for a private eye, doing surveillance and research, and had dropped 100 lbs' (Quittner 1994). The connection between Mitnick's not 'touching' computers and modems and his weight loss is presented as mini-narrative in and of itself, a narrative that suggests both a causal connection between his lack of access to technology and his weight, as well as the broader suggestion that technology is, itself, somehow harmful to the body. While the first connection is obvious on the face of things, the second is a bit more elusive.

The connection of technology to the body in Mitnick's case is through the theme of addiction. Hacking, according to the judicial system, is akin to 'substance abuse' (the actual term deployed by Mariana Pfaelzer, the sentencing judge for US District Court in Mitnick's case). The judge's decision was the result of the tactics of Mitnick's attorney who argued 'that his client's computer behaviour was something over which his client had little control, not unlike the compulsion to take drugs, drink alcohol or shoplift' (Hafner and Markoff 1991: 343). As a result, Mitnick was sentenced to a one-year prison term with six months of rehabilitation to be served in a halfway house. After leaving prison, Mitnick went to:

> a small residential program that emphasizes the twelve-step Alco-holics Anonymous model for treatment. When he entered the program, he remained aloof from the others at first, asserting that his problem was unique and no one else could understand it. He was cold and emotionally remote. For the first several weeks, in what his counselor called a classic example of denial, Kevin con-tinued to maintain that he could stop at any time he wanted. Eventually, he came to accept the facts of his compulsion and his counselor said she believed he had changed his behavior.
>
> (Hafner and Markoff 1991: 343)

Mitnick continued attending meetings for codependent children and children of alcoholics following his release from the halfway house (ibid.: 344).

What is interesting about this treatment is the manner in which the law and the structures of punishment remain blind to the social dimensions of technology. In Mitnick's case, the computer is viewed as an object which is essentially *negative* in character. It is not a value-neutral tool, one which can be used beneficially or maliciously. It is positioned not as a *substance*, but as a *dangerous substance*. Computers are likened to drugs and alcohol. The shift is subtle but important, it betrays an underlying anxiety and hostility towards technology. It is also, most likely, the reason why the plea was successful.

The problematic nature of drugs, has centred (at least since Plato's time) on the undecidability of their nature. Drugs have traditionally been regarded as 'substances' which when taken had the ability to either poison or to cure.[9] Only recently, in the wake of national hysteria, have drugs taken on a fundamentally negative symbolic valance. There are at least two reasons for this transformation. First, the national campaigns dating from the mid-1970s and 1980s, have heavily coded drugs as dangerous, deadly and addictive. And second, in the wake of HIV and AIDS, drugs have begun to lose their positive valance. HIV has created a rhetoric of viral infection that has rendered the positive symbol of the drug impotent. These two movements – the first signifying the destructive, essentially negative, power of drugs, the second, the medicinal impotence of healing drugs – have had the effect of rendering the *undecidable* nature of drugs *decidable*.

The equation of technology with drug addiction is a powerful one. It is also the means by which technology is attached to the body and out of which is constructed the activity of hacking not as a malicious or even intentional activity, but, instead, as an obsessive disorder resulting from physical contact with the object of the obsession. Mitnick's 'treatment' consists of not 'touching' a computer or modem, suggesting that it is the physical contact with technology, rather than the actual usage of it, that produces the addiction. Again, the body, particularly its physicality, plays a crucial role in the construction of the hacker. Technology itself is written as a drug and the hacker is written as an addict. As Mike Godwin of the Electronic Frontier Foundation puts it, 'The great ones are all obsessed, which is what it's about.'[10]

As a result of the discourse surrounding hacking and the body, the most interesting definitions of computer crime are to be found in the nomenclature used to describe hackers during actual investigations and 'manhunts'. It is during these times that the characterizations of the 'cyberbody' take on heightened importance and emphasis. There is a mechanism for describing hackers in terms of computer crime during these periods of pursuit which deploys a well-embedded narrative that fosters clear perceptions of who the hacker is and what they pose. It is commonly framed in the basic 'cops and robbers' vernacular, where the hacker is often described in criminal, but non-violent terms. Those who pursue him are often characterized as 'sleuths', 'trackers' or 'hunters'. The hacker is a 'cyberthief' or, for high drama, a 'master cyberthief', and the pursuit invokes the language of the hunt ('tracking', 'snaring', 'tracing', or 'retracing'). Often this narrative will feature the hacker as a 'fugitive' who 'eludes' and repeatedly, they will be described (once apprehended) as being 'caught in their own web'. In some cases, hackers are even given honorific titles such as 'Prince of Hackers' or 'Break In Artist'.

What is most compelling about these narratives is the manner in which the metaphors of the hunt are enacted. The hunt is not, as one might immediately suspect, a strategy of depersonalization – the hacker is not reduced to some animal form which is tracked, hunted and captured or killed. In fact, the discourse of the hacker is less about the hunted and more about the hunter. As we read about the hunt, we uncover two dynamics. First, the drama of the hunt itself, which always seems to hold a particular narrative fascination, and second, the narrative of the hunters themselves, who, in order to catch their prey must learn to think like them. Part of our fascination is with the act of repetition, which we live out vicariously, through the hunt. We watch as the hunter learns to think like the hunted and it is through *that* process that information about the hacker's motives, intentions and world view are disclosed.

The drama of the 'hunt' is an extremely familiar narrative and it presumes a great deal of information: the activity is adversarial, there is a hunter and a hunted, and a game-like quality which relies on deception, sleight of hand, illusion and misdirection. Indeed, the notion of a 'trap' relies, at its heart, on the act of deception. It must look like something appealing, when in fact it presents great danger. The manner in which the hunt is described, and often enacted, is also about how one thinks, particularly how the hunted thinks. Will they be smart enough to see the trap in advance? Will they outsmart the hunter? The structure of the hunt, then, is primarily a battle of intelligence, a test of skill, rather than physicality or even will.

Accordingly, the hunt is always about thinking the thoughts of the other. If the hunter is to succeed, they must understand the hunted better than the hunted understands the hunter. As a result, the hunt begins to exist in a world of its own, a world which possesses a game-like quality. John Markoff, after helping get him arrested, explains his reaction to Kevin Mitnick actually being sent to jail: 'It felt odd to me. It was as if it had all been a game, and all of a sudden the game was over and everybody realized this is the real world.'[11] The sense of 'real worldness' can be traced to the moment when Federal Agents knocked on Kevin Mitnick's door and placed him under arrest. The game lost its game-like quality the moment a body was made present.

In this sense, we must also understand the hunt as a hunt for the body. In the case of Kevin Mitnick, everything that was needed to make the arrest and prosecute the case was already known, documented and recorded. Given the manner in which Mitnick's body figures into the narrative of his relationship to technology, it shouldn't be surprising that his 'Wanted' poster reads, under the heading 'Miscellaneous Information': 'Subject suffers from a weight problem and may have experienced weight gain or weight loss.'[12]

Conclusions

In examining the body as the primary locus for the juridical construction of the hacker, it becomes readily apparent that the notion of 'virtual' crime problematizes the law at its most basic level. Perhaps as important, the non-corporeal nature of hacking has yet to be grasped and understood by both law enforcement and the mainstream media. As a result, hackers are continually defined in corporeal terms in an effort to reattach the act of hacking to a physical presence.

In tracing out the history and technologies of punishment, it becomes clear that contemporary juridical norms are continually being outstripped by this new breed of criminality. As a result, outmoded standards of legality and characterizations of criminality are forced upon hackers and in the process retroactively reconstruct their activities as 'criminal'. As the law is reconfigured to meet the challenges of the next generation of cybercrime, one of the primary areas which will need to be rethought is the relationship between the body and the emerging digital frontier, a frontier where secrecy has become the standard by which the value of information is guaranteed.

Notes

1 *Hackers* (United Artists, 1995).
2 *United States v. Edward Cummings*, Nos 95–320, 8 June 1995.
3 See, for example, Title 18, United States Code, Section 1029(b)(2).
4 It also refers to items which allow the hacker to hide his or her identity, a point which will be taken up later in the discussion of panopticism.
5 This problem is also at the heart of the origins and debate over the implementation of cryptographic systems. Cryptography can be read, in this context, as a way to negotiate these questions of identity in a more sophisticated and complex manner.
6 Interestingly, 'cyberspace' is a term that emerged from cyberpunk literature in the early 1980s, and was popularized by John Perry Barlow (one of the inventors of the Well). Bruce Sterling attributes the popularization of Gibson's terminology to Barlow's usage of it, claiming that it was the term 'as Barlow employed it, [that] struck a useful chord, and this concept of cyberspace was picked up by *Time*, *Scientific American*, computer police, hackers, and even constitutional scholars' (Sterling 1992: 236).
7 While there are documented cases of hackers engaging in serious computer crime, more often the efforts of law enforcement are aimed at cracking down on fairly innocuous behaviour. For an instance of the former, see Stoll (1989); for an analysis of the latter, see Sterling (1992).
8 Letter from Marc J. Stein, US Probation Officer, to Kevin Lee Poulsen, 22 May 1996. Poulsen's saga continued after his release.
9 On this point, particularly, see Jacques Derrida's essay 'Plato's Pharmacy' in *Dissemination* (Derrida 1981).
10 Godwin, in Fine (1995).
11 Interview with John Markoff, 19 January 1995.
12 US Marshals Service, NCIC entry number NIC/W721460021.

3 Hackers – cyberpunks or microserfs?

Paul A. Taylor

> I got thinking about sin, or badness, or whatever you want to call it, and I realized that just as there are a limited number of consumer electronics we create as a species, there are also a limited number of sins that we can commit, too. So maybe that's why people are so interested in computer 'hackers' – because they've invented a new sin.
>
> (Coupland 1995: 357)

Introduction

Hacking is an intrinsically contentious area of investigation. The meaning of the term has evolved over time but is still applied somewhat variably to a complex mix of legal and illegal activities ranging from legitimate creative programming techniques to illicit lock-picking and manipulation of worldwide phone/computer systems.[1] In his seminal study *Hackers: Heroes of the Computer Revolution*, Levy (1984) describes three generations of hackers who exhibited to various degrees qualities associated with hacking's original connotation of playful ingenuity, an ingenuity epitomized by the earliest hackers who were the pioneering computer aficionados at MIT's laboratories in the 1950s and 1960s. These form Levy's first generation of hackers defined as those who were involved in the development of the earliest computer programming techniques. The second generation is defined as those involved in bringing computer hardware to the masses with the development of the earliest PCs. The third generation refers to the programmers who became the leading lights in the advent of computer games architecture. The phrase *hacker* is now predominantly used to describe an addition to Levy's schema: the fourth generation of hackers who illicitly access other people's computers.

This chapter seeks to highlight those elements of the first four generations of hackers that form the basis of the fictional representations of a putative fifth generation. The two poles of the vestigial fifth generation are represented in the defining cyberpunk work *Neuromancer* (Gibson 1984) and the zeitgeist novel *Microserfs* (Coupland 1995), giving rise to this chapter's title: Hackers – cyberpunks or microserfs? These two contrasting portrayals illustrate the inherent ambivalence with which society confronts the issue of technological change: we seek to control it but fear being controlled by it instead. Both cyberpunk fiction and the real-life activity of hacking are shown to highlight two specific aspects of societal concerns over technology: first, computers are presented as an invasive force that continually threaten to dehumanize its would-be virtuosos, whilst second, control over the ultimate direction of computer technology developments has been subsumed to the requirements of the highly abstract and impersonal system of late capitalism.

Hacking fiction

Neuromancer (1984) is the seminal example of the recent genre of science-fiction known as cyberpunk. It depicts hackers in a futuristic guise as anarchic, mercenary and technically savvy mavericks who seek (with generally limited success) to reappropriate the technology of advanced capitalism for their own ends. *Microserfs* (1995) is a contemporary fictional analysis of the giant US computer firm Microsoft. It depicts hackers as gifted but 'geekish' and obsessive computer programmers. The frenetic pace of *Neuromancer* is allied with its setting in a dystopian urban milieu where both nature and humans are intimately connected to technology in various invasive forms. Overseeing such rapidly changing and technologically saturated environments are the impersonal zaibatsus, huge largely Japanese multinational conglomerates, one of which is ultimately found to be run by an artificial intelligence (AI) construct. *Microserfs* provides a more contemporary account of similar themes. The narrator obsessively questions the relationship of himself and his fellow programmers to their bodies which are persistently conceived of in terms borrowed from computing. This merging of bodies and machines culminates at the end of the novel where the narrator's mother suffers a stroke and is kept alive by technologically complex life-support machines. It uses the particular working patterns prescribed by Microsoft to highlight more general technological issues. These include the effect technology has on our relationship to our bodies and the way it encourages subordinance to highly formalized systemic structures, whether they be in the microcosmic form of the code programmers produce, or the macrocosmic form of the larger corporate code which regulates the programmers' work (and to a large extent their private) lives.

Fear and hyperbole

> I'm coming close to believing that the computer is inherently anti-human – an invention of the devil.
>
> (Weizenbaum 1976: 125)

> In the hothouse atmosphere of media hype, our favorite nerds blossomed into mythic Hackers: a schizophrenic blend of dangerous criminal and geeky Robin Hood. Chalk it up to an increasingly bi-polar fear and fascination with the expanding computer culture.
>
> (Hawn 1996: 1)

Modern technological times can be described as increasingly vulnerable to a wide range of viral and other security-transgressing threats to social well-being.[2] Western society has recently experienced cyanide-laced Tylenol, glass shards in baby food, benzyne in mineral water, computer viruses, AIDS, chemical poisoning on the Tokyo subway, the millennium bug and repeated publicity describing the potential for widespread destruction to technological infrastructures from determined cyber-terrorists. Ironically, perceptions of what could be termed techno-vulnerability are often expressed with recourse to body-based forms of expression and they have arguably helped to fill the void left by the end of the Cold War and its associated fears of military threat from the Soviet Bloc:

> The form and content of more lurid stories like *Time*'s infamous story, 'Invasion of the Data Snatches' (September 1988), fully displayed the continuity of the media scare with those historical fears about bodily invasion, individual and national, that are endemic to the paranoid style of American political culture [and] the paranoid, strategic mode of Defence Department rhetoric established during the Cold War. Each language repertoire is obsessed with hostile threats to bodily and technological immune systems; every event is a ballistic manoeuvre in the game of microbiological war, where the governing metaphors are indiscriminately drawn from cellular genetics and cybernetics alike.
>
> (Ross 1991: 76)

The breadth of such feelings of vulnerability is illustrated by the following excerpt from an edited collection of articles devoted to providing a predominantly left-wing critique of the values inherent in 'microcybernetic consumerism':

> The disturbing prospect is that opposition to the microcybernetic consumerist dictatorship will then find its only effective location deep underground, in the hands of zealots or fanatics who are content to destroy without bothering to dialogue. And microcybernetic technology is particularly vulnerable to just such a sort of opposition; as we have seen, hackers generally get caught only when they become brazen; and a determined band of computer nihilists, endowed with patience as well as skill, could even now be ensconced deep in the system, planting their bugs, worms and bombs.
>
> (Ravetz in Sardar and Ravetz 1996: 52)

Hacking has been subject to a large amount of hyperbole. The usual levels of media hype have been compounded by the fact that the activity relates, in the eyes of the public, to the recondite area of computing. Exacerbating the process still further is the anonymity and the non-physical nature of their computer intrusions. The combination of these factors makes a heady brew for those wishing to sensationalize the issue. Elements of the hacking community contribute their own brand of rhetoric to the mix with the adoption of colourfully threatening group names such as *The Legion of Doom*, *Bad Ass Mother Fuckers* and *Toxic Shock*. Pre-existing societal feelings of technological vulnerability may be exaggerated by the hype surrounding hacking but such hype itself merely reflects more deep-rooted fears about technological change in general.

Cyberpunk – technology hits the streets

A factor that has contributed to a general atmosphere of hyperbole in the public's perception of hacking has been its close association with the genre that has come to be known as cyberpunk, the novel *Neuromancer* being its most famous example. The esoteric technical complexity of computer intrusion has found an expressive medium in this radical new genre. Gibson's work and the wider cyberpunk oeuvre has played a significant role in creating a cultural expression for the democratization of science and technology. Cyberpunk in its heyday sought to identify and then imaginatively fictionalize the pace and extent of the technological trends of the 1980s. Whereas 'traditional' science fiction (SF) tends to use time-frames projected far into the future, cyberpunk fiction has distinguished itself by reflecting much more closely contemporary concerns:

> The cyberpunks are perhaps the first SF generation to grow up not only within the literary tradition of science fiction but in a truly science-fictional world. For them, the techniques of classical 'hard SF' – extrapolation, technological literacy – are not just literary tools but an aid to daily life. They are a means of understanding, and highly valued.
>
> (Sterling 1986: ix)

The cyberpunk author Bruce Sterling points out that our perennial fear of and fascination with new technologies has coincided with a zeitgeist shift that cyberpunk has sought to describe. Technology, although increasingly complex, is simultaneously becoming increasingly intimate and physically invasive. This is due, amongst other factors, to the trend to miniaturization and the increasingly invasive forms technology takes. It is now more readily accessible and manipulable than in previous times when it was more easily subjected to institutionalized control:

> times have changed since the comfortable era ... when Science was safely enshrined – and confined – in an ivory tower. The careless technophilia of those days belongs to a vanished, sluggish era, when authority still had a comfortable margin of control. For the cyberpunks, by stark contrast, technology is visceral. It is not the bottled genie of remote Big Science boffins; it is pervasive, utterly intimate. Not outside us, but next to us. Under our skin; often, inside our minds. Technology itself has changed. Not for us the giant steam-snorting wonders of the past: the Hoover Dam, the Empire State Building, the nuclear power plant. Eighties tech sticks to the skin, responds to the touch: the personal computer, the Sony Walkman, the portable telephone, the soft contact lens.
>
> (Sterling 1986: xi)

In a Chandleresque-style cameo, a bar-stool occupying protagonist of the Gibson short story *Burning Chrome* mixes an inhaler with his alcohol to create a personalized 'high'. Gibson's character accompanies his action with the observation that: 'Clinically they use the stuff to counter senile amnesia, but the street finds its own uses for things'

(Gibson 1986: 215). The latter phrase could be used as an emblematic motto for the way in which the cyberpunk genre fictionalizes not only the ubiquitous ingenuity with which hackers seek to approach technology in its various forms (not simply computers) but also hacking's desire to obtain a certain degree of 'street-cred':

> The elitist class profile of the hacker prodigy as that of an undersocialized college nerd has become democratized and customized in recent years; it is no longer exclusively associated with institutionally acquired college expertise, and increasingly it dresses street-wise.
>
> (Ross 1991: 89)

Hacking has spread far from its origins in the academic cloisters of places such as MIT, it has now become more associated with an urban aesthetic (whether this is in practice largely illusory or not).

Hackers, cyberpunk fiction and the pace of change – flux and blurred boundaries

> Nature has all along yielded her flesh to humans. First we took Nature's materials ... Now Bios is yielding to us her mind ... we are taking her logic ... The world of our own making has become so complicated that we must turn to the world of the born to understand how to manage it ... Yet as we unleash living forces into our created machines, we lose control of them. They acquire wildness and some of the surprises that the wild entails ... The world of the made will soon be like the world of the born: autonomous, adaptable, and creative, but, consequently, out of our control. I think that's a great bargain.
>
> (Kelly 1994: 2–5)

The advent of the information revolution with its pace of change and the paradigm shift it has induced heightens perennial concerns about technological change and our ability to control it. Chip Tango a 'midnight irregular' and archetypal hacker provides a real-world example of the enthusiastic embracing of technological flux espoused by techno-utopian writers such as Kevin Kelly and portrayed in cyberpunk fiction:

> He takes for granted that computer technology is out of control, and he wants to ride it like a surfer rides a wave. The opportunities

for fouling up the world through computer power are unlimited, but he thinks that people like him are useful agents in establishing a balance, a sense of humaneness and humor ... when presented with a scenario of a world which increasingly uses information in an oppressive Orwellian manner, [he] replied, 'I'm not worried for a minute about the future. If the world you describe is going to happen, man, I can fuck it up a lot faster than the world we live in now!'

(Vallee 1984: 150–151)

Ironically, however, with their finger on the cultural pulse of the information zeitgeist even cyberpunks may struggle to keep pace with the rapidity of technological change. Istvan Csiscery-Ronay, Jr, has termed this constant struggle 'retro-futuristic chronosemiitis, or futuristic flu'.[3] In *Neuromancer*, even Case, the otherwise technologically savvy cyberpunk, is not immune to the difficulty of keeping abreast of change:

The one who showed up at the loft door with a box of diskettes from the Finn was a soft-voiced boy called Angelo. His face was a simple graft grown on collagen and shark-cartilage polysaccharides, smooth and hideous. It was one of the nastiest pieces of elective surgery Case had ever seen. When Angelo smiled, revealing the razor-sharp canines of some large animal, Case was actually relieved. Toothbud transplants. He'd seen that before. 'You can't let the little pricks generation-gap you', Molly said.

(cited in Markley 1996: 84)

A more prosaic example of the information technology generation gap is provided by the father–son relationship of Robert Morris Senior and junior. The elder at the time of his following statement was Chief Scientist at the US National Computer Security Centre:

The notion that we are raising a generation of children so technically sophisticated that they can outwit the best efforts of the security specialists of America's largest corporations and the military is utter nonsense. I wish it were true. That would bode well for the technological future of the country.

(Lundell 1989: 11)

In a rather ironic twist of fate, this assertion proved to illustrate more than Morris originally intended. The statement was uttered five years before his own son caused widespread disruption of the Internet when he released in November 1988 a self-replicating program that came to be known as The Internet Worm. This ironic father and son example neatly illustrates the end of the days when once, in the previously cited words of Bruce Sterling, the authorities had a comfortable margin of control. Robert Morris Senior, a key figure in the computer security establishment, was not even aware of the technical ability of his own son.

Sterling in his preface to Gibson's collection of short stories, *Burning Chrome*, vividly summarizes the way in which cyberpunk captures the zeitgeist of constant change:

> In Gibson's work we find ourselves in the streets and alleys, in a realm of sweaty, white-knuckled survival, where high tech is a constant subliminal hum, like a deranged experiment in social Darwinism, designed by a bored researcher who kept one thumb permanently on the fast-forward button. Big Science in this world is not a source of quaint Mr Wizard marvels but an omnipresent, all-permeating, definitive force. It is a sheet of mutating radiation pouring through a crowd, a jam-packed Global Bus roaring wildly up an exponential slope. These stories paint an instantly recognizable portrait of the modern predicament.
>
> (Gibson 1986: 11)

In the context of this modern predicament the protagonists of cyberpunk fiction frequently give the sense that even though they may be literate in the workings of the technologically saturated environments they inhabit, they have little control over their own eventual fates and are constantly struggling to assert their individuality in the face of the identity-threatening technological systems they nevertheless yearn to immerse themselves in.

Technological intimacy – cyberpunks meet microserfs

> Further personality fragmentation and a breakdown of empathy lead to 'cyberpsychosis'. Behind this idea lies a long history of anxieties about 'dehumanization' by technology; a quintessentially humanist point of view which sees technology as an autonomous, runaway force that has come to displace the natural right of individuals to control themselves and their environment.
>
> (Ross 1991: 160)

The fictional representations of hacking analysed in this chapter derive their creative impetus by exploring, in the sharp relief afforded by the medium of the novel, the key issues highlighted by those who seek to interact with a range of technologies at an above-average level of intensity and intimacy. Levy foresaw cyberpunk's depiction of the human/machine symbiosis with his observation that 'Real optimum programming, of course, could only be accomplished when every obstacle between you and the pure computer was eliminated – an ideal that probably won't be fulfilled until hackers are somehow biologically merged with computers' (Levy 1984: 126). He describes how to some extent at least the earliest hackers achieved this feeling by attaining, 'a state of pure concentration ... When you had all that information glued to your cerebral being, it was almost as if your mind had merged into the environment of the computer' (ibid.: 37). Jacques Vallee (1984) similarly describes such a process with relation to a hacker called Chip Tango:

> He never speaks of 'using a machine' or 'running a program'. He leaves those expressions to those engineers of the old school. Instead, he will say that he 'attaches his consciousness' to a particular process. He 'butterflies his way across the net, picking up a link here, an open socket there'.
>
> (136)

A continual redefining of both the body and the wider natural world is a distinguishing feature of cyberpunk's fictionalized and futuristic portrayal of hacking life. *Neuromancer* begins with the sentence: 'The sky above the port was the color of television, tuned to a dead channel' and cyberpunk's 'relaxed contempt for the flesh' is evident from the frequency with which the boundaries separating organic bodies from technology and even other species are transgressed within the genre. Neil Stephenson's *Snowcrash*, for example, features a radioactive guard-dog, whilst Jeff Noon's *Vurt* and *Pollen* include dog/cat–human and zombie–human hybrids. These extreme fictional entities in cyberpunk fiction serve as a vehicle to symbolize societal fears of the invasive power of the various technologies hackers enjoy identifying themselves with so much. Despite the fact that cyberpunks clearly represent a highly modernized form of the maverick spirit of the Western cowboy, cyberpunk fiction is riddled with examples of the negative consequences of their intimate relationship with technology and we shall now see how such examples have resonance in the real world and the way in which the relationship of hackers with technology is presented as unhealthily obsessive, addictive and dehumanizing.

Hackers, addiction and the prison of flesh

> he'd cry for it, cry in his sleep, and wake alone in the dark, curled in his capsule in some coffin hotel, his hands clawed into the bedslab, temperfoam bunched between his fingers, trying to reach the console that wasn't there ... For Case, who lived for the bodiless exultation of cyberspace, it was the Fall. In the bars he'd frequented as a cowboy hotshot, the elite stance involved a certain relaxed contempt for the flesh. The body was meat. Case fell into the prison of his own flesh.
>
> (Gibson 1984: 11 and 12)

One of the most vivid fictional examples of the purportedly addictive qualities of hacking is the above excerpt from Gibson's *Neuromancer*. The major reason for the 'relaxed contempt for the flesh' shown by cyberpunk characters is their affinity with the rich data environment known as the matrix (with the psychoanalytical/oedipal overtones the womb-related Latin root of this phrase implies). For real-world hackers a similar, if less marked, affinity is shown for 'the system' whether that be complex phone or computer networks:

> There's a real love–hate relationship between us and the phone company. 'We don't particularly appreciate the bureaucracy that runs it, but we love the network itself', he says, lingering the world love. 'The network is the greatest thing to come along in the world.'
>
> (Colligan 1982)

The affinity to enter and then be at one with the impersonal system can be seen as a highly addictive experience:

> The hacker wants to break in. Breaking in is the addictive principle of hacking ... It produces anxiety, as it is a melancholic exercise in endless loss ... The experience of the limit that cyberspace affords is an anxious, addictive experience in which the real appears as withdrawal and loss ... The matrix is too complex and fragmented to offer itself to any one unifying gaze ... Hence, the attraction of the cyberspace addiction: to jack in is briefly, thrillingly, to get next to the power; not to be able to jack in is impotence. Moreover, the cyberspace addiction, the hacker mystique,

posits power through anonymity ... It is a dream of recovering power and wholeness by seeing wonders and by not being seen. But what a strange and tangled dream, this power that is only gained through matching your synapses to the computer's logic, through beating the system by being the system.

(Moreiras in Conley 1993: 197–198)

The obsessive body-neglecting qualities of cyberpunk's fictional depiction of what is involved by mentally 'jacking into' the matrix of information is similar to the imagery of close identification and even addiction used by real-life hackers:

> I just do it because it makes me feel good, as in better than any-thing else that I've ever experienced. Computers are the only thing that have ever given me this feeling ... the adrenaline rush I get when I'm trying to evade authority, the thrill I get from having written a program that does something that was supposed to be impossible to do, and the ability to have social relations with other hackers are all very addictive. I get depressed when I'm away from a networked computer for too long. I find conversations held in cyberspace much more meaningful and enjoyable than conversing with people in physical-reality real mode ... I consider myself addicted to hacking. If I were ever in a position where I knew my computer activity was over for the rest of my life, I would suffer withdrawal.
>
> (*Maelstrom* cited in Taylor 1993: 107)

> rushing through the phone line like heroin through an addict's veins, an electronic pulse is sent out, a refuge from the day-to-day incompetencies is sought ... a board is found. 'This is it ... this is where I belong.'
>
> (*The Mentor – Phrack* Vol. 1, Issue 7)

The image of flesh as a prison is a particularly forceful expression of an uneasiness hackers have with their bodies. Levy (1984), for example, describes how the hackers of MIT typically paid little attention to their bodily needs or physical appearance whilst absorbed by their activity. This lack of interest in bodily matters periodically and perversely culminated in an annual ugliest geek on campus competi-tion run by the hacker community. This disregard of hackers for their bodies which receives its most dramatic expression in the dehumaniz-ing concerns contained within cyberpunk fiction is also a key element of Coupland's account of Microsoft's workers in the more socially realistic novel *Microserfs*. The narrator makes the following observations:

> I don't even do any sports anymore and my relationship with my body has gone all weird. I used to play soccer three times a week and now I feel like a boss in charge of an underachiever. I feel like my body is a station wagon in which I drive my brain around, like a suburban mother taking the kids to hockey practice.
>
> (Coupland 1995: 4)

> When I was younger ... I went through a phase where I wanted to be a machine ... I honestly didn't want to become flesh; I wanted to be 'precision technology' – like a Los Angeles person.
>
> (ibid.: 72 and 73)

> I want to forget the way my body was ignored, year in, year out, in the pursuit of code, in the pursuit of somebody else's abstraction. There's something about a monolithic tech culture like Microsoft that makes humans seriously rethink fundamental aspects of the relationship between their brains and bodies – their souls and their ambitions; things and thoughts.
>
> (ibid.: 90)

> We were all wearing laundry-junk clothes and we looked like scare-crows flailing about. Why are we so hopeless with our bodies?
>
> (ibid.: 76)

Although Coupland's work does not contain the extreme blurring of bodily boundaries present within cyberpunk, this basic theme provides the novel's denouement as the mother of the narrator suffers a stroke which is described in terms of a computer system crash:

> Mom's functions may one day be complete and may be one day partial, but as of today there's nothing but the twitches and the knowledge that fear is locked inside the body. Her eyes can be opened and closed, but not enough to semaphore messages. She's all wired up and gizmo'ed; her outside looks like the inside of a Bell switchbox. What is *her* side of the story? The password has been deleted.
>
> (ibid.: 365)

Co-optation, addiction and the Otaku

> We're still not sure what happened to the pirate flag that once flew
> over Apple Computer's headquarters but we do know that what was
> once a nerd phenomenon backed by an idealistic belief in the freedom
> of information became the powerful aphrodisiac behind sexy initial
> public offerings. Che Guevara with stock options.
>
> (Hawn 1996: 2)

We have seen above how hackers and their fictional representatives
intimately identify and interact with both abstract communication
systems and more prosaic artefacts. In addition, at a more metaphorical
level hackers have been accused of identifying too closely with the code
of capitalism. Instead of using their technical proficiency in order to
control the worst excesses of corporate-driven technological progress
and redirecting it to more counter-cultural ends, they are instead
charged with reinforcing its values as their ingenuity is co-opted by
corporate concerns:

> the hacker cyberculture is not a dropout culture; its disaffiliation
> from a domestic parent culture is often manifest in activities that
> answer, directly or indirectly, to the legitimate needs of industrial
> R and D. For example, this hacker culture celebrates high produc-
> tivity, maverick forms of creative work energy, and an obsessive
> identification with on-line endurance (and endorphin highs) – all
> qualities that are valorised by the entrepreneurial codes of silicon
> futurism ... The values of the white male outlaw are often those of
> the creative maverick universally prized by entrepreneurial or
> libertarian individualism ... teenage hackers resemble an alienated
> shopping culture deprived of purchasing opportunities more than
> a terrorist network.
>
> (Ross 1991: 90)

The ambivalence of hackers' claims to be a counter-cultural force are
mirrored in what has been identified as an inherent contradiction of
cyberpunk literature. Cyberpunks are presented as anarchic opponents
to established corporate power yet the genre is marked by the
frequency with which the cyberpunk's human agency is subsumed to
the greater ends of their corporate hirers. They fail frequently to
redirect corporate power to more humane ends and this is perhaps due
to the ultimate conflation of the cyberpunks/hackers and corporations'
desire for technological experimentation. Hackers and cyberpunks only

wish to surf the wave of technological innovation, but corporations constantly seek to co-opt that desire for their own ends.

> There is … a tension in cyberpunk between the military industrial monster that produces technology and the sensibility of the technically skilled individual trained for the high tech machine … Even the peaceful applications of these technologies can be subordinated to commercial imperatives abhorrent to the free thinking cyberpunk. There is a contradiction between the spirit of free enquiry and experiment and the need to keep corporate secrets and make a buck. Cyberpunk is a reflection of this contradiction, on the one hand it is a drop-out culture dedicated to pursuing the dream of freedom through appropriate technology. On the other it is a ready market for new gadgets and a training ground for hip new entrepreneurs with hi-tech toys to market.
>
> (Wark 1992: 3)

A dramatic example of both the alienating and co-opting aspects of hacker behaviour is provided by the phenomenon of the Otaku who have various hacker attributes. The phrase is used to describe a Japanese subculture who are noticeable by their preference for interacting with machines over people and their penchant for collecting, exchanging or hoarding what for non-Otaku would seem trivial information such as the exact make of socks worn by their favourite pop-star. The most publicized Otaku to date is Tsutomu Miyazaki who abducted, molested and mutilated four pre-teen Tokyo girls in a serial killing spree. The quality of alienation associated with Otaku culture is inadvertently indicated in one reaction to this case from an Otaku seeking to distance Miyazaki from the movement:

> 'Miyazaki was not really even an otaku', says Taku Hachiro, a 29-year-old otaku and author and author of Otaku Heaven … 'If he was a real otaku he wouldn't have left the house and driven around looking for victims. That's just not otaku behavior. Because of his case, people still have a bad feeling about us. They shouldn't. They should realize that we are the future – more comfortable with things than people,' Hachiro said. 'That's definitely the direction we're heading as a society.'
>
> (Greenfeld 1993: 4)

Along with this alienated aspect of the Otaku is their amenability to co-optation by corporate culture:

'The otaku are an underground (subculture), but they are not opposed to the system per se,' observed sociologist and University of Tokyo fellow Volker Grassmuck ... 'They change, manipulate and subvert ready-made products, but at the same time they are the apotheosis of consumerism and an ideal workforce for contemporary capitalism ... Many of our best workers are what you might call otaku,' explained an ASCII corp. spokesman. 'We have over 2,000 employees in this office and more than 60 percent might call themselves otaku. You couldn't want more commitment.'

(Greenfeld 1993: 3 and 4)

It is this over-willingness of hackers to identify with *the system* be it a complex telephone/computer network or the regimented and codified corporate framework that Microsoft provides for its employees that Coupland describes as lying behind the gradual enervation of the human spirit implied by the eponymous soubriquet 'Microserfs'. The highly intelligent computer programmers working at Microsoft's headquarters in Seattle become effectively indentured to the process of producing abstract code and increasingly divorced from the physical world and their own bodies.

Ubiquitous hacking

Despite the above concerns over the ultimately unhealthy nature of hackers' relationship with both technology and the economic system which seeks to profit from their technological proficiency, they remain a potent symbol of control in a world of constantly changing technology. 'True' hackers exhibit technological ingenuity that is manifested as an idiosyncratic attitude to a wide range of technological artefacts, not just computer systems. They are intrigued by the ability to explore the configuration of computer networks and the underlying instrumentality of all types of systems and artefacts, computer systems merely being those most amenable to control at a distance:

In my day to day life, I find myself hacking everything imaginable. I hack traffic lights, pay phones, answering machines, micro-wave ovens, VCRs, you name it, without even thinking twice. To me hacking is just changing the conditions over and over again until there's a different response. In today's mechanical world, the opportunities for this kind of experimentation are endless.

(Kane 1989: 67)

Hacking is also viewed by its practitioners as a mind-set evident in scientific and technological endeavours in general, not just computing; for example, gene-splicing in this model is seen as a form of biological hacking. The common underlying theme to all activities that could be classed under the broad term hacking is their instrumental yet unorthodox approach, as described by Ralph, a Dutch hacker:

> Hacking not only pertains to computers but pertains to any field of technology. Like if you haven't got a kettle to boil water with and you use your coffee machine, then that in my mind is a hack. Because you're using the technology in a way that it's not supposed to be used. Now that also pertains to telephones, if you're going to use your telephone to do various things that aren't supposed to be done with a telephone, then that's a hack. If you're going to use your skills as a car mechanic to make your motor do things it's not supposed to be doing, then that's a hack. So for me it's not only computers it's anything varying from locks, computers, telephones, magnetic cards, you name it.
>
> (Taylor 1993: 78)

A humorous example of such a ubiquitous approach was provided by Kevin Poulsen who, serving a prison sentence for his hacking exploits said: 'I've learned a lot from my new neighbors ... Now I know how to light a cigarette from an outlet and how to make methamphetamine from chicken stock' (Fine 1995). Such pragmatic technological ingenuity is redolent of the previously cited possible motto of cyberpunk: 'the street finds its own use for things'.

Cultural lag

> What we have today, instead of a social consciousness electrically ordered ... is a private subconsciousness or individual 'point of view' rigorously imposed by older mechanical technology. This is the perfectly natural result of 'culture lag' or conflict, in a world suspended between two technologies.
>
> (McLuhan 1964: 108)

Widespread fear of the extent and pace of technological change and the contrasting manner with which hacking and cyberpunks are associated with street level technological savvy highlight the extent to which hackers can be viewed as key illustrators of the phenomenon of the *culture lag* described by Marshall McLuhan. Hackers are a sub-cultural group that go against the norm by seeking to avoid the demonization of technology. They are arguably the prototypical denizens of the interstices that exist between old social mores and the cultural implications of new technologies. John Perry Barlow and the Electronic Frontier Foundation assert their wish to avoid 'a neo-Luddite resentment of digital technology from which little good can come ... there is a spreading sense of dislocation, and helplessness in the general presence of which no society can expect to remain healthy' (*Computer Underground Digest* Vol. 1, Issue 13). Hacking provides a possible escape route from such resentment and has been viewed in the mode of a postmodern counter-cultural response to the seemingly inevitable advance of new technology, hackers are seen as constituting:

> a conscious resistance to the domination but not the fact of technological encroachment into all realms of our social existence. The CU represents a reaction against modernism by offering an ironic response to the primacy of technocratic language, the incursion of computers into realms once considered private, the politics of the techno-society, and the sanctity of established civil and state authority ... It is this style of playful rebellion, irreverent subversion, and juxtaposition of fantasy with high-tech reality that impels us to interpret the computer underground as a postmodernist culture.
>
> (Meyer and Thomas 1990: 3 and 4)

This somewhat elevated postmodern status afforded to hackers is predicated upon a cultural malaise that they are not so much immune to as more able to cope with than the rest of society:

> The tie between information and action has been severed ... we are glutted with information, drowning in information, we have no control over it, don't know what to do with it ... we no longer have a coherent conception of ourselves, and our universe, and our relation to one another and our world. We no longer know, as the Middle Ages did, where we come from, and where we are going, or why. That is, we don't know what information is relevant, and what information is irrelevant to our lives ... our defences against information glut have broken down; our information immune system is inoperable. We don't know how to reduce it ; we don't know how to use it. We suffer from a kind of cultural AIDS.
>
> (Postman 1990: 6)

Uncertainty and ethical ambiguity in the information age

The uncertainty that has accompanied the advent of the information age is manifested in the ambiguous ethical status of some computing activities and society's vacillating responses to the maverick qualities that seem to be at a premium in the hard-to-adapt-to hi-tech world of constant change. In the post Cold War world new security fears increasingly centre around the threat posed by cyber-terrorists yet the corollary also exists: the tacit pride felt in one's own electronic cognoscenti. The Israeli hacker Ehud Tenebaum (aka the Analyser), for example, was accused of being responsible for the 'most systematic and organised attempt ever to penetrate the Pentagon's computer systems' (*The Guardian* Online section 26 March 1998: 2). Whilst Tenebaum was under house arrest in the Israeli town of Hod Hasharon, the US authorities were seeking to use his apprehension as a deterrent to other hackers: 'This arrest should send a message to would-be hackers all over the world that the United States will treat computer intrusions as serious crimes', said US attorney general Janet Reno. 'We will work around the world and in the depths of cyber-space to investigate and prosecute those who attack computer networks' (ibid.: 2).

However, Israeli public figures have taken a much more conciliatory attitude to Tenebaum's activities and their implications:

> If there is a whiff of witch-hunt swirling around Washington, then in Israel Tenebaum's popularity seems to rise by the day. Prime minister Netanyahu's first comment on the affair was that the Analyser is 'damn good', before quickly adding that he could be 'very dangerous too'.
>
> (ibid.: 2)

Tenebaum's lawyer Zichroni further argued: 'It appears to me he brought benefit to the Pentagon ... in essence he came and discovered the Pentagon's coding weaknesses' ... adding sardonically that 'the US authorities should maybe pay Tenebaum for his services' (ibid.: 2 and 3).

Whilst such comments may be interpreted as a lawyer's tongue-in-cheek defence of his client, the way in which the unethical aspects of Tenebaum's actions are blurred by their potential pragmatic uses to industry and national security is illustrated by the fact he was subsequently asked to appear before the Knesset's committee for science and technology research and development.

Conclusion

> On the one hand, the popular folk hero persona offered the romantic
> high profile of a maverick though nerdy cowboy whose fearless raids
> upon an impersonal 'system' were perceived as a welcome tonic in the
> grey age of technocratic routine. On the other hand, he was some-
> thing of a juvenile technodelinquent who hadn't yet learned the dif-
> ference between right and wrong; a wayward figure whose technical
> brilliance and proficiency differentiated him from, say, the malad-
> justed working-class J.D. street-corner boy of the 1950s.
>
> (Ross 1991: 84)

This account of hackers and their fictional counterparts has thus
sought to highlight the various ambivalences that seem to inevitably
accompany our perceptions of those who exhibit technological mastery
and ingenuity. The dark and perennial appeal of such tales as Faustus
and Frankenstein is based upon a notion contained deep within our
culture: knowledge is often obtained only at a price. The price in
Microserfs is a loss of self-awareness and an ingrained patina of
geekishness, whilst cyberpunk literature portrays a frenetic, individu-
alistic and ultimately dehumanized world. More positively, the
cyberpunk account of the increased dissemination of science and
technology to the street describes the democratisation of technology,
power over which has historically been held by emblematically white-
coated scientists. To this extent real-world technological sub-cultures
such as hackers are portrayed as part of a welcome countervailing trend
whereby technological power can be reappropriated by the people.
Levy (1984), for example, explicitly describes the first generation of
hackers as a group of computer users and program developers who
played a crucial part in the undermining of the quasi-sacerdotal
position of the lab-coated technicians who controlled the punch-cards
that conveyed instructions to the first computers.

With the dissemination of hi-tech to the streets, however, also
comes the concomitant loss of some of the previous certainties
epitomized by those reassuring authority figures in white coats.
Characters in cyberpunk exhibit a visceral enjoyment in their
interactions with technology, yet the majority of cyberpunk action is
set in dystopian social settings of exponential change where society is
frequently feral and in which technological ingenuity needs to be
closely aligned with day-to-day survival skills. The dysto-
pian/liberating ambivalence apparent in cyberpunk portrayals of
hacking is thus arguably a literary expression of an equally ambivalent

present-day feeling about the social significance of hackers. On the one hand, the maverick nature of the hacker spirit can be viewed as a healthy example of the technological ingenuity required to prosper in the hi-tech world, yet on the other, hackers personify the enervating pitfalls that face those who seek to redirect corporate control of technological progress to more humane ends. It remains to be seen whether a 'third way' can be found between the anarchic individualism of cyberpunk and the empty regimented corporatism of *Microserfs*.

Notes

1   For the specific purposes of this chapter the contested elements of the fourth generation's ethical and legal legitimacy are side-stepped so that hacking is simply and broadly defined as 'the exhibition of technological ingenuity'. This limited and thereby more inclusive definition of hacking is necessary in order to develop the argument that an analysis of hacking serves to illustrate wider social attitudes to the broad issue of technological change without becoming enmeshed in the ethical debates and minutiae of its evolutionary history.
2   Cf. Woolgar and Russell (1990).
3   Cited by David Brande in Markley (1996: 85).

4 Attitudes towards computer hacking in Russia

Alexander E. Voiskounsky, Julia D. Babaeva and Olga V. Smyslova

Historical overview

Computer hackers seem to represent one of the smallest samples of the globe-wide population, and one of the most esoteric, since the logic of their actions is universally recognized as incomprehensible. Very few people can boast they know a hacker personally – in fact hackers resemble a sort of a secret organization. As an invisible college, they have no definite location, no central or ruling body, and almost no coordination in general. At the same time hackers have gained a reputation as one of the most intensely talked about and widely discussed groups, both in special forums and in the mass media. Their power is perhaps much overestimated, and yet in the information society we pay a special rent to this non-organized, if not fully anarchic, group: a sort of a tax is added to the cost of almost every computerized system, the money has to be spent on so-called computer security. Institutions and corporations are encouraged to pay more and more in attempts to guarantee security; the latter is never believed to be safe enough. The ever-growing costs are justified, since the evil actions of computer hackers (or else phreakers, crackers, carders, computer pirates, etc.) have evidently proved that they might be really harmful and, if successful, cause even more tiresome and unexpected costs.

Hackers and their historical predecessors (phreakers, or 'telephone pirates') have for a long time used low-circulation specialized journals and/or bulletin boards to exchange views and to inform the members of this highly dispersed group about recent actions (called 'achievements'), and usually attach the protocols of these villain actions. The general public applied the term to computer experts as well, learning the term 'hacker' from Joseph Weizenbaum's 1976 book. This is the case, at least in the USA (Turkle 1984).

The idea of giving a special name to the most qualified computer experts, who are intrinsically devoted to the profession, who have the best possible knowledge of programming techniques and methods, who have developed many of the most elaborate techniques, and who work hard to supply end users with the most needed and valuable items of software, seems to be quite natural. Since a small influential group of super-qualified computer programmers has arisen in computing centres throughout the world, the term 'hacker' has become popular both inside and outside the USA. This is true for Russia (then the Soviet Union) as well. The term became widely known in 1982 when Weizenbaum's (1976) book was translated into Russian (Weizenbaum 1982). From the translator's footnote (ibid.: 164) the Russian readers of the book learned that, first, persons resembling those described by Weizenbaum could be observed (though not too often) in Soviet computing centres, and second, that in the Russian computer programming jargon there seems to be no equivalent to the word 'hacker'. For this reason the term has been transliterated in the Russian variant of the Weizenbaum (1976) book (Weizenbaum 1982).

It is perhaps worth mentioning that the transliterated word does not contradict the norms of Russian pronunciation, and is constructed in terms of production: the verbal word-stem with the ending -er forming a noun is one of usual models of transliteration in the modern Russian language. From that time on, professionals in information technology used the term 'hacker', though it stayed almost entirely unknown to the general public in the Soviet Union for another half a decade. It seems also worth mentioning that the practice of global computer telecommunications, and especially the Internet, was entirely unknown in the USSR until the 1990s. During the 1980s local area networks were used at most.

Computer hackers were known in Russia as 'soloists', as described by Weizenbaum (1976), who does not report computer-mediated communications within the hackers' community. Turkle who started her research two years after Weizenbaum's (1976) book was published, mentions that hackers widely use e-mail and listserves (Turkle 1984). But her book has never been translated into Russian, and the term 'hackers' in Russian computer programming jargon is used in the way it is understood and described by Weizenbaum: it refers exclusively to extremely talented and hard-working experts in various computer applications, who are usually non-communicative, idiosyncratic, and engaged in global projects. The short list of the parameters that Turkle (1984) uses to characterize hackers ('mastery, individualism, nonsensuality') is not formulated in these words, though the connotations are similar.

People's attitudes towards 'Soviet hackers' (a rather rarely used name) were mostly positive: they were welcomed as competent consultants, as hard-workers, and as experts in efficient computer usage (due to the overall shortage of the most needed computer resources – memory span, operation rate, access time, etc. – the efficient usage of existing resources has been vital for most organizations). Since no PCs were available in the USSR until the end of 1980s, all computer programmers, including hackers, were attached to organizations – usually to larger or smaller computing centres which owned mainframes. Eager to have longer access to the mainframes, many of them voluntarily used to work over night when the schedule was less busy.

Inside the organizations, computer experts, including hackers, have been connected rather closely: the main goal was the efficient adaptation of the brandname (IBM, DEC, Wang, etc.) operating systems and software packages in order to make them workable on the Soviet mainframe, computers analogous to those of brand name producers, mainly IBM. Adaptation required precise work by system programmers of program code and accurate changes. Intrusion into program code in order to make these changes was analogous to hacking. Thus, during the late 1960s and 1970s the most qualified computer programmers – all of them employed by the government – were earning their salaries performing hacking-like activities.

When and if hackers performed illegal actions or disobeyed instructions for computer use, positive attitudes towards them changed immediately. One of the first known court trials against a computer programmer took place in the USSR in 1983: the man was prosecuted for his actions that caused a break of several hours on an assembly line at a car factory. Minor and non-documented illegal actions have been performed by hackers in order to extend their access time to the mainframe computer: system administrators have had to correct the 'broken' (i.e., the unauthorized changes in) working schedules. Soviet hackers carry out illegal money transfer very rarely because the banking system in the USSR has not been dependent on electronic transactions of money orders, and in a minor degree only on electronic accounting. Since no copyright-protected software has been available, no illegal piracy actions could be performed or prosecuted. With no access to global computer networks, the temptation to create computer viruses has not been strong.

During the years of Soviet 'perestroika' (beginning with 1985) an entirely new mode of behaviour gained popularity. As a consequence, a great many of the terms used previously in Russia in a restricted (professional) context acquired additional connotations. Mostly, these terms were professional terms inherent in financial or information technology spheres. The idea of hacking and the word 'hacker' have also acquired popularity. At that time, several generations of high-school graduates and schoolchildren who have had classes in informatics at school (with very little, if any, access to PCs, which were highly primitive at the time) were advanced enough to join the worldwide groups of teenagers interested in computer applications and to begin hacking – mostly by way of cracking, gaining unauthorized access to computer systems.

Around this time the practice of writing and distributing computer viruses and anti-virus programs impelled some professionals – including law experts – to use the terms 'hackers/hacking' as terms equivalent to computer criminals and illegal action (Baturin 1987). At the same time the advanced Russian teenagers felt interested in the fundamentals of the ideology worked out by some creative groups within the computer hacker community. These are the ideas that computer software should be distributed freely, that the information contained in the governmental, corporate and private databases should be publicly available, and that security systems should be abolished. Neophite hackers were drawn to the hackers' ideology, their anti-war attitudes and anti-military actions, and the underground way of life, particularly the Burroughs-like esoterics, the Leary-like psychedelic happenings and the Gibson-like fantasy underlying this way of life, etc.

By 1987 computer hacking had become a popular theme of discussion and the mass media published original and/or translated papers on computer hacking. At first the authors needed to supply readers with explanations of the term but, as the years passed, it became widely recognized and comprehended. In the authors' collection there is a copy of an explanation given in a popular youth paper *Komsomolskaya Pravda* (10 December 1987): a hacker is said to be synonymous with a computer criminal who gains unauthorized access to distant archives and databases in order to steal secret data, and especially money from bank accounts and from credit cards; hackers are smart at mathematics and information technologies, they are mostly outside politics, but being computer hooligans they might be vulnerable to abuse by this or that political group.

It is not surprising that these explanations were being corrected as information about the way of life outside the 'iron curtain' became widely available. Perhaps the strongest impact on this generation of teenagers who understood the terms 'hacking/hacker' (and the words 'Internet', or 'virtual reality', etc.) was provoked not by printed or electronic media but by popular American movies. In the period of 1987–9 the term 'computer hacker' became popular in mass surveys of school-age children (males, as a rule) as a probable future profession/occupation. Of course this reply was characteristic of relatively advanced teenagers, usually those who have had some access to computers, either at home or, more often, at the parents'/relatives' workplace. During the last ten years (1989–99) attitudes towards computer hacking have undergone marked change.

State of the art overview

Current information about the actions of computer hackers (that are usually performed overseas) is now widely available in Russia. Traditional and electronic media provide readers, subscribers and WWW surfers with reviews and descriptions of those actions performed by Russian and foreign hackers, as well as with detailed technical protocols of computer attacks, if these protocols are made available. The 'hacking news' genre represents an increasing discourse of publications in Russia. General audiences prefer verbal descriptions of current sensational performances by hackers/crackers/carders, etc., and of the security personnel's attempts to arrest and prosecute hackers. The technically advanced audience enjoys the protocols of computer attacks, the lists of poorly administered websites, Intranet and LANs that might be used for unauthorized penetrations, and descriptions of new sorts of software for hacking.

In the late 1980s and 1990s the traditional scope of printed periodicals coming from the old (i.e., Soviet) period was greatly diversified. A variety of newborn periodicals have come to life, among them special journals and weekly papers related to different aspects of information technologies. Some of them are produced by Russians, the others are the translations of American (and sometimes European) journals. Typically, they include both articles that have been translated into Russian and articles that have been originally written in Russian. These periodicals include *Computerra* (www.cterra.ru), *Interface* (ceased), *World of PC* (www.pcworld.ru), *Qwerty* (ceased), *Computerworld Russia* (www.computerworld.ru), *PC Magazine* (www.newman.ru), *LAN* (www.lanmag.ru), *Seti* (networks, www.networld.ru), *Softmarket* (ceased), *Planeta Internet* (http://www.netplanet.ru), *Zhurnal.ru* (ceased), *Mir Internet* (www.piter-press.ru), *Chip* (http://www.chip.kiev.ua), *Mir Bezopasnosti* (demos.security.journal), *Computerpress* (www.cpress.ru/russian/), *Monitor* (ceased), *Connect* (www.connect.ru), *Internet* (www.inter.net.ru), *Hard'n'soft* (www.hardnsoft.ru).

Electronic papers (with no hard-copy equivalent) publishing daily and weekly reviews for a mass audience need to be mentioned, too. Among the most respected and popular are the newspaper *Gazeta* (www.gazeta.ru) and the collection of daily digests and reviews *Vechernii Internet* (http://www.cityline.ru/vi/). These papers covering items of general interest – sensations, politics, economics, sport, movies, fiction, etc. – include a heading for the Internet-related papers and news. All the hard-copy and electronic papers and journals supply the readers with updated news on computer hacking and hackers both inside and outside Russia (perhaps with a special interest in cracking, since news of this is seen as the most sensational). For example, detailed information on the hostile opposition between Mitnick and Shimomura has been provided many a time and in many sources.

This popular, i.e. non-technical, flow of information has been amplified with several books translated from English. These are the well-known books: *Hackers* by John Markoff and Kathy Hafner (Markof and Hafner 1996), *The Cuckoo's Egg* by Clifford Stoll (Stoll 1996), and the second edition of *The New Hacker's Dictionary* compiled by Eric Raymond (Raymond 1996). It is a paradoxical coincidence, that these three books were independently translated and issued by the three different publishers almost at the same time, and all three happened to be available for Russian consumers within a short interval – several months only.

During the 1990s wider audiences, consisting primarily of Russian teenagers, got to know, and usually admired, popular American movies – among them *WarGames* (1983), *The Net* (1995), *Hackers* (1995), and some other movies less related to computer hacking but dealing intensely with the information technologies (for example, a serial *Virtual Reality*). For a much wider audience – far beyond the community of computer hackers – some fiction and fantasy novels have been recently translated, including novels by William Burroughs *The Ticket that Exploded* (Burroughs 1998a, 1999), *Naked Lunch* (Burroughs 1998b), *The Soft Machine* (Burroughs 1999) and *Nova Express*, (Burroughs 1998a, 1999). A report on psychedelic experience by Timothy Leary and his collaborators, based on the *Tibetan Book of the Dead* and published in 1964, has been translated into Russian, at first unofficially distributed, and recently published (Leary *et al.* 1999).

These novels and provocative quasi-research volumes seem to supply some additional (it might be called in a way theoretical, eclectic as it is) understanding of the underground way of life that is/was traditional for an influential minority group of the ideologists within the worldwide community of hackers – those who are intellectually and/or practically interested in psychedelic happenings, in cyberpunk ideas, and in the anarchist-like revolutionary liberation movement of the old-days – beatniks, hippies and/or Yippies (Youth International Party). Gibson's *Neuromancer* is not yet available as a hard-copy book, though WWW surfers have easy access to the text translated into Russian (kulichki.rambler.ru/moshkow/GIBSON/gibson01.txt).

During the second half of the 1990s, technical publications on methods of computer hacking and, on the other side, on various computer security issues were available in Russia. In recent years, hard-copy publications (books and journal articles), both written by Russians experts and translated from foreign languages, have been published (Grusho and Timonina 1996; Platonov *et al.* 1997; Vakka 1997; Zegzhda and Ivashko 1998). Articles are welcome in most of the journals and papers dealing with the information technologies. Among the books translated into Russian there is an electronic version of Bruce Sterling's *The Hacker Crackdown: Law and Disorder on the Electronic Frontier* (Sterling 1992). Original publications in Russian on legal aspects of secure usage of information technologies include Krylov (1997) and Petrakov (1997) and others.

In 1999, the first issue of the hard-copy technical journal *Hacker* (100 pages) was published (URL: www.xaker.ru). It is expected to become the major specialized source for all those who are experts in hacking and all newcomers to the field. In a critical response (not a review, formally) to the first issue (http://www.russ.ru/journal/netcult/99–02–19/baby.htm) it is argued that the journal will be mostly useful for those who are not going to hack full time and are not altogether devoted to this sort of activity. Since the slang of the younger generation is heavily used in the journal, the target group evidently will be the newcomers with rather low qualifications in the technology of computer attacks.

During the same period of time, several conferences on computer security have been held; many universities throughout Russia have announced courses in the computer security field. Some of them are equipped and supported by international companies – brand names in the information technologies field. Theoretical and applied issues of so-called information warfare are discussed, original system theory models are worked out and presented (Rastorguev 1998). Political and military aspects of information technologies' usage as a major component of modern (sixth generation) warfare has been stated and discussed at an international conference Information Technologies and Political Power held on 26–28 January 1999 in Moscow.

No wonder these activities have parallels in electronic publications.

A Russian language echo-conference on computer hacking is running on the BBS-based network FIDO. The same groups that publish and promote hard-copy books/journals dedicated to computer hacking, administer websites that are enthusiastically visited by Russian speaking hackers (and those interested in hacking experiences) both from Russia and from the other newly independent states of the former Soviet Union – among the most advanced in information technologies' usage and applications are the Ukrainians. Numerous websites publishing data useful to hackers can be discovered throughout the Russian segment of the web. To retrieve them, one can use several originally Russian search engines such as Rambler (www.rambler.ru), Yandex (www.yandex.ru), Aport (www.aport.ru), Au (www.au.ru), etc. – or else the Cyrillic version of the AltaVista (www.altavista.com).

The major Russian website in the field that gained the most solid reputation and contains the full range of the hacking related issues (phreaking/cracking/carding, etc.) is located at: http://www.hackzone. ru. It includes an archive of weekly reviews; relevant papers – both translated and in Russian; a webguide with links to the pertinent newsgroups, ftps, FAQs and websites containing the archives of the software needed for web attacks and for different ways of hacking activities; a description of the laws of the Russian Federation dealing with the full range of information activities; an e-journal *HackZone*; FAQs and recommendations for the newbies; special forms of humour; updated lists of the hacked sites; a 'clubboard' – a space for club-like activities; a visitor's forum, etc.

The site is well known and intensely visited. In a competition held via the web in 1998, this very website has been elected as the winner in the area of 'Public Recognition' (the voters are self-selected web-surfers). The same website has shared the second place in the same competition for 'Informational Site' – in this area the voters are the professionals in information technologies and in web design. The information about the appraisal of the site http://www.hackzone.ru is available in the December 1998 issue of the journal *Mir Internet* (www.piter-press.ru).

Actions of Russian hackers are too diverse to report on them in full. Of all the hackers' subgroups, the phreakers seem to be the less numerous in Russia, due to the fact that Russian phone lines are mainly non-digital, and in general far from being modernized, compared to the developed countries that have entered the information society. Besides, the Russian population of the owners of mobile phones is rather small; thus the business of pirating mobile phones and of criminal reselling the 'free' mobile phone numbers seems to be not too competitive (though certainly profitable). It's worth mentioning that the 'Russian Phreackers' Site' (mypage.goplay.com/phreack/) is actually located outside Russia though the owners report they are planning to move the website to Russia.

Compared to phreakers, groups of criminal hackers as computer pirates/crackers turned out to be much more numerous in Russia. The majority of organizations and all the private desktop computer owners throughout Russia seem to have no budget to purchase the most needed software (both operating systems and applied programs) from producers and legal providers. To be able to exploit computers, the programmers have to be competent in cracking the safety systems in order to copy operating systems and applied computer programs and to adapt them in an unauthorized way on as many computers as needed. Computer users or programmers need not perform this themselves, since everybody is able to purchase pirated copies of updated software. These are easily accessible, and the costs are extremely low. These sets of illegal software incorporate all sorts of the programs, including illegal Russian translations of the new computer games, and of course the newest updated programs needed for hacking.

The anti-pirate actions performed jointly by Russian customs, police, intellectual copyright agencies and legal producers/providers of software are not efficient enough. China and the Eastern Europe area (including mainly Russia, Bulgaria, Poland and the Ukraine) are widely believed to be the world's greatest producers and importers of illegal software. Particularly in Russia, 'a blossoming hacker culture has begun to thrive on cheap, widely available hacking software' (Dougherty 1999). In the same publication it is reported that the 'street peddlers' sell software specifically for creating viruses and generating credit card numbers for 'just a little more than $3' (ibid.).

Special journals, forums, echo-conferences, FAQs, and webguides supply the newbies – newcomers to the community of Russian hackers – with the lists of drawbacks and faults in the various security systems; the technical descriptions and protocols of hacking are also easily available. No wonder the primary (or primitive, the experts would say) level of hacking skills is now swiftly and effectively growing. This is one of the reasons that the population of Russian hackers is growing rapidly. Another reason is that for teenagers in Russia hacking, and especially cracking, is a preferred way of self-realization. It is the way they try to gain a reputation of being smart and risky. One more reason is that being affiliated with a reference group of hackers is prestigious and exceptional, and thus highly appreciated by teenagers. Finally, cracking or carding is a means to earn money, either as an occupation or as an opportunity for free shopping at virtual e-commerce shops – paid by nobody at all or by the real credit card owners.

Hackers' group activities

Rather little is known about individual hackers not affiliated with groups. A brief review of current group actions will be given below.

A growing team of Russian hackers is busy with the 'distributed.net' project trying to crash the RC5 codes – the international project is initiated by the RSA (http://www.rsa.com) ready to pay to a winner a premium of US$10,000. The Russian team – called the 'HackZone Team' – is organized and administered by managers of the HackZone website (http://www.hackzone.ru), and it is acting in close cooperation with a German 'Werwolf' group (www.werwolf.de).

A well-organized, highly competent hacker group called United Crackers League (UCL) reports (http://www.ucl.ru) that from 29 March 1999 it ceased any illegal activity, and a new group is now being organized based on the former UCL – the United Copyprotection/Cryptography Labs (UCLabs). Comments in the special press (Shipilov 1999) add to this the information about the recent arrest of Andrej Leshutin (nickname Leshy), an active member of the UCL and regarded as one of the most competent and talented Russian crackers. Leshy is said to be accused of fabricating (and distributing) computer infections. This news was met with fierce disapproval by numerous members of the hackers' community and the lively discussion has been removed from the website guestbook to the specially organized forum (http://www.computerra.ru/forums/hackers). While the discussion proceeds, highly critical views are being addressed to the security and cyberpolice bureaux.

A small group of hackers calling itself 'Russian Antifascist Frontier' (RAF) modified on 13 February 1999 the homepage of the Russian nationalistic fascist website http://www.ruspatriot.com (Karsanova 1999; Nosik 1999). The RAF has placed the text on the hacked homepage saying that they are not going to let the fascists freely express their views on the Internet. The RAF members are planning to go on opposing fascist-like websites in the Russian-language segment of the Net (Karsanova 1999). It is mentioned in the published comments (Nosik, 1999) that several other websites organized and supported by the different wings of the 'red-brown' (i.e., fascist/racist/nationalistic) movement have disappeared, since the providers (namely, HyperMart in the USA and BizLink in Russia) no longer provide resources to these groups. Russian networkers' attitudes and estimations of the RAF action are ambivalent, since even marginal groups have the right to express their views in cyberspace. There is nevertheless an indication that the Russian fascists have launched, from late 1998 an aggressive style of propaganda; the RAF action is to be comprehended as the adequate counterattack (Nosik 1999).

The most massive and enthusiastic actions of Russian hackers seem to have taken place in spring 1999 as a response to the crisis in Kosovo, when NATO made the decision to bomb selected targets in Yugoslavia. Many Russians were against this decision and hackers declared a cyberwar on NATO (mostly American) websites. The full account of the day-to-day activities can be read in the Russian daily electronic paper *Gazeta.Ru* (http://www.gazeta.ru). On the HackZone website limited-time surveys are administered: the majority (3,059 persons) of self-selected respondents affirmed the idea of attacking NATO information servers and report they are eager to participate in the action; much fewer give negative reactions (347 persons); even fewer (297 persons) feel positive but are not willing to participate in attack. At the same time respondents believed that such attacks will be favourable for both Yugoslavia and Russia (2,708 persons), believe it will do harm to both (451 persons), or feel ambivalent (798 persons), or will be hardly noticed (311 persons). Counting on the number of respondents and on the contents of the guestbook and forum discussions, the majority of the voters are only interested in hacking activities, but are not competent hackers themselves.

In the FIDO echo-conference (fido7.mo.job) someone proposed a $100 prize to anyone who illegally entered a NATO server and changed its content to an anti-war proclamation. The attack takes two main forms: illegal access to the selected servers and viruses, and spamming activities aimed at overloading the servers. In Russia it is widely believed that the NATO server in Brussels (http://www. nato.int) crashed for several hours, and that the White House server (http://www.whitehouse.gov) has been out of order as long as thirty-six hours. A group of teenage hackers called Chaos Hackers Crew (CHC) is active in anti-NATO attacks: an interview with a representative of this group has been published in an electronic paper *Gazeta.ru* (Leibov 1999). The young man turned out to have been apolitical before the crisis in Kosovo. He had very limited knowledge about the reasons NATO was bombing Yugoslavian targets, and the sites the CHC chose for its attacks had nothing to do with the military ones (for example, a Chinese site was mistakenly attacked).

There are different views on the effectiveness of the hackers' attacks against the NATO information structures. The very idea that hackers should react when any political aggression takes place is not new: for example, 'the Indonesian Government is being blamed for a highly-organized attack on computers in Ireland which brought down the East Timor virtual country domain' (Nutall 1999). Needless to say, Serb hackers are trying to do their best to cripple NATO websites by e-mailing spam, pings, and virus infections (Diederich 1999; Boodhoo 1999). The US officials believe that the 'sophisticated and organized' attacks on the Pentagon computer systems might denote the start of the cyberwar and that the Russians might be partly responsible for that, though they assume it is quite possible that 'the probes are coming from other countries that are simply routing through Russian computer addresses to disguise their origin' (Starr 1999).

Legal issues of computer hacking in Russia

The most widely known criminal episode of computer hacking in Russia is the Vladimir Levin case. It is widely reported that in 1994 Levin from St Petersburg managed to illegally transfer US$10 million from the US Citibank to several bank accounts. The bank really lost only US$400,000 since the transaction of the rest of the money was blocked by the bank security system. Levin was arrested in London in 1995 and tried in the US and is in prison now.

The whole affair is legendary in Russia. One of the most popular legends says that Levin is not a hacker himself; he happened to buy very cheaply the secrets of illegal intrusion into the Citibank from a very competent and creative computer programmer known in St Petersburg under the nickname Protozoid.

Perhaps the most important point in the Levin case is that officially, while staying in Russia he could not be accused: there were no statements on computer-related crime in the criminal code in Russia until 1997. Being modernized now, the Russian criminal code includes several major statements: article 272 regulates the cases of illegal access to computerized information; article 273 regulates the cases of creation, usage, and distribution of dangerous programs (mainly computer viruses and logical bombs); article 274 regulates the cases of incorrect exploitation of computers and computer networks.

Applying the updated legislation, the newly organized cyberpolice (http://www.cyberpolice.ru) arrested the abovementioned hacker Leshy. The police officers are perhaps more successful prosecuting carders – those who generate phone or credit cards and perform distant shopping from the foreign shops and use illegal cards for payments, or pay for the Internet account with a fictitious or generated phone card. For example, on 18 November 1998 Pavel Sheiko, aged 18 was found guilty by a Moscow court of illegal carding (Verbitskaya 1999). Sergej Pakhmutov, a computer programmer employed in the local division of Sberbank, was found guilty by the Rostov-on-Don (European part of southern Russia) city court of illegal modification of banking information system (anon. 1999). Ilya Gofman (nickname SpyBull), 21, known as a gifted viola playing student in Moscow, stole from a USA e-zine over $20,000 and in September 1998 he was imprisoned in Moscow. As a result of his illegal access to the e-zine he managed to give orders to the electronic accounting system to transfer money to the specially indicated accounts in Moscow banks. The owner of the accounts, Vladimir Voznesensky, 19, from Mytischi (near Moscow), and Artem Fidelman, 19, a Moscow student and a computer networker (both never met Gofman face-to-face), cashed the stolen money and passed it to SpyBull via an anonymous depository (Demchenko 1998). On 19 January 1998 Sergej Goyarchuk, 19, a student, was found guilty by the city court of Juzhno-Sakhalinsk (Sakhalin Island, far eastern Russia, neighbouring Japan) of illegal access to the mailboxes of corporate and private e-mail users (URL: http://qwerty.nanko.ru/ security/crime/rushak.htm). As a rule, judges find hacking cases difficult. Those accused of cybercrimes (carding, hacking, etc.) are usually put on probation, not in prison, indicating that the Russian courts consider this sort of crime relatively minor.

Though modernized, the criminal code of the Russian Federation contradicts the US law regulating information technology usage. The actual example is the conflict e-mail communication 'Macromedia, Inc. vs Ivanopulo'. The conflict started on 26 February 1999 when Steve Wozniak, the Macromedia anti-piracy manager, in a personal message addressed to a Russian computer programmer, Ivanopulo, demanded that Ivanopulo should remove from his website Macromedia copyright-protected software. In subsequent communication Ivanopulo, first, denied the accusation of theft, arguing that he downloaded a trial version, meaning he was a legal user, and, second, argued that the Russian law does not prohibit disassembly and reverse engineering of programs. The cracks on the website Ivanopulo says are for educational purposes only, to let the interested colleagues know that the protection schemes used are insufficient. Any attempts to use the software downloaded from the www.artcon.ru website are illegal. Ivanopulo, who is not intending to use it, feels no responsibility for those who might try to perform illegal actions. In several messages

Wozniak rejects the idea that Ivanopulo has undertaken an intellectual exercise, telling him he is only teaching others how to steal software.

Attitudes of non-hackers to computer hacking

The research aimed at the Russian non-hackers' (layperson's) attitudes towards computer hacking and towards hackers (both Russians and non-Russians) was carried out in February and March 1999. To the best of the authors' knowledge, this is the first research of this sort held in Russia and in the former Soviet Union. A group of students specializing in ergonomics and information systems at the Moscow Aviation Technologies University have been assisting in the fieldwork.

Research methodology and procedure

The research method involved interviewing teenagers and adults on their attitudes towards hackers and hacking. The procedure consisted of administering a structured questionnaire (fourteen open-ended questions). All the questions have undergone probation during the pilot stage (January 1999). The open-ended questions have been chosen in order to let the respondents verbally formulate the reasons for their responses. These formulations are expected to be useful in future research planning – presumably for constructing closed questions. The responses were fixed in a written form either by respondents themselves or by the interviewers. The responses were subjected to content-analysis. Most respondents formulated several reasons at once, so after responses have been classified, the total percentage of the reasons turned out to be more than 100 per cent.

The total number of respondents was 180, all Muscovites or settled near Moscow. This sample consists of two groups: schoolchildren (85 respondents, 36 females and 49 males) from 13.5 to 17 years old, and grown-ups (95 respondents, 42 females and 53 males) from 18 to 63: the core of the latter group are the respondents whose age is between 22 and 30 (71 respondents, 33 females and 48 males). The respondents have been interviewed mostly at their workplace or at school.

Research results and discussion

All the respondents (but for 2.8 per cent of schoolgirls) report they have heard about hackers previously. The two major sources of knowledge about hackers are reported: media and friends/acquaintances; a small group of schoolboys (12.2 per cent of younger males) added a third source, i.e., the Internet. Available knowledge makes only partial reference to the practice: about half (49 per cent) of respondents were not able to imagine they might become a victim of hacker's actions. Of the rest, 2.9 per cent are quite sure that this situation will never happen to them, and 48.1 per cent have showed enough experience and/or imagination to report that a hacker might send a virus to their PC, rob money from their bank account, or steal and use their password for an Internet connection. Thus, for about a half of the respondents the knowledge about hackers' actions is declarative knowledge, and for about another half of the respondents this knowledge is procedural, since they are able to refer it to self-related problem situations.

When asked whether they believe that the hackers are all alike, the respondents gave different replies (see Table 4.1). The schoolboys seem to be the least likely to believe that hackers are all alike; it is worth remembering that this very age group and gender is the most attracted to the pleasures of computer hacking. Few reasons have been formulated by respondents in order to explain their positions. Hackers have been called all alike, since they all are 'possessed by computers', 'their characters are alike', or 'they have the same aims'; adults mention two more reasons: 'solitude' and 'one-sided development of a personality'. On the contrary, hackers have been called all different, since they have 'different aims', 'different characters', 'different social status', or 'use different methods'; schoolchildren add to the list 'different competence level' and 'different profit' (the last one noted by boys only).

It is rather curious, but some respondents believe hackers are psychologically (characters and/or aims) different, and some believe they are identical in characters and/or aims. This obvious contradiction might be caused by the fact that no respondent is likely to be personally acquainted with several hackers, though some of them report they know a hacker personally (16 per cent adult women; 17 per cent girls; 37.5 per cent adult men; 22 per cent boys).

Moreover, the majority of respondents (54 per cent) show no prejudice towards making friends with hackers; 24 per cent would not

Table 4.1   Responses of non-hackers given to the supposition that the hackers are all alike (%)

Age/gender	'Yes, all alike'	'No, differ'	'Don't know'
Adult females	21.2	69.7	9.1
Adult males	31.2	64.6	4.2
Schoolgirls	31.4	57.1	11.4
Schoolboys	8.2	79.6	12.2

like to be on friendly terms with a hacker; 12 per cent report it makes no difference to them; 10 per cent have no definite opinion. The first group (tending positively towards being friendly to a hacker) includes more adults (60.5 per cent) than school age children (50.6 per cent), and the reasons declared are: interesting communication that leads to acquiring new knowledge about information technologies, and making use of the hacker's abilities and knowledge. The second group (tending negatively) includes 29.6 per cent adults and 24.7 per cent schoolchildren; the reasons declared are the disharmony of interests, and the conviction that hackers are criminals. The third group (friends' profession/interests make no difference) includes 7.1 per cent adults and 12.9 per cent schoolchildren; the fourth group (no definite opinion) includes 2.8 per cent adults and 11.8 per cent schoolchildren. No gender differences are presented as to the possibility of being on friendly terms with hackers; age differences might be explained by the fact that adults feel surprisingly more positive towards making friends with hackers than younger respondents do, and that the latter seem to be less certain (they have no definite opinion, or are indifferent) in their attitudes towards the possibility of being friendly with a hacker than the older ones.

When asked of the possible reasons for becoming a hacker and performing hacking actions, respondents propose different reasons which have been classified and content-analysed. One set of reasons includes 'self-assertion', 'intellectual curiosity', and 'strive for real-life conflicts' – all of them have been united and classified as 'Personal Drives'. A group of reasons includes 'being a computer fan' and 'professionally interested in computers' – these have been united and called 'Professional Interests'. One more group of reasons includes 'passionate', 'venturous', and 'striving for the unattainable' – this class of reasons has been defined as 'Strive for Risk'. 'Money Problems' is a class of reasons combining such reasons as 'short of money', 'greedy', and 'money-maker'. Reasons saying that hackers are simply bored or have leisure time with nothing to do has been called 'Free Time Hobby'. Some respondents have expressed a reason that hackers are 'hooligans', 'demolishers', 'ruiners', etc. – this class of reasons has been called 'Criminal Accentuation'. Someone's (i.e. older hackers') influences – presumably of negative character – have been called 'Negative Influences' (see Table 4.2).

It's noteworthy that the adult females overestimate (as compared to the other groups of respondents) hackers' personal drives, their strive for risk, and money problems (in the latter case the schoolboys do the same). Contrary to the younger respondents, some adults believe that

Table 4.2   Possible reasons for being a hacker declared by non-hackers (%)

Age/ gender	Personal drives	Profes- sional interests	Strive for risk	Money problems	Free- time hobby	Criminal accentua- tion	Negative influences
Adult females	57.6	27.3	33.1	45.5	6.1	9.1	0
Adult males	43.8	37.5	14.6	22.9	10.4	14.6	0
School- girls	48.8	28.5	14.3	28.6	0	0	2.9
School- boys	48.9	32.6	14.3	40.9	18.4	0	0

the reason for being a hacker is a criminal accentuation in their character. Males rank the professional interests of hackers higher than females, and often enough believe – contrary to females – that the main reason for hacking is that it's a hobby (i.e., a leisure time with activity where there is nothing particular to do).

To compare the classified data characterizing schoolgirls and schoolboys respectively, it should be noted that no girls believe the reason for being a hacker is 'short of money' – 28.6 per cent of them believe the reason is 'money-making'. The boys believe the 'short of money' reason is four times as important as the 'money making' reason (32.7 per cent vs 8.2 per cent). The group of adults shows no peculiarities and/or disharmony of this sort.

Older and younger respondents react somewhat differently to the question on the characteristics that are absolutely necessary for successful hackers. It is of interest that there are no gender differences in the replies to this question. Respondents mentioned such character-istics as 'high professional level' (with no ingredients of this quality), 'high intellectual level', 'strong will', 'special traits of character' (no peculiarities are indicated, but for a 'special temperament'), and 'unusual appearance'. Only one (younger) respondent believes there is nothing at all special about hackers (see Table 4.3).

Table 4.3   Characteristics of a successful hacker reported by non-hackers (%)

Age	High professional level	High intellect	Strong will	Special traits of character	Unusual appearance
Adults	9.4	24.4	14.6	48.8	1.2
Children	8.1	41.6	13.0	26.0	8.1

It can be concluded that adults rank high traits of character, while the younger respondents find nothing special with the character, but rank intellectual abilities of hackers very highly, and, curiously enough, believe that hackers have a 'special' and unusual appearance.

It is a common view that most of the hackers lack close company, are poorly understood by mates and adults and have got some problems in human to human communication. Of adults, 37.9 per cent (and only 16.7 per cent of schoolchildren) believe this is true, while 55.8 per cent of adults (and even more – 61.9 per cent of schoolchildren) disbelieve it, and 6 per cent of adults (21.4 per cent of schoolchildren) report this 'might be/might not be' true. Thus we can conclude that the numbers of adults and children who do not definitely oppose the idea that computer hackers are poor communicators are about the same: 44.2 per cent of adults and 38.1 per cent of schoolchildren. The other conclusion is that schoolchildren are much less definite in assuming this idea than adults are.

Even though females are largely underrepesented within a hackers' community, it is rather interesting to note that there are no significant age and gender differences in the respondents' views on the respective question. As many as 10.6 per cent of adults (and 10.5 per cent of schoolchildren) oppose this view, the latter believe that there are few females among hackers. The reasons put forward to explain this evident bias include: 'females' interests are outside hacking', 'females' personality traits are specific', 'lack of professional and intellectual abilities', and 'females are apt to escape difficult problems'. Neither those who disagree with this idea, nor those who believe that females lack intellect and professional knowledge, put forward ideas that one should distinguish biological and psychological gender, and that the levels of feminine/masculine traits should be measured. Thus, it is a commonplace that peculiarities of interests, personality traits, intellectual abilities and professional knowledge restrict the number of females competent in hacking.

Media usually present hacking as equal to or close to crime. Nevertheless, most respondents believe that cybercrime should be distinguished from ordinary crime. This view is reported by 61.4 per cent of adults and 78.6 per cent of schoolchildren; the reasons put forward to justify this position are: 'no physical aggression' (adults and schoolchildren express it equally often), 'impunity' (schoolchildren mention it twice as often as adults), 'no contact to a victim' (about equally often), 'non-spontaneity and well thought-outness of cybercrime' (adults report it thrice as often as schoolchildren). At the same time 35.7 per cent of adults and 16.6 per cent of schoolchildren consider cybercrime equal to any other crime (adults give reasons: 'cybercrime is ordinary theft', or 'moral harm is the same', or 'criminal code makes no distinctions'); 2.9 per cent of adults and 4.8 per cent of schoolchildren have no definite views. Thus schoolchildren who are more likely to understand their mates being hackers tend to differentiate ordinary crimes and computer crimes; the impunity of the latter is specially stressed by schoolchildren. As expected, adults give more differentiated views than the younger respondents.

Hackers are usually presented as defending the idea that all the information sources should be freely accessible; they are known to fight against secrets and security systems. When asked of their views, respondents differentiate the problem. The data are presented in Table 4.4.

As expected, the schoolchildren seem to be close to the views expressed by hackers. Twice as often, when compared to adults, they report that they cannot tolerate any secret information and/or the politics of security. At the same time they report four times as often, compared to adults, that they have no definite opinion at all on this problem. The pieces of entirely secret information that the respondents mention they can reconcile themselves with (i.e., 'some secrets are possible') are: personal data, medical files, military (defence) secrets, financial information, commercial secrets, information collected by governmental bodies in order to make reasonable decisions. This is the list of secrets the minority (23.8 per cent) of the younger respondents are able to reconcile themselves with.

Computer hackers keep declaring that by illegal intrusions into computers and information systems they motivate computer programmers and security experts to be competent, precise and careful. Is it a really good excuse for the hackers' activity? This question has been proposed to the respondents. The attitudes expressed by respondents are shown in Table 4.5.

It can be concluded that males, both older and younger, are more apt – compared to females – to approve of and justify the hackers' illegal actions, the explanation being that these actions make others

Table 4.4   Attitudes towards secret information expressed by non-hackers (%)

Age	'No secrets'	'Secrets are necessary'	'Some secrets are possible'	'It's the same for me'
Adults	12.7	40.9	44.6	1.8
Schoolchildren	27.5	41.6	23.8	7.1

Table 4.5   Non-hackers' attitudes towards the idea that evil actions of
hackers motivate computer experts to be careful (%)

Replies	Adults		Schoolchildren	
	Females	Males	Females	Males
Yes	53	63	50	65
No	40	37	38	24
Don't know	7	0	12	11

more precise and careful. Only 7 per cent of adult females seem to have
no definite opinion on that problem.

One of the most significant questions to be investigated in the
research is whether hackers in Russia and abroad differ a lot or have
much in common. Most respondents (76 per cent of adults and 62.2
per cent of schoolchildren) believe the hackers differ, and they have
proposed some possible reasons for these differences. These reasons are:
different intellectual and professional abilities (the latter means
abilities regarding computer usage and programming) different
personality traits (no details available); different aims of the Russian
and non-Russian hackers' activities; different equipment available (i.e.,
hackers from abroad are believed to possess the newest upgraded
hardware); different traditions of obeying/disobeying the law; different
possibilities in making hacking profitable (i.e., easier access to bank
accounts and credit cards, etc.) (see Table 4.6).

The younger respondents are less certain in their choice (the 'don't
know' option); when they are certain they are less likely to explain the

Table 4.6   Non-hackers' views on the possible differences between hackers in
Russia and outside Russia

Age	Differ in:								Don't differ	Don't know
	1		2	3	4	5	6	7		
	(a)	(b)								
Adults	14.0	4	10.0	5.0	14.0	3.0	9.0	17	20.0	4.0
Children	8.5	0	6.1	3.7	9.8	1.2	11.0	22	26.8	11.0

Key:
1   Abilities: (a) intellectual; (b) professional
2   Personality traits
3   Aims
4   Equipment
5   Attitudes towards law
6   Possibilities
7   No explanations

choice (the 'no explanations' option). At the same time they are more certain that hackers do not differ at all, and are less certain that there are any differences.

Almost all the respondents – Muscovites from 13.5 to 63 – recognize the word 'hacker' and have at least limited knowledge about the forms of their activities. Thus the social changes are very rapid: about 4–5 years ago the terms 'Internet' or 'hacker' were known only to a few people in Russia. Connotations of the word 'hacker' are drawn mostly from mass media, though some respondents knew hackers personally, and hackers are not altogether mixed with cybercriminals. The term is not yet well-structured, older and younger respondents have slightly differing connotations. The Russian hackers are widely enough believed to differ from the 'outer world' hackers.

Attitudes of hackers to computer hacking

The description of the hackers' attitudes is drawn from the three main sources. The first is the guestbook of the Moscow cyberpolice website (www.cyberpolice.ru). In total, 68 guestbook messages are available in April 1999, some of them shape the problems beyond the scope of cybercrime or computer hacking (comment on the website's design, or give greetings to the administrators of the new website, or complain on the hackers' evil actions, etc.), and are thus irrelevant to the aims of the current research project. The rest of the messages, over 50, have been analysed.

The second source is a discussion of the various problems related to hackers and hacking that took place on the website www.zhurnal.ru/ hack-zone/webboard/index.htm during the period of time from November 1996 to April 1997. These discussions contained 225 messages. Two years have passed since the discussions took place, and the declared positions have never been updated. Due to that reason the results of this discussion will be observed only briefly.

The third source is an interview held by a Russian journalist Vadim Fedoseev on 12 February 1999 via the Internet. The interviewees were hackers; some of them responded to several questions only; total number of questions was 29. The core of respondents were 5–7 hackers who gave replies to the majority of the questions. We will discuss the responses of this core group of hackers.

The messages that are available on the cyberpolice website guestbook refer mostly to the hacking/cracking/carding experience. All the messages available in early April 1999 have been analysed. In one third of the guestbook messages the cyberpolice activity in exposing hackers (more specifically – carders) and convicting them of stealing goods/ money from e-shops is approved and supported. In two-thirds of the guestbook messages the activity of the cyberpolicemen is disapproved of, sometimes very actively and aggressively. The arguments are that the police in Russia have too many urgent tasks (protecting people from street hooligans and robbers, seeking killers, etc.) to be too concerned with exposing those who are loyal to the property owners inside Russia but steal from the overseas e-shops or hack the distant websites and information systems. Since the victims of these crimes are usually the Americans (owners of credit cards and of companies), why should Russian policemen work hard to protect the foreigners' property, when they have a lot to do to protect their countrymen?

The guestbook visitors argue that one needn't blame a hacker when he 'purchases' software in a typically hacker's way: using a false credit card, or not paying at all. The possible reasons are: first, producers – Microsoft especially – overestimate the costs of software products; second, software and the database information must be free; third, qualified computer experts need all the newly updated versions of modern software, but there are too few legal ways in Russia to earn enough money to pay for that; and fourth, the foreigners, especially Americans and American companies are rich enough (as compared to Russian computer programmers and small/medium-size companies) and will hardly notice the losses; if they do notice, insurance companies will cover the losses.

These views originate from Cold War times and are thus old-fashioned. Surprisingly, they coincide pretty well with the current (March and April, 1999) appraisal of political Russian-American opposition due to the crisis in Kosovo. This sort of mentality seems to be characteristic of both laypeople and advanced computer hackers: numerous examples of the unexpected rebirth of patriotic feelings in the hackers' community are given in the previous sections of the paper. Hopefully, this feeling of infantile irresponsibility, as well as the remnants of the ideology of confrontation in general will fade and disappear sooner or later.

In about half of the guestbook messages computer-mediated theft is defended; it is declared to be inevitable until the Russian economy is in deep crisis, and the most qualified and hard working individuals, as well as small and medium-size companies do not earn enough to be able to purchase the needed goods, particularly software and hardware products. Really competent hackers, their occupation being risky as it is, in any case would never be caught, the guestbook visitors peremptorily declare. To defend this view the visitors refer to inefficient law enforcement and incompetent cyberpolice in Russia. The young men who are already exposed and convicted of cybercrime are scornfully called lamers, not hackers. The cyberpolice are said to be successful with lamers only – hackers need not feel any danger.

The other group of guestbook visitors is equally emotional in arguing that theft is always illegal, and hackers, being criminals, should be sentenced and imprisoned. Cybercrime is believed to be equal to an ordinary crime and should be punished, according to the criminal code. Those who prefer to generate false credit cards to steal goods, or use pirate versions of software are persistently recommended to work harder and more productively. As a result, they will find that they are able to purchase the needed products legally. Several anonymous visitors announce they are going to stop hacking and inquire of cyberpolice website administrators, whether they can escape punishment for the prior illegal actions.

In the discussion that took place on the website www.zhurnal.ru/ hack-zone/webboard/index.htm in 1996–7 a greater variety of problems were debated. The total number of discussants is not certain. As many as 87 persons submitted one message only, 14 persons submitted two messages each, 6 persons three to four messages each, 2 persons seven messages each, and 1 person ten messages. Possibly, some of them submitted more messages using a different nickname each time, and if so, the total number of discussants is even smaller. Not all of the messages were relevant; sometimes the declared views were neither supported nor opposed, but simply ignored by discussants.

Some discussants were trying to introduce organizational or specifically technical issues, proposing for example to get united in a team for hacking this or that target, or else to estimate the currently availability of hacking instruments. Several messages were aimed at establishing personal contacts, or else at consulting on technical problems. These contacts and/or consultations likely took place, maybe via the IRC. Irritated victims of the hackers' actions had also sent messages. About 10 per cent of messages were entirely humorous and contained nothing but jokes. The rest of the messages, the pertinent ones, have been analysed.

First let us note the entirely positive views on hacking. Being intellectually curious, hackers are believed to facilitate computer programmers' research activity: they verify and test security methods, and make program codes available to interested professionals. It is stressed that hackers should not be mixed with pirates and crackers, i.e. those who are exclusively interested in destroying and stealing information. Although the hackers are capable of doing the same, their reputation is quite different, since they are known as competent computer programmers, devoted to the profession. Hackers have created the most useful operating systems, applied programs, and high-level languages. In other terms, this group of discussants recalls the older Weizenbaum-like description of hackers. The so-called 'alternative hacking' is also appreciated. It means that instead of hacking selected websites, alternative websites are constructed that resemble the originals but which contain quite different information created by an 'alternative hacker'. Another positive view of hackers is based on the idea that by ensuring free distribution of information, hackers are in a way human rights advocates. Robin Hood-like, consistently liberal or anarchic political views motivate hackers to oppose any inclination to keep information blocked and any attempts to regulate and establish control over media (it is well known that the Internet is often functioning as a medium). Finally, some discussants declare, by providing free access to the hidden data hackers oppose the political restoration of communism and totalitarianism.

Not surprisingly, the population of discussants is inclined to justify hackers. For example, hacking is defined as an illegal action (as a crime and a theft) in six messages only. The alternative views are presented in much greater variety. The discussants also proposed working stimuli and actual inducements for hacking, among them: a strive to overcome the other crackers and to be ranked at the top (and, possibly, best-paid) consultant in the problem area of computer programs' and information systems' security; active self-assertion, very likely compensating for inferiority complexes; a desire to belong to a reference group of top level experts in computer programming; a challenge, i.e. an urge to hack/crack a definitive computer program/website/security system; a desire to 'punish' incompetent and inefficient system administrators and/or security professionals; a desire to be ranked high in profession, and thus be distinguished from lamers, i.e. unsuccessful and non-curious end users – hackers usually seem to disdain less competent colleagues.

Actually, very few disputes occurred in the framework of the so-called discussion: although a lot of opposite views were forwarded, most of them were completely ignored. Hypothetically, the majority of the participants (as many as 87 persons contributed one message each) visited the website only once – evidently, to declare their views. In case they visited it again, they discovered that the other discussants completely ignored their contribution, and thus they felt they were not provoked to produce new messages (if only using another nickname), and had obviously no inclination to initiate any dispute.

Very few political arguments were declared during the discussion. At that time (late 1996–early 1997), soon after Yeltsin was re-elected as President, a short period of political stability was observed in Russia. In generally, the themes of political resistance and opposition were more common both for the cyberpolice website guestbook, discussed above in this section, and for the web interview held in February 1999.

The interviewer – Vadim Fedoseev – has managed to cover most of the popular topics widely believed to be typically intrinsic to hackers. Geographical location and age of the interviewees is not known; the core group includes three hackers specializing in illegal penetrations into distant LANs and information systems, one software pirate, one creator of viruses, and one carder. The specialization is not too strict, since the hackers report they are doing their best to acquire and update 'universal' professional habits. Two hackers of the core group members believe that not all the information should be widely accessible (military defence information, and some personal data should not); four hackers stand for free access to every piece of information.

All the interviewees report they are quite experienced in 'punishing' numerous security experts and system administrators, and report they feel satisfied with these actions. It is significant that most of the interviewees report having had enough experience in fighting against other hackers/spammers/crackers/phreakers, etc. who happened to hack/destroy/spoil/steal, etc. some resources – information/programs/websites/traffic, etc. – that the interviewees' friends, close colleagues and/or clients own or need. The interviewees anticipate that though the overall number of hackers will stay relatively the same, the number of their victims will be rapidly increasing alongside with the growth of the cyberspace population. The interviewees disagree with the Robin Hood-like romantic descriptions of their motives: they insist that the actual motives include getting money, cognitive interests, and the prospect of becoming famous. Moreover, five of the seven hackers report their actual motivation to be fairly evenly divided (maybe, fifty–fifty) between gaining money and satisfying cognitive interests; one more hacker reports he would agree to commit routine hacking which has not the slightest interest for him but which will bring reasonably good money; and one hacker has ranked cognitive interests higher than money (earlier, he confesses, money has been a more crucial problem for him).

Responding to the questions, some hackers seem to articulate a basic immorality. Hackers presented themselves as an elite group participating in a worldwide information warfare; most of the Internet users will never notice the struggle that is going on; if any of them is hurt by chance, the elite persons will feel no sympathy for him/her. The cyberwar morality dictates that one's own information sources are not to be hacked, but hacking and destroying the other persons' and organizations' sources is believed to be moral. This confrontational morality is expressed rather eloquently and is further expanded: the elite hacker is engaged in fighting against the rich owners of all the imaginable goods and supplies. Thus the cyberwar seems to be close to a sort of intellectual expropriation, which is close to an anarchist ideology.

Hackers report they do not believe the real world to be equal in any way to the virtual reality of computer networks: various pleasures are available in real life (including sex and having beer), and hackers feel much less powerful there. An increased standard of living in the real world might be achieved, the interviewees report, through crime and they suggest that cybercrime is less dangerous than other forms of criminal activity. Successful hacking of money from banks, they insist, depends partly on being moderate. If the cost of investigation needed to trace the thief exceeds the stolen sum, then the security is not working efficiently. Any hacker might be caught – this depends first on the sum stolen, and second, on the budget of investigation. When hacking money from banks, the goal should be to find drawbacks in the security system. Instead, such investigations result in extended and intricate tracings, which only serve to increase the cost of the investigation.

Few hackers report being patriotic. In the virtual world, they insist, no borderlines are available or meaningful. Some interviewees did not like the idea of leaving Russia, others would prefer to sooner or later to move abroad. At the same time most of the interviewees would prefer to hack from within Russia. They explain this position in some detail: all the needed software is easily available in Russia, and pirated versions are available cheaply, legal regulations for hacked programs and data are less sophisticated in Russia than in the older democracies, cyberpolice are less competent, since the officers earn much less than they do abroad, and those who are not paid enough will never, the hackers believe, be really successful. It is widely believed, and the interviewees stress it, that the Russian system and web administrators are smarter and more responsible than foreign ones, due to that fact that hackers prefer to penetrate the foreign websites and information systems (hypothetically, the foreign banks as well, although this view was not touched on in the interview).

The three sources discussed in this section present differing images of hackers; this fact derives from the heterogeneity of the population of hackers in Russia. Yet they partly coincide: hackers are intellectually curious, smart, good learners, aggressive, self-assertive, risky, disdainful towards lamers, possibly perverted in moral norms, have a peculiar mixture of cosmopolitan and patriotic views, poor communicators and polemicists, and devoted to cyberspace problems while having strong interests in real life.

Hackers vs computer fans on hacking

During 1997–8 two groups of high-school and college age students – hackers and computer fans who identify themselves as non-hackers – were interviewed. This was a part of an ongoing project. Alongside with the other questions, both groups were asked to formulate the principal characteristics of hackers – those distinguishing hackers from all the others, especially from computer experts (non-hackers) of the same qualification. The hackers' group includes subscribers (mostly adults – university students' age and older) to the newsgroups and echogroups on hacking, and high-school students – pupils of the 'Hackers' School'. The latter is functioning officially, but is not well-known in Moscow. The total number of interviewees in the hackers' group is 38. The non-hackers' group includes 'computer fans' – advanced students of the technical universities and institutes, and high-school students attending a kid's club 'Computer', in which advanced computer experts are being trained. Those trained in the club would not call themselves hackers. The total number of interviewees in the non-hackers' group is 32. No differentiation between hackers (i.e., cracking/carding/phreaking, etc.) were mentioned during the interviews. The interviews were conducted by O. Smyslova for her master's thesis under the supervision of A. Voiskounsky.

Both groups believe the following characteristics to be necessary for successful hacking:

- high enough (not necessarily *very* high) intellect – strict, algorithmic, and precise;
- advanced abilities to collect information from technical books and manuals;
- cognitive motivation: general intellectual curiosity, enthusiasm in solving ever new problems, and interest in structural analysis of computer products;
- a need for professional communication, either face-to-face or

computer-mediated, with colleagues – over half of the interviewees report they engage in non-professional communication as
well;

- abilities to acquire and collect any knowledge on computer
  programs and security, on methods of hacking (penetration, etc.)

Several computer fans (15 per cent) report that hackers have a special
sense of humour and are eager to mock and perform practical jokes.
The members of the same group (19 per cent) believe hackers struggle
to be distinguished, and generally are fond of revealing their abilities.
They also mention (31 per cent) a widely shared point of view that
hackers are supposed to have problems in their early childhood – these
problems restrain them from contacts with those who feel no interest
in computers.

The latter point contradicts reports given by hackers themselves: 55
per cent of them reject the idea that they are poor narrow-theme
communicators. They say they have a wide enough circle of friends,
and they communicate within this circle on various themes. At the
same time 45 per cent of them confess that their closest friends are
computer programmers.

One point should be specially stressed. Two-thirds of the hackers
mention cognitive motivation as a very significant characteristic of
their activity. In the non-hackers group, only 22 per cent (three times
less) mention motivation. This is probably one of the main points of
differentiation between hackers and equally competent in computer
usage non-hackers.

When asked to compare computer hackers in Russia and abroad, the
interviewees proposed different views: Russians and foreigners are
equal in their capabilities, Russians are more advanced, and lastly,
foreigners are more advanced. But the most popular view expressed in
the both groups is that Russians are more advanced. The explanations
given include two popular views: first, that the lack of access to the
most updated hardware and software products in Russia forces Russian
experts in computer programming to seek – and to find – creative
solutions; and second, that education in technical sciences and
mathematics is of a higher level in Russia, compared to ordinary (i.e.,
non-top level) universities outside Russia. Summing up, over half of
the interviewees believe that Russians hackers have a better education,
and some of them have 'privilege'. Due to the lack of the needed
resources they have been forced to discover quite new ways in hacking.
Thus, both computer fans and computer hackers of all ages tend to
give preference to Russians hackers.

Conclusions

Attitudes towards computer hacking in Russia are influenced mostly by the mass media, and the dominant attitudes are rather positive. Hackers constitute a very diverse population and, not surprisingly, they are characterized in various ways. The more competent the respondents are in computer usage, the closer their characteristics to the characteristics produced by hackers themselves. Computer-mediated forms of communication seem to push some hackers to aggravate (sometimes even to demonize) their behaviour, their capabilities, and their personality traits. In face-to-face interviews the hackers are rather likely to stress the characteristics that bring them close to computer experts who do not tend to identify themselves with hackers.

Acknowledgments

Research reported in this chapter is supported by the Russian Foundation for Basic Research, grant 99–06–80159, and by the Research Support Scheme of the Open Society Support Foundation (Soros Foundation), grant 443/1998.

5 The new spectacle of crime

Gareth Palmer

> Surveillance practices are not so much a threat to the 'privacy' of an
> individual subject, but are actually involved in the very constitution
> of subjects.
>
> (Lyon 1998: 100)

Introduction

It could be argued that documentary on television owes its existence to
the purpose and sense of mission guiding two Scots – John Grierson
and John Reith. What inspired both men was the need to develop a
new and articulate citizenship for the twentieth century. Grierson
helped to form the British Documentary Movement in the 1930s with
an evangelistic fervour to reveal, and in so doing celebrate, the
working man. Documentary was to explain the complexity of
twentieth-century life in order to make people fit for democracy
(Hardy 1979). It was a similarly patrician brand of thinking that
inspired the first Director-General of the BBC, John Reith. For him
the aim of the BBC was to inform, educate and entertain in that order.
Grierson's formal innovation coupled with Reith's political sense
created the environment in which documentary developed at the centre
of public service broadcasting.

Several writers have suggested that television is 'arguably the
dominant media institution of the modern public sphere' (Scannel
1989; Thompson 1990; Dahlgren 1995: 7). In many senses documentary fulfils Habermas' criteria of the public sphere in that it provides
information for rational and informed debate amongst the citizenry by
organizing itself as the bearer of public opinion (Habermas 1989/
1962).

While it was protected from commercialism documentary could
investigate all manner of subjects without the taint of the market. When

commercial television began in the 1950s, legislation worked to protect documentary which soon developed landmark series such as *Special Enquiry* and *World in Action*, each of which went on to spark debates which brought prestige to the form and celebrated its public function.

While Verstraeten (1996) reminds us that public sphere and public service are not the same thing it is reasonable to argue that documentary's role to rationally inform the public backed up by a relatively autonomous broadcasting body remain important principles for any informed democracy.

However what we were faced with in the 1990s was a new situation in which documentary could no longer be relied upon to perform this democratic and informative function. This destabilization was partly due to the introduction of the market into broadcasting. But we should also consider a variety of factors which are changing both the meaning of citizenship and the public sphere.

Television documentaries have become symptomatic of a climate in which 'public service' has to be financially viable and information has become a commodity. This chapter focuses on the implications of these changes in representations of the police in three new sub-genres of documentary.

Programmes such as *Real TV* include often humorous footage of incidents involving police alongside other workers. By contrast *Cops*, *Highway Patrol*, *LAPD*, *X-Cars* and *Police!Camera!Action!* all present the police as heroic figures struggling with law-breakers in dangerous cities. In a third variation programmes such as *Crimebeat* and *Crimewatch UK* betray a public service heritage while also serving to actively extend the meaning of policing by featuring a blend of commercial forces and encouraging public participation. Each of these genres has developed from cooperation between the police and broadcasters. The implications of this for documentary, citizenship and the public sphere are the sub-themes of this chapter.

I will begin by providing a background to the production and consumption contexts for these programmes. I will then analyse them: as texts constructing a new citizenship where disciplinary technology is deployed to fashion missing communities, as spaces for performances by the police, and as sites for the circulation of discourses on crime.

Television changes

In the past twenty years there have been changes in our understanding of the production and consumption of television which are intimately related to cultural shifts in our burgeoning information society.

In terms of production the major change has been the introduction of the market. On a global level this has entailed internationalization and digitization. This has led to a standardization of programming style in an effort to maximize audiences with the subsequent neglect of local programming. Digitization has meant the proliferation of many more channels through the new technologies of satellite and cable, with a similarly homogenizing effect.

On a local level both the British Conservatives and the American Republicans introduced legislation which broke forever the old conditions under which television was made and ushered the market into all levels of broadcast activity. Perhaps the clearest example of this change would be to compare the introduction of Channel Four in Britain in 1982 with its public service brief to cater to minorities, with the introduction of Channel 5 in 1997 – a lifestyle channel with no such restriction. In America the sustained attack on PBS and the active encouragement of commercial forces which mitigated against documentary have also considerably changed conditions for the form (Price 1995).

The changes have entailed new conditions for media workers in which 'efficiency' is the watchword. Producers are required to create more television in a shorter period of time. Casualization has made for a less qualified staff working for lower pay in conditions of increasing insecurity (O'Malley 1994).

The market has also informed the debate on programme quality. Consumer sovereignty has worked to dethrone the old claims to the high ground made by those at august institutions such as the BBC. Rupert Murdoch provides the people with what they want.

Another more discrete revolution has taken place within government relations with the media. The Thatcher government centralized information, paying particular attention to news management. Journalists writing under new time pressures felt themselves rushed and began reproducing government PR rather than using the information as merely another source of information. In both Britain and America there was a streamlining of information management in which 'spin doctors' took on the responsibility of selling the government's message (Franklin 1997; Altschull 1995).

In terms of consumption, research by both academics and the industry analysed the audience 'to a point of near-invisibility' with considerable complications for both sectors. David Morley's ethnographic studies of the audience demonstrated how the TV was not simply read and understood but integrated into the fabric of everyday life (Morley 1980). Hall worked on how messages were encoded and then accepted/negotiated or opposed while being decoded (Hall 1974). Writers have discussed the ways in which marginalized and forgotten groups use texts in a variety of unplanned and self-validating ways (Ang 1996). The notion that television produced information that empowered 'semiotic bricoleurs' reached its zenith (or nadir depending on one's point of view) with John Fiske's work where the polysemy of the image freed viewers to make their own meanings. This served to marginalize any study of the production context (Fiske 1987).

These new conditions for television served as a moving framework for documentary's own identity crisis as it fought to preserve its value as guarantor of the real and organizing element in the public sphere. These insecurities may be based on the fact that documentary has long been established as an enemy of the right. In the 1980s Thames Television *Death on the Rock* dealing with the unlawful shooting of three suspected IRA terrorists was broadcast despite veiled government threats. The Broadcasting Acts of 1990 and 1996 which stipulated, amongst other things, the necessity for balance within each programme certainly put paid to this sort of crusading journalism (Franklin 1997).

The new documentaries are perfect 'brands' for the new broadcasting climate. They are relatively cheap to make, they incur little in the way of costs in terms of researchers and a high percentage of the footage originates with the police. As prime-time thirty-minute programming their success is well-documented (Corley 1998: 86).

But such programming also illustrates a shift in emphasis from a public service orientation to provide citizens with information to programming where the priority becomes the need to entertain and to shock in the name of the law. The classic signifiers of documentary such as sober tone, ragged camera-style, anchormen-narrators and the celebration of victimhood are utilized to marshal communities through fear rather than offering an even-handed account of crime for audiences to debate.

Whether the police are presented as humorous, violent or friendly what is significant for those concerned with the function of documentary in democracy is that the editorial role which maintained a critical distance between the journalists and their subjects has been exchanged for a ring-side seat at the action. Rather than discussing the multiplicity of factors responsible for the mushrooming of crime the journalistic function has been relaxed as TV aids the police in the capture and identification of miscreants.

These programmes may be cheap illustrations of what critics call the tabloidization of television but it would be wrong to dismiss them as merely police PR. They work in four interrelated ways:

- as conduits for the police in their attempts to fashion a community which has begun to abandon its own informal surveillance functions because of new technologies;
- as demonstrations of the new policing where the boundaries between public and private responsibility for law and order are breaking down;
- to normalize surveillance by carrying the disciplinary technology into the suburban arena;
- as illustrations of and contributions to the informal networks of information and power that circulate between various groups – police, audience and criminals.

These four themes will be explored in the following sections.

Citizenship and CCTV in the city

> Our society is not one of spectacle but of surveillance ... We are much less Greeks than we imagine. We are ... in the panoptic machine, invested by its effects of power, which we bring to ourselves since we are a part of the mechanism.
>
> (Foucault 1977: 217)

One of the epochal shifts that has taken place in the past twenty years has been the change in the definition of citizenship. In this neo-liberal age market ideologies define the individual's connection to welfare and participation as a private choice rather than a public concern. Citizenship is thus defined by the new accountability in which one's ability to consume and gain access to information is paramount. Lack of either spending power or information can lessen one's citizenship and can lead to a state of non-belonging. The public are those without the means to become private (Golding 1990). The *zoon politikon* is no longer defined by participation in the city but by his or her ability to be set apart from it.

In this new climate the distinctions between left and right are breaking down. The public sphere where such crisis might be discussed is, it is argued, being filled by ICTs such as the Internet. Rather than competing for this space the new documentaries discussed here have simplified issues by defining citizenship through the law and order discourse. This perspective is alarmingly close to the British government's own 'Together we'll crack it' campaign in the erroneous belief that communities acting together will identify and help solve crime.

The new documentaries offer us models of good citizenship where the criminal is figured as 'other' and the city is a dangerous place where the middle-class plan of order is forever threatened by crime.

> The fear is that the machine is breaking down by itself, and that outside in the chaos of urban life, in the desolate city streets abandoned to the predators, lies the ultimate horror – chaos, disorder, entropy.
>
> (Cohen 1988: 210)

Paul Virilio has written of how the city has used video surveillance to increase its span of visualization (Virilio 1980). The city here is predictable, routine, a place of achievement, of energy channelled into order. We share an understanding of the rules and welcome their smooth operation as we watch from fortress-homes apparently safe from the city out there. Our watching has become a habit and our surveillance a custom. The details of the crime are subject to our viewing – an examination in which individuals are placed within the field of surveillance.

In those programmes which feature the police as heroic or concerned public servants such as *Cops*, *LAPD* or *Crimebeat* the form is strictly adhered to. An agenda is set out at the beginning in the form of clips featuring 'what's to come'. After some dramatic music we are greeted by a calm model of order – either a police officer or a national news anchor. The steady mode of address deployed by trusted commentators working within legitimized documentary frameworks hails us as law-abiding citizens appalled at the criminal coded as a furtive grainy figure from the fringes. Our participation is intended to feel like a measured intervention into public affairs. Follow-up shows such as *Crimewatch* and *Crimebeat* foreground the role of the public in solving crimes and in doing so help to validate the network of communication that transmission activates.

The form itself is significant for it works to reassure the public that crime is manageable and measurable. Order is imposed upon order and the limits are safely patrolled. The criminal is reduced to a jumble of signs – mug-shots, fingerprints and faded photographs. S/he is easily made sense of and dismissed as 'other'.

Clarke offers a distinction between active and passive citizenship with the former defined as little more than mere status with 'minimal political activity, obedience to and protection of the state that doesn't necessarily involve rights' (Clarke 1996: 46). It is this easy, relatively safe definition of citizenship that is being invoked in these new documentaries. As the officer/narrator turns to face us it is clear that we are being addressed not as mere viewers but as citizens. The sacrifices and dangers encountered by officers 'out there' in the city reminds us of our obligations as citizens. Our putative membership is activated by looking out and phoning in. The closing words serve both as a threat – you have been warned – and as an uneasy source of comfort in the police's apparent success.

The citizen can greatly enhance his or her own citizenship by embracing the technology. Private security has become one of the fastest growing businesses in Britain and America. This may be linked to the 1995 survey of British Social Attitudes which revealed 'increased public support for police surveillance measures in climate of rising fear of crime' (Coleman and Sim 1996). When these two tendencies are combined it is clear that we are adopting a new attitude to surveillance, which these documentaries are not merely reflecting but contributing to.

Social control theorists inspired by Foucault argue that we are living in a new age in which disciplinary technology fashions subject populations (Rose 1989; Gandy 1993). The panopticon has been taken as a model for the way in which both body and soul are controlled. They argue that disciplinary technologies are changing the meaning of everyday life by entering into us and fashioning our subjectivity. We self-discipline in the name of a new and forceful rationality. In such a world the distinctions between the private and the public are collapsing. The rise of digital networks has further exacerbated these tendencies. We now live in a superpanopticon in which 'the population participates in its own selfconstitution as subjects of the normalizing gaze' (Poster 1990: 97).

In those programmes which seek to extend the meaning of policing such as *Crimewatch* and *Crimebeat* CCTV is presented as the 'magic bullet' technicist solution to crime. It is cost-effective, weather-proof and needs no specialist training. Commercial partnerships also seem to legitimize the use of CCTV as a surveillance measure in the quest for efficiency and savings to be passed on to the good consumer (although their recorded data are also available to the police). The government are anxious to build such communities of interest and have encouraged such collaborations between commercial forces, police and community with the CCTV City Challenge. CCTV forms a central plank in the government's own law and order strategy (Coleman and Sim 1996).

However one consequence of this surveillance is the virtual disenfran- chisement of those people who do not fit the ideal model consumers designed by such groups. 'Those individuals caught on camera become part of a "muted group" ... silenced and chastised, whose guilt is beyond reasonable doubt because the camera never lies' (Coleman and Sim: 1996).

These documentaries do not point out that the deployment of CCTV cameras could be seen as a threat to civil liberties. They do not suggest how criminal activity may be displaced by the technology rather than eradicated. It may be argued that CCTV is a symptom rather than a healer of crime. That such arguments are rarely heard may be because of 'empirically defined standards of public interest (which are) replacing a more ethically derived definition of the public interest' (Gandy 1993: 11).

The installation of such systems sets up asymmetries of power with the viewing of our communities being conducted by remote unknown individuals. The argument often deployed during the programmes is that such technologies help to build communities. Yet they do so by criminalizing those who live on the fringes – the poor, ethnic minorities, the underclass. This helps marginalize uneconomic strangers. To be good citizens in this intersecting mesh of glances is to be measurable and predictable consumers.

One entire episode of *Police!Camera!Action!* was taken up with the journey of a parcel containing a human organ through town. The tension of the show came from whether the police would 'make it' in time. Yet what was laid out for the viewer was how the police had extraordinary control over the complexity of the city. Here was a city grid they could master as a perfect model of imposed order.

In *Cops* the typical sequence begins with the distraught victim/ callers phone message. The sound of their voice and the police response is played over footage of the rush to the crime scene which is itself overlaid by conversation of the officers. At the scene walkie-talkie messages are still audible while the shaky camera records the action. Caption-crawler provides further details. This dense mapping of information gives an impressive sense of progress and order over the apparent complexity of crime. And yet there is little rest before the next crime tests the forces of law and order once more.

CCTV is the mediating technology working between citizens, commercial forces and police in the city. On one level its adoption by documentary works to normalize its function. By proving through visible evidence that dangerous criminals have been apprehended due to the technology the programmes legitimize this deployment as well as justifying its own use of police footage as a public service. Yet it also serves to encourage subjects to gain membership of the community by a willingness to become law-abiding. To be an 'active audience' means taking on the gaze in their own neighbourhoods and, in doing do, extending the meaning of policing. When public responses are connected up to other centres of communication we have a super-panopticon in which fewer and fewer acts can escape. Such documentaries mobilize dominant discourses on law and order which echo the state's investment in disciplinary technology. What is being offered here is passive citizenship in place of civic participation. It remains to be seen whether anticipatory conformity is reinforced by such programming.

Performing/policing

> The new media and police have an instrumental affinity in reproducing order and an ideological affinity in acknowledging order.
>
> (Ericson *et al.* 1989: 12)

Over the last twenty years the old antipathy between the police and the media has faded away to be replaced by a happier, more mutually rewarding relationship.

These more positive images on our screens are the result of four interrelated factors: (1) increased police awareness of the importance of good public relations leading to a professionalization of presentation; (2) new levels of co-operation between police and media in the detection of crime; (3) the increasing opportunities for the police to use the media to fashion their image and (4) new working relationships between the media and the press forged as they both attempt to reach a lost community of viewers.

The police realize that the media need them more than they need the media. The latter are in a subordinate position as the police have all the access to information as frontline fighters and primary definers of crime.

Some journalists consider their work to be closely related to the aims of the police. In *Negotiating Control* Ericson *et al.* investigated the Canadian police system and found two types of crime reporter. One group comprised those 'on the inside' privy to sensitive information and treated to discreet tip-offs because they could be trusted. It is this inner circle who, when experiencing a conflict of values between those of their own profession and those of the police's, usually allowed the police culture to prevail. The opposing group comprised those journalists of a more independent mind who would not naturally turn to the police as their first point of contact when investigating a crime. This split discovered by Ericson *et al.* illustrates the divide that is apparent between the old brand of television documentary and the new breed. It is this latter type that illustrate no independence of mind or critical distance that are the source of the discussion here.

What we see in these new police documentaries are various levels of performance – some more pronounced than others but all turned into the fact of performance by being broadcast. The first type of performance considers the presentation of crime itself:

> For the purpose of public knowledge, public affairs employees settled on the facts of crime, and in the process gave these facts their performative character' (Fiscman 1980). That is, crime was constructed not as it happened but as it was produced by the force bureaucracy as they wanted it understood publicly.
>
> (Ericson *et al.* 1989: 143)

It should be stressed that the performances we see in *LAPD*, *Cops* or *Real Stories of the Highway Patrol* are the result of close working agreements between producers and police at all levels of production. The police understand the value of such positive representations and are happy to take part in reconstructions which cannot help but glamorize their work for a jaded public. Performative elements such as music and dynamic editing serve to connect the police to their more romantic fictional brothers and sisters.

Within the new documentary framework three roles can be discerned in the performances of the police. In 'jokey' formats like *Real TV* and sometimes *Crimebeat* we see the beat officer as part of the community, a friendly face working to reassure the public. This might be the policeman who visits schools as part of an outreach programme into the community. The regular appearances of certain officers on *Crimewatch UK* or the giving of nicknames to police in *Crimebeat* is television's re-creation of this function. Humanizing officers stresses their ordinary qualities, and makes them more like other people. In such ways are they dissociated from power.

In *Cops* and *LAPD* the police are presented as agents of the technology in pursuit of dangerous criminals. Here the discussion is between the policeman as expert and the narrator or presenter learning about the power of a given technology which serves as a sort of warning.

Here the viewers are permitted to glimpse power behind closed doors. In these performances the police are given the opportunity to comment 'casually' on the limitations of legal processes or describe law-breakers as 'evil' without the remarks criticized or editorialized. In their wish to step beyond the limitations of the system for the good of all (us) the police here are closer to the stereotype of television drama.

The third performance which helps to mediate between the two is that of the self-reflexive actor. This performance is a more subtle one and occurs when the officer is seen reflecting on his 'performance' in the reconstruction of a crime. Here s/he demonstrates a self-awareness which may also be read as a symptom of the disciplinary technology. As a public servant what we see here is a model of the self-discipline necessary to deal with the most difficult situations. The officer explains history through a sort of legitimized self-writing which also appears to be the most revelatory of police work. Such self-surveillance may also relate to the officer's career:

> the development of career ladder as crucible for new forms of surveillance ... the elaboration of notions of the career was centrally tied up with issues of discipline and control.
>
> (Savage 1998: 70)

These performances are all framed by reminders of the law. In *LAPD* and *Cops* a disclaimer is issued which states that 'All persons featured are innocent until proven guilty'. A further signifier of the law framing the performance is the digitization of faces. This effect creates a space between the public and the criminal. In that space the police are able to exercise power and preserve anonymity. This also works to create a mystique around crime.

The movement between these police performances reproduces the tension between the technologically enhanced centralizing of power and a rhetoric which seeks to extend policing into the community. The police understand the need to reach the community but they also need to centralize this power to manage their resources more efficiently. The split between technological agent of the state and community policeman illustrates the public relations dilemma faced by the forces of law and order. These new documentaries reflect this crisis by showing how efficient and human the police really are despite the pressures. Yet they cannot do it all alone.

> It's getting so complicated now that unless we can encourage the community to come forward and report a mysterious thing or get

involved in neighbourhood watch we can't stay on top of crime and the problem itself.'

(Ericson et al. 1989: 104)

It is this reaching out to the community in place of actual contact that we see operationalized in the new programming. The potentially inhumane aspects of the technology is softened – either by humorous mishaps (in *Real TV*) or by stressing the role of ordinary folks becoming heroes in capturing criminals (in *Crimebeat*).

For all their raw edges and poor quality sound these scraps of police footage have been placed with much forethought. The idea of filming car crimes is an old one and was started by the Kings Lynn police force in England. It was only later that commercial producers picked up the idea. It was only short step from this to celebrating police technology. A large part of these programmes is devoted to illustrating how effective these technologies are in capturing criminals and in this respect they serve as a warning and as a threat. They seem to extend the technological loop first expressed in the CCTV footage and then further elaborated on the ground.

In *Crimebeat* it is clear from the direct address of national newsreader Martyn Lewis that the community has to work together to guarantee its own safety. This performance as 'concerned objective journalist' is also important in framing the efforts of the police and granting them further legitimacy (Palmer 1998). As he warns us, the police cannot always be there so it is up to the community to bind together in schemes such as Neighbourhood Watch. In reporting these successes the programmes are seeking to prove how the natural surveillance of the already existing community 'works'. To this end the programme offers information, sometimes in booklets – a very public service function – in order to assist this process. But while this seems a return to the old 'natural' ways of safeguarding the community's members this message is overlaid with a technological one about the 'objective' eye looking over the neighbourhood that could undermine it. The combination of the friendly policeman onscreen coupled with the proven ability of the technology helps to normalize a technology that may seem at first have seemed intrusive. But are the communities activated by such programming and related initiatives? 'The research on Neighbourhood Watch also shows that the public are reluctant or unable to make much of an impact in policing their areas or in helping the police to do it for them' (Bennett 1994: 125).

The programmes inadvertently illustrate the tension between public and police perceptions of their role. While local communities feel comforted by the bobby on the beat the police favour a more technologically oriented approach (Walklate 1991; Rawlings 1991). Due to the new economic logic CCTV is presented as a labour-saving device which has to displace traditional police work. As a result, coming into the lounge through the television is the closest to the community most police get.

A two-step movement is being performed in these community-related programmes. On the one hand are reminded of the traditional virtues of 'our' police force. But the rhetoric stresses the fact that the crisis is now so bad that once again we have to act as a watching community, to take on the meaning of 'police' ourselves. Yet we watch in an increasingly surveilled community. The technologically oriented signs of policing stress their power, accuracy and ubiquity. It is made very evident that nothing can escape the gaze. The community we take back in the act of surveillance was 'always' ours. The new technology restores us as the natural guardians. And yet we cannot help but know through the revelations that are the programme's unique selling point that our own gazes may be monitored. As we watch they may watch. As one presenter put it 'You never know when real TV might happen.'

What makes this urgent for those concerned with documentary's declining role is that the police do have considerably extended powers in which the technology aids them to manipulate rather than coerce, to tag rather than imprison: 'Home office has allowed the police to plant bugging devices on people's property without recourse to any procedures set out in any Act of Parliament or found in any decision of the courts.' (Gearty and Ewing 1997: 7). We are unlikely to learn this in the new sub-genre of documentaries.

Tensions watching the spectacle

> Inside synopticon, which devours this news, the material is purged of everything but the purely criminal – what was originally a small fragment of a human being becomes the whole human being ... The executions in Paris in 1757 become, as a spectacle, peanuts compared to the executions (real or metaphoric) on the screens of modern television.
> (Mathieson 1997: 231)

Foucault's use of the panopticon has its limitations when applied to television. In this new 'viewer society' we also operate within a synopticon in which we, the many, are witness to the crimes of the few thus reversing the asymmetry of the gaze. This is not to deny the existence of the panoptical machine. Indeed it is the panoptic machine that operates through CCTV and related Neighbourhood Watch schemes. However the synopticon redoubles the circuit of power by turning crime into spectacle. To what extent does this spectacle differ from past depictions?

There are certainly continuities between portrayals of crime in programmes such as *Cops* and *LAPD* and fictional works such as *NYPD Blue*. These documentaries are dramatic in structure and in their identification of heroes and villains in which the good is unambiguously good and personified in the brave officer and the bad is typically, predictably bad. Those most often caught on camera are also the stereotypical villains of drama – young men, the underclass and those from ethnic minorities. The viewer is offered the excitement of drama coupled to the social purpose of documentary. When these programmes are considered alongside others such as *Justice Files* we are presented with an impressive picture of an all-encompassing system efficiently punishing deviance.

It need hardly be added that such programming works against the documentary ethos by confirming stereotypes rather than exploring the cracks and fissures in the system which introduces the ambiguity vital to healthy debate.

The public service tradition represented by *Crimebeat* and *Crimewatch UK* work in two ways. In one sense they target the criminal as deviant and patrol the boundaries with the same vigilance as their American cousins. Yet the focus in the newer breed of programming such as *Crimebeat* and *Police!Camera!Action!* is on the role of a technology which turns the gaze inward.

When these programmes feature ordinary folk caught speeding they excite a double measure of fear (of capture) and disgust (at the transgressors) and, as such, offer new possibilities for the personalization of crime. The programmes become a revelation of capillary power which operates 'firstly through the elaboration of techniques of bodily control, and secondly, through the construction of new forms of self-monitoring subjectivity. Surveillance operates on the body and on the soul' (Savage 1998: 67).

By focusing on modest previously hidden crimes such as speeding we learn of the technologies' ability to implicate 'us' in criminality. In this is the dull compulsion of the format. New criminals are created via the visible evidence on which we can all agree but the criminal here could be us. To view is to learn of the power of the law working through ever-more efficient technologies. Our role as good citizens and consumers is to welcome them.

A recent broadcast of *Crimebeat* explored the issue of credit card fraud.

Footage was shown of shoplifters caught on camera. One particular sequence demonstrated how quickly the police linked with the shop and the credit-card controllers to arrest a couple. But, as the narrator pointed out, the efficiency of this system can be improved on if, for example, we print our photographs on our cards or adopt the French practice of incorporating micro-chips. Both practices are presented as having dramatically decreased fraud and as such make good sense. However the civil liberties issues coupled with the implications such data storage has for government agencies are not explored. Good citizenship is intimately connected to sound commercial sense. It would be too much to suggest broadcasters and state collude but such programming might be seen as an example of governance which 'helps to aim, shape and guide the conduct of the population' (Carrabine 1998).

Some criminologists have argued that we are undergoing a shift from the old to the new penology. Simply put this is a move from a concern with origins and causes of crime in socio-specific environments to a concern with behaviours, with monitoring the movements of suspect individuals. If the old penology offered therapy and analysis the new penology is best represented by electronic tagging so that criminals can be seen and monitored at all times (Cohen 1988). It has been argued that the distinction being drawn here is too strong and that there are continuities between the two approaches (Coleman and Sim 1996; Carrabine 1998). However what we see acted out in these public-service-oriented documentaries is the widening of the Net which itself implies an ever more vigilant self-policing by the individual in order not to be misrecognized as a criminal. The increasing deployment of databases reinforces the surveillance already at work in the city: 'the database imposes a new language on top of those already existing and that it is an impoverished, limited language, one that uses the norm and constitutes individuals and defines deviants' (Poster 1990: 95).

The spectacle of crime celebrated in these new documentaries is intended to work in a similar way to expose the criminal to public scrutiny. The punishment is to be shown. In those programmes which feature the public being made criminal by the technology it is not a judicial punishment that is being activated but shame – a powerful normalizing disciplinary agent in suburbia and a force for reintegration that reinforces the self-control within the imagined community:

> The purpose is intentionally and openly to penalize unacceptable action, to prevent repetition and to deter others by making examples of those who infringe the rules.
>
> (Worrall 1997: 26)

In *Cops* and *LAPD* we are offered a glimpse of a power more usually hidden. If, as Foucault suggests, power is now capillary, 'exercised within society rather than from above it', spectacular car chases and robberies resulting in capture offer us the excitement of drama legitimized as a display of necessary police power. The efficient deployment of new technologies for modest crimes represent a reminder that we also have to police ourselves and others.

The power of CCTV and the new databases is that they lead to the emergence of new objects of knowledge, new abnormalities which then have to be treated. It is because this power is so subtle that we are not aware of it as a force but through programmes such as these it works to operate through us. The possibilities for guilt offered here complicate the pleasures of the spectacle and confirm its ability to mobilize a series of discourses around good citizenship.

Signs of resistance?

This pessimistic scenario should not lead us to take a technologically deterministic view of these developments. As a source for television and as contemporary cultural phenomena, surveillance through CCTV and the interlinked databases have to be placed in the social and political context in which they operate.

The programmes discussed here make up a small percentage of the schedule in Britain and America but they do stress the dilemmas of documentary. Flagship series such as *Panorama*, *Dispatches* and *60 Minutes* continue to perform the brand of critical analysis that is part of television's noble tradition. Yet the *Guardian*'s recent exposé of two documentaries by Carlton illustrates the effects of cost cutting on some producers. Granada's imminent replacement of the relatively heavy-weight *World In Action* illustrates the fact that the market continues to enforce considerable pressures.

Although we may be heartened by the knowledge that viewers may be able to negotiate, refuse and oppose the meanings offered to them by television we also have to acknowledge that legislation has eroded documentary's capacity to be an oppositional force for change.

It is difficult to deny that these new documentaries are propaganda for technologies which will further curtail our civil rights. They are part of the 'strategic rationalization of technology' whose aim is to 'identify, classify and assign individuals on the basis of a remote, invisible, automatic and comprehensive sensing of personhood' (Gandy 1993: 3).

We have seen that power is not a top-down operation but one

complicated by its dispersion and activation through individuals who are able to resist. The citizen subject is produced and reproduced by a variety of discourses yet the empirical work performed on surveillance systems confirms the complexity of these operations. The stubborn fact of human agency works to buckle the elegant metaphor of the 'web' so often proposed. People refuse, they set up alternative networks, they behave illogically (Coleman 1998). Often without intending to they escape measurement and control. Writers in Britain and America have identified moments of resistance (Lyon 1994; Berko 1992). Hoaxes are taking place that disrupt this panoptic machine. It would be useful to see some documentaries about them.

Another area of resistance may lie in new patterns of identity-formation taken up by self-determining subjects. Some writers have suggested that we can adapt the technology to take part in our own self-construction (McGrath 1998). Surveillance has been challenged by gay activists who seek to bring displays of sexuality into the public arena as a means of challenging the panopticon to 'refuse what we are' (Simons 1995: 50).

Yet these signs of resistance should not permit us to escape some fundamental questions of power. The viewer proposed here is neither a docile body nor a free agent. He or she is a result of governmentality which 'constructs individuals who are capable of choice and action' but which seeks to shape them 'as active subjects, and seeks to align their choices with the objectives of governing authorities' (Carrabine 1998). The viewer is actively persuaded to embrace the technology. The rapid increase in home surveillance systems would suggest that s/he has done so. Although the individual may feel empowered by the rhetoric of CCTV a new brood of information agencies are creating circuits of communication which 'are the supports of an accumulation and a centralization of knowledge; the play of signs defines the anchorages of power ... the individual is carefully fabricated in it, according to a whole technique of forces and bodies' (Foucault quoted in Poster 1990).

The new documentaries discussed here contribute to a model of citizenship which connects public well-being to consumerism and technologically enhanced strategies of policing. Citizens are offered entertainment with only a tenuous connection to the documentary ideal. Our gaze is narrowed as we stare at spectacles of crime that confirm the prejudices learnt elsewhere in television's spectrum. What is celebrated here is the controlling function of the technology. Audiences activated in these documentaries are being asked to help the police track down criminals. The intended product is the idealized lost community. There is scant evidence of it returning.

Such programming demonstrates a synergy between the police and the media which cannot be good for public service television in the long term. It may help to lose any respect the populace still has for the media. It will help to further undermine documentary. This may 'liberate' the form in a new direction. The signs are however that it will not.

Finally such programming is useful in that it explicates the media's role in shifting, defining or exploring the boundary between the private and public spheres. The new documentaries visualize a relatively fixed moment in fluid displays of power – through the intersecting gazes of all participants on screen and at home, in the productive performances of the disciplinary technology and through the actions of the agents of the law. The co-terminus product of these transmissions is to cause to arise new objects of knowledge which are then fed into our definitions of the deviant and help to maintain a distance between them and us – the good citizens.

Part II

Privacy, surveillance and protection

Themes and issues identified

The rapid development of ICTs has raised questions about individual privacy, government and corporate surveillance, and the need to balance the privacy of individuals with law enforcement's ability to fight crime. Accordingly, ICTs are making possible both new ways to commit crimes as well as new crimes themselves.

The value of information is based, in large part, on the ability to keep it proprietary. This part explores three different dimensions of secrecy in relation to the development of new ICTs. First, these essays examine the importance of keeping business information secret, and the corresponding value attributed to information based primarily on its secret nature. Second, these essays explore the manner in which secrets are kept, primarily through the technology of encryption, exploring both the broad ranging questions of how encryption can and should be used, as well as the possibilities of the criminal misuse of encryption to hide or disguise criminal activity. Third, the theme of privacy is explored in relation to both the government's and law enforcement's ability to deter and prosecute crimes as well as the individual's rights to privacy and freedom from surveillance.

These three issues are interrelated in complex ways. In all cases, however, two central themes emerge. First, with the emergence of new ICTs, freedom and security are based, fundamentally, on the ability to maintain a degree of confidentiality regarding information. Second, perhaps the most difficult problem that ICTs present is one of balancing issues of privacy and surveillance. As ICTs develop and information collection and management strategies become more nuanced and complex, the ability to collect, organize and disseminate information will pose new threats to individuals' privacy. As government agencies and law enforcement are better able to use ICTs to monitor activities, profile behaviours and disseminate information, ICTs become a powerful tool for law enforcement.

Additionally, ICTs often create problems for personal privacy as unintended consequences. Inherent in issues of data collection, for example, are issues of individual privacy, where information collected for one purpose (such as advertising) may end up being used for a different purpose (law enforcement or surveillance). The power of ICTs for data collection, organization, storage and retrieval all pose new threats to and challenges for the preservation of personal privacy. With the increase of the power of ICTs, questions also arise about the right to privacy, particularly in relation to the increased need for security and crime prevention. At what point, to what degree, and in what ways do those suspected or accused of crimes give up their right to privacy?

With the development of increased surveillance technology, there is also a parallel increase in the number of ICTs, such as encryption, which promote and insure secrecy and privacy. The degree to which these ICTs are controlled, made accessible to law enforcement and criminals, and subjected to export regulation are certain to be some of the most contested arenas of legal and policy debate in the coming years. How are we, in the coming years, to balance the need for an individual's privacy with the ability to use new ICTs to commit crime or hide criminal activity from law enforcement?

The essential question remains one of balance: How do we find the appropriate uses for ICTs which both allow law enforcement to do their job fighting crime, while preserving the integrity of individual rights and privacy in a new information society? The following essays address this question by examining the roles of ICTs in contexts of their use and misuse by government, industry criminals, and law enforcement.

6 Hiding crimes in cyberspace[1]

*Dorothy E. Denning and
William E. Baugh, Jr*

Introduction

The growth of telecommunications and electronic commerce has led to
a growing commercial market for digital encryption technologies.
Business needs encryption to protect intellectual property and to
establish secure links with partners, suppliers and customers. Banks
need it to ensure the confidentiality and authenticity of financial
transactions. Law enforcement needs it to stop those under investigation from intercepting police communications and obstructing
investigations. Individuals need it to protect their private communications and confidential data. Encryption is critical to building a secure
and trusted global information infrastructure for communications and
electronic commerce.

Encryption also gives criminals and terrorists a powerful tool for
concealing their activities. It can make it impossible for law enforcement agencies to obtain the evidence needed for a conviction or the
intelligence vital to criminal investigations. It can frustrate communications intercepts, which have played a significant role in averting
terrorist attacks and in gathering information about specific transnational threats, including terrorism, drug trafficking and organized
crime (White House 1995). It can delay investigations and add to
their cost.

The use of encryption to hide criminal activity is not new. The
April 1970 issue of the *FBI Law Enforcement Bulletin* reports on several
cases where law enforcement agencies had to break codes in order to
obtain evidence or prevent violations of the law. None of the cases,
however, involved electronic information or computers. Relatively
simple substitution ciphers were used to conceal speech.

Digital computers have changed the landscape considerably. Encryption and other advanced technologies increasingly are used, with
direct impact on law enforcement. If all communications and stored

information in criminal cases were encrypted, it would be a nightmare for investigators. It would not be feasible to decrypt everything, even if technically possible. How would law enforcement agencies know where to spend limited resources?

We address here the use of encryption and other information technologies to hide criminal activities. Numerous case studies are presented for illustration. We first examine encryption and the options available to law enforcement for dealing with it. Next we discuss a variety of other tools for concealing information: passwords, digital compression, steganography, remote storage, and audit disabling. Finally, we discuss tools for hiding crimes through anonymity: anonymous remailers, anonymous digital cash, computer penetration and looping, cellular phone cloning and cellular phone cards.

Encryption in crime and terrorism

This section describes criminal use of encryption in four domains: voice, fax and data communications; electronic mail; files stored on the computers of individual criminals and criminal enterprises; and information posted in public places on computer networks.

Voice, fax, and real-time data communications

Criminals can use encryption to make their real-time communications inaccessible to law enforcement. The effect is to deny law enforcement one of the most valuable tools in fighting organized crime – the court-ordered wiretap. In March 1997, the director of the Federal Bureau of Investigation, Louis J. Freeh, testified that the FBI was unable to assist with five requests for decryption assistance in communications intercepts in 1995 and twelve in 1996 (US Congress 1997a). Such wiretaps can be extremely valuable as they capture the subjects' own words, which generally holds up much better in court than information acquired from informants, for example, who are often criminals themselves and extremely unreliable. Wiretaps also provide valuable information regarding the intentions, plans and members of criminal conspiracies, and in providing leads in criminal investigations. Drug cartels and organizations rely heavily on communications networks: monitoring of these networks has been critical for identifying those at the executive level and the organizations' illegal proceeds. Communications intercepts have also been useful in terrorism cases, sometimes helping to avoid a deadly attack. They have helped prevent the bombing of a foreign consulate in the United States and a rocket attempt against a US ally, among other things (ibid.).

There is little case information in the public domain on the use of communications encryption devices by criminal enterprises. The Cali cartel is reputed to be using sophisticated encryption to conceal their telephone communications. Communications devices seized from the cartel in 1995 included radios that distort voices, video phones which provide visual authentication of the caller's identity, and instruments for scrambling transmissions from computer modems (Grabosky and Smith 1998).

We understand that some terrorist groups are using high-frequency encrypted voice/data links with state sponsors of terrorism. Hamas reportedly is using encrypted Internet communications to transmit maps, pictures and other details pertaining to terrorist attacks. The Israeli General Security Service believes that most of the data are being sent to the Hamas worldwide centre in Great Britain (IINS 1997).

The lack of universal interoperability and cost of telephone encryption devices – several hundred dollars for a device that provides strong security – has likely slowed their adoption by criminal enterprises. The problems to law enforcement could get worse as prices drop and Internet telephony becomes more common. Criminals can conduct encrypted voice conversations over the Internet at little or no cost. This impact on law enforcement, however, may be balanced by the emergence of digital cellular communications. These phones encrypt the radio links between the mobile devices and base stations, which is where the communications are most vulnerable to eavesdroppers. Elsewhere, the communications travel in the clear (or are separately encrypted while traversing microwave or satellite links), making court-ordered interception possible in the switches. The advantage to users is that they can protect their local over-the-air communications even if the parties they are conversing with are using phones with no encryption or with incompatible methods of encryption. The benefit to law enforcement is that plaintext can be intercepted in the base stations or switches. Although there are devices for achieving end-to-end encryption with cellular phones, they are more costly and require compatible devices at both ends.

Hackers use encryption to protect their communications on Internet Relay Chat (IRC) channels from interception. They have also installed their own encryption software on computers they have penetrated. The software is then used to set up a secure channel between the hacker's PC and the compromised machine. This has complicated, but not precluded, investigations.

Electronic mail

Law enforcement agencies have encountered encrypted e-mail and files in investigations of paedophiles and child pornography, including the FBI's Innocent Images national child pornography investigation. In many cases, the subjects were using Pretty Good Privacy (PGP) to encrypt files and e-mail. PGP uses conventional cryptography for data encryption and public-key cryptography for key distribution. The investigators thought this group favoured PGP because they are generally educated, technically knowledgeable and heavy Internet users. PGP is universally available on the Internet, and they can download it for free. Investigators say, however, that most child pornography traded on the Internet is not encrypted.

One hacker used encrypted e-mail to facilitate the sale of credit card numbers he had stolen from an Internet service provider and two other companies doing business on the web. According to Richard Power, editorial director of the Computer Security Institute, Carlos Felipe Salgado Jr had acquired nearly 100,000 card numbers by penetrating the computers from an account he had compromised at the University of California at San Francisco. Using commonly available hacking tools, he exploited known security flaws in order to go around firewalls and bypass encryption and other security measures. Boasting about his exploits on Internet Relay Chat, Salgado, who used the code name SMAK, made the mistake of offering to sell his booty to someone on the Internet. He conducted online negotiations using encrypted e-mail and received initial payments via anonymous Western Union wire transfer. Unknown to him, he had walked right into an FBI sting. After making two small buys and checking the legitimacy of the card numbers, FBI agents arranged a meeting at San Francisco airport. Salgado was to turn over the credit cards in exchange for $260,000. He arrived with an encrypted CD-ROM containing about 100,000 credit card numbers and a paperback copy of Mario Puzo's *The Last Don*. The key to decrypting the data was given by the first letter of each sentence in the first paragraph on page 128. Salgado was arrested and waived his rights. In June 1997, he was indicted on three counts of computer crime fraud and two counts of trafficking in stolen credit cards. In August, he pleaded guilty to four of the five counts. Had he not been caught, the losses to the credit card companies could have run from $10 million to over $100 million (Power 1997).

We were told of another case in which a terrorist group that was attacking businesses and state officials used encryption to conceal their messages. At the time the authorities intercepted the communications, they were unable to decrypt the messages, although they did perform some traffic analysis to determine who was talking with whom. Later they found the key on the hard disk of a seized computer, but only after breaking through additional layers of encryption, compression and password protection. The messages were said to have been a great help to the investigating task force. We also received an anonymous report of a group of terrorists encrypting their e-mail with PGP.

Stored data

In many criminal cases, documents and other papers found at a subject's premises provide evidence crucial for successful prosecution. Increasingly, this information is stored electronically on computers. Computers themselves have posed major challenges to law enforcement, and encryption has only compounded these challenges.

The FBI found encrypted files on the laptop computer of Ramsey Yousef, a member of the international terrorist group responsible for bombing the World Trade Center in 1994 and a Manila Air airliner in late 1995. These files, which were successfully decrypted, contained information pertaining to further plans to blow up eleven US-owned commercial airliners in the Far East (US Congress 1997a). Although much of the information was also available in unencrypted documents, the case illustrates the potential threat of encryption to public safety if authorities cannot get information about a planned attack and some of the conspirators are still at large.

Successful decryption of electronic records can be important to an investigation. Such was the case when Japanese authorities seized the computers of the Aum Shinrikyo cult – the group responsible for gassing the Tokyo subway in March 1995, killing twelve people and injuring 6,000 more (Kaplan and Marshall 1996). The cult had stored their records on computers, encrypted with RSA. Authorities were able to decrypt the files after finding the key on a floppy disk. The encrypted files contained evidence that was said to be crucial to the investigation, including plans and intentions to deploy weapons of mass destruction in Japan and the United States.

In the Aum cult case, the authorities were lucky to find the key on a disk. In other cases, the subjects turned over their keys. For example, the Dallas Police Department encountered encrypted data in the investigation of a national drug ring which was operating in several states and dealing in the drug Ecstasy. A member of the ring, residing within their jurisdiction, had encrypted his address book. He turned over the password, enabling the police to decrypt the file. Meanwhile, however, the subject was out on bond and alerted his associates, so the decrypted information was not as useful as it might have been. The detective handling the case said that in the ten years he had been working on drug cases, this was the only time he had encountered encryption, and that he rarely even encountered computers. He noted that the ecstasy dealers were into computers more than other types of drug dealers, most likely because they are younger and better educated. They were using the Internet for sales, but they were not encrypting electronic mail. The detective also noted that the big drug dealers were not encrypting phone calls. Instead, they were swapping phones (using cloned phones – see later discussion) to stay ahead of law enforcement (Manning 1997).[2]

In many cases, investigators have had to break the encryption system in order to get at the data. For example, when the FBI seized the computers of CIA spy Aldrich Ames, they found encrypted computer files, but no keys. Fortunately, Ames had used standard commercial off-the-shelf software, and the investigator handling the computer evidence was able to break the codes using software supplied by AccessData Corporation of Orem, Utah. The key was Ames's Russian code name, KOLOKOL (bell). According to investigators, failure to recover the encrypted data would have weakened the case. Ames was eventually convicted of espionage against the United States (CSI 1997).[3]

Code breaking is not always so easy. In his book about convicted hacker Kevin Poulsen, Jonathan Littman reported that Poulsen had encrypted files documenting everything from the wiretaps he had discovered to the dossiers he had compiled about his enemies. The files were said to have been encrypted several times using the 'Defense Encryption Standard' [sic]. According to Littman, a Department of Energy supercomputer was used to find the key, a task that took several months at an estimated cost of hundreds of thousands of dollars. The effort apparently paid off, however, yielding nearly ten thousand pages of evidence (Littman 1997).

A substantial effort was also required to break the encryption software used by the New York subway bomber, Edward J. Leary. In that case, the result yielded child pornography and personal information, which was not particularly useful to the case. Investigators, however, retrieved other evidence from the computer that was used at the trial. Leary was found guilty and sentenced to ninety-four years in jail.

Timeliness is critical in some investigations. Several years ago, a Bolivian terrorist organization assassinated four US Marines, and AccessData was brought in to decrypt files seized from a safe house. With only twenty-four hours to perform this task, they decrypted the custom-encrypted files in twelve, and the case ended with one of the largest drug busts in Bolivian history. The terrorists were caught and put in jail (CSI 1997). In such cases, an effort that requires months or years to complete might be useless.

In other cases, the ability to successfully decrypt files proved unessential, as when a Durham priest was sentenced to six years in jail for sexually assaulting minors and 'distributing child pornography (Akdeniz). The priest was part of an international paedophile ring that communicated and exchanged images over the Internet. When UK authorities seized his computers, they found files of encrypted messages. The encryption was successfully broken. However, the decrypted data did not affect the case.

Even when decrypted material has little or no investigative value, considerable resources are wasted reaching that determination. If all information were encrypted, it would be extremely difficult for law enforcement to decide where to spend precious resources. It would not be practical or even possible to decrypt everything. Yet if nothing were decrypted, many criminals would go free.

Some investigations have been derailed by encryption. For example, at one university, the investigation of a professor thought to be trafficking in child pornography was aborted because the campus police could not decrypt his files. In another case, an employee of a company copied proprietary software to a floppy disk, took the disk home, and then stored the file on his computer encrypted under PGP. Evidently, his intention was to use the software to offer competing services, which were valued at tens of millions of dollars annually (the software itself cost over a million dollars to develop). At the time we heard about the case, the authorities had not determined the passphrase needed to decrypt the files. Information contained in logs had led them to suspect the file was the pilfered software.

At Senate hearings in September 1997, Jeffery Herig, special agent with the Florida Department of Law Enforcement, testified that they were unable to access protected files within a personal finance program in an embezzlement case at Florida State University. He said the files could possibly hold useful information concerning the location of the embezzled funds (US Congress 1997b).

Herig also reported that they had encountered unbreakable encryption in a US Customs case involving an illegal, worldwide advanced fee scheme. At least 300 victims were allegedly bilked out of over $60 million. Herig said they had encountered three different encryption systems. Although they were able to defeat the first two, they were unsuccessful with the third. The vendor told them that there were no backdoors. 'Although I have been able to access some of the encrypted data in this case,' Herig said, 'we know there is a substantial amount of incriminating evidence which has not been recovered' (ibid.).

In early 1997, we were told that Dutch organized crime had received encryption support from a group of skilled hackers who themselves used PGP and PGPfone to encrypt their communications. The hackers had supplied the mobsters with palmtop computers on which they installed Secure Device, a Dutch software product for encrypting data with IDEA. The palmtops served as an unmarked police/intelligence vehicles database. In 1995, the Amsterdam police captured a PC in the possession of one organized crime member. The PC contained an encrypted partition, which they were unable to recover at the time. Nevertheless, there was sufficient other evidence for conviction. The disk, which was encrypted with a US product, was eventually decrypted in 1997 and found to be of little interest.

There have been a few reported cases of company insiders using encryption as a tool of extortion. The employees or former employees threatened to withhold the keys to encrypted data unless payment was made. In these cases, encryption is not used to conceal evidence of crimes, but rather to intimidate the organization. We are not aware of any extortion attempts of this nature that succeeded.

The use of encryption by the victims of crime can also pose a problem for law enforcement. At hearings in June 1997, Senator Charles Grassley told of an 11-year-old boy in the Denver area who committed suicide after being sexually molested. The boy had left behind a personal organizer, which investigators believed might contain information about the man whom his mother believed molested him. The organizer was encrypted, however, and the police had been unable to crack the password. The investigation had been on hold since February 1996.

In April 1998, the FBI's Computer Analysis Response Team (CART) forensics laboratory started collecting data on computer forensics cases handled at headquarters or in one of the FBI's field offices. As of 9 December, they had received 299 examination reporting forms, of which twelve (4 per cent) indicated use of encryption.[4] This is slightly lower than CART's estimate of 5–6 per cent for 1996 (Denning and Baugh 1997). There are at least three possible explanations. One is that the 1996 estimate, which was made before the FBI began collecting hard data, was somewhat high. A second is that as computers have become more common and user friendly, they are increasingly being used by criminals who lack the knowledge or skills to encrypt their files. Hence, the percentage of computer forensics cases involving encryption is staying about the same or decreasing even as the total number of forensics cases (and encryption cases) is growing. A third is that the early reports are skewed; as more come in, the percentage could approach 5–6 per cent.

Public postings

Criminals can use encryption to communicate in secrecy through open fora such as computer bulletin boards and Internet websites. Although many people might see the garbled messages, only those with the key would be able to determine the plaintext.

This technique was used by an extortionist who threatened to kill Microsoft president and chief executive officer Bill Gates in spring 1997.[5] The extortionist transmitted his messages to Gates via letter, but then asked Gates to acknowledge acceptance by posting a specified message on the America Online Netgirl bulletin board. Gates then received a letter with instructions to open an account for a Mr Robert M. Rath in a Luxemburg bank and to transfer $5,246,827.62 to that account. The money was to be transferred by 26 April in order 'to avoid dying, among other things'. Gates was reminded that 26 April was his daughter's birthday. The letter came with a disk, which contained an image of Elvira and the key to a simple substitution cipher. Gates was told to use the code to encrypt instructions for accessing the Rath account via telephone or facsimile. He was then to attach the ciphertext to the bottom of the image and post the image to numerous image libraries within the Photography Forum of America Online (AOL). The graphic image with ciphertext was uploaded to AOL at the direction of the FBI on April 25. Figure 6.1(a) shows the image as posted and Figure 6.1(b) gives the translation code.

Although Gates complied with the requests, he did not lose his money. The extortion threat was traced to Adam Quinn Pletcher in Long Grove, Illinois. On 9 May, Pletcher admitted writing and mailing the threatening letters (there were four altogether) to Gates.

Law enforcement options

The majority of investigations we heard about were not stopped by encryption. Authorities obtained the key by consent, found it on disk, or cracked the system in some way, for example, by guessing a password or exploiting a weakness in the overall system. Alternatively, they used other evidence such as printed copies of encrypted documents, other paper documents, unencrypted conversations and files,

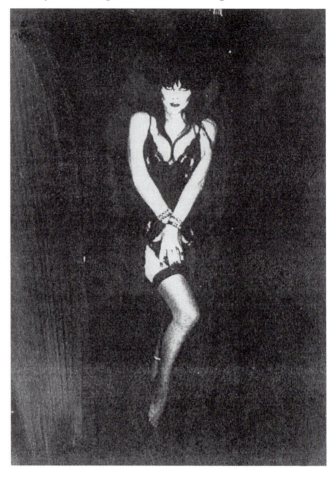

DQKURO XOKOGQBO IR BRCOPDNRGX
© > GRO OIJQGI VMOETLOK
B %#/©, BRCOPDNRGXWEBBO, BRCOPDNRGX
YL > ©© */% @%@% />>%
    > ©© */% @%@% />//
GNDOGM VTLBOEPOG
QTTM *> ~- ©@>/ >~
TNIO IQPERV
GG DEGML / * / ©
    NWOGVOQV YGNIRTMENKV
    ©%@©© GOIPNKI JQF, GOIPNKI, JQ #->/%

Figure 6.1(a)   Image and code from Gates extortion case

TRANSLATION CODE:

Alphabet		Numeric
A *(Q)*	N *(K)*	1 *(©)*
B *(D)*	O *(N)*	2 *(%)*
C *(T)*	P *(Y)*	3 *(*)*
D *(I)*	Q *(U)*	4 *(@)*
E *(O)*	R *(G)*	5 *(/)*
F *(H)*	S *(V)*	6 *(<)*
G *(X)*	T *(M)*	7 *(~)*
H *(L)*	U *(R)*	8 *(-)*
I *(E)*	V *(W)*	9 *(#)*
J *(S)*	W *(J)*	0 *(>)*
K *(Z)*	X *(C)*	
L *(B)*	Y *(F)*	
M *(P)*	Z *(A)*	

NOTE: You may use punctuation marks as they would normally be applied.
To ensure that the correct message is relayed, it is extremely crucial that
you encode your message precisely!!!

Figure 6.1(b)   Translation code from Gates extortion case

witnesses and information acquired through other, more intrusive,
surveillance technologies such as bugs. We emphasize, however, that
these were cases involving computer searches and seizures, not
wiretaps. This section discusses the options available to law enforcement for dealing with encryption.

Getting key from subject

In many cases, subjects have cooperated with the police and disclosed
their keys or passwords, sometimes as part of a plea bargain. One
hacker who had encrypted his files with the Colorful File
System confessed to his crimes and revealed his CFS passphrase:
'ifyoucanreadthisyoumustbeerikdale--**oragoodcypherpunk'. He (Erik)
wanted to speed the process along. The decrypted files contained
evidence that was important to the case.[6]

A question that frequently arises is whether a court can compel the
disclosure of plaintext or keys, or whether the defendants are protected
by the Fifth Amendment. Philip Reitinger, an attorney with the
Department of Justice Computer Crime Unit, studied this question

and concluded that a grand jury subpoena can direct the production of plaintext or of documents that reveal keys, although a limited form of immunity may be required (Reitinger 1996). He left open the question of whether law enforcement could compel production of a key that has been memorized but not recorded. He also observed that faced with the choice of providing a key that unlocks incriminating evidence or risking contempt of court, many will choose the latter and claim loss of memory or destruction of the key.

In *People v. Price* in Yolo County, California Superior Court prosecutors successfully compelled production of the passphrase protecting the defendant's PGP key. In this case, however, the key was not sought for the purpose of acquiring evidence for conviction, but rather to determine whether the defendant's computer should be released from police custody. He had already been convicted of annoying children and wanted his computer back. The police argued it should not be released as there was reason to believe it contained contraband, specifically PGP-encrypted files containing child pornography. This determination was based on the existence of a pair of files named 'Boys.gif' and 'Boys.pgp' (when PGP encrypts a plaintext file, it automatically gives the ciphertext file the same name but with the extension '.pgp').[7]

The defendant was unsuccessful in arguing a Fifth Amendment privilege. The prosecution argued that the contents of the file had already been uttered and, therefore, were not protected under the 5th Amendment. As long as prosecutors did not try to tie the defendant to the file by virtue of his knowing the passphrase, no incrimination was implied by disclosing the passphrase.

To handle the passphrase, a court clerk was sworn in as a special master. An investigator activated the PGP program to the point where it prompted for the passphrase. He left the room while the defendant disclosed the passphrase to the special master, who typed it into the computer. The investigator was then brought back into the room to hit the Enter key and complete the decryption process. As expected, child pornography fell out. The judge then ordered the computer, its peripherals, and all diskettes destroyed. The defendant argued that the computer contained research material, but the judge admonished him for commingling it with the contraband.

Getting access through a third party

Some encryption products have a key recovery system which enables access to plaintext through a means other than the normal decryption process. The key needed to decrypt the data is recovered using information stored with the ciphertext plus information held by a trusted agent, which could be an officer of the organization owning the data or a third party. The primary objective is to protect organizations and individuals using strong encryption from loss or destruction of encryption keys, which could render valuable data inaccessible.

Key recovery systems can accommodate lawful investigations by providing authorities with a means of acquiring the keys needed. If the keys are held by a third party, this can be done without the knowledge of the criminal group under investigation. Of course, if criminal enterprises operate their own recovery services, law enforcement may be no better off. Indeed, they could be worse off because the encryption will be much stronger, possibly uncrackable, and the criminals might not cooperate with the authorities. Moreover, with wiretaps, which must be performed surreptitiously to have value, investigators cannot go to the subjects and ask for keys to tap their lines. Key recovery systems could also encourage the use of encryption in organized crime to protect electronic files, as criminal enterprises need not worry about loss of keys.

Because of the potential benefits of key recovery to law enforcement, the Clinton administration encouraged the development of key recovery products by offering an export advantage to companies making such products. Beginning in December 1996, products with key recovery systems were readily exported with unlimited key lengths. The advantage, however, is no longer great. In September 1999, the administration announced significant liberalizations for a variety of products, including non-recoverable products of any key length.

Breaking the codes

It is often possible to obtain the key needed to decrypt data by exploiting a weakness in the encryption algorithm, implementation, key management system, or some other system component. Indeed, there are software tools on the Internet for cracking the encryption in many commercial applications. One site on the World Wide Web lists freeware crackers and products from AccessData Corp. and CRAK Software for Microsoft Word, Excel, and Money; WordPerfect, Data Perfect, and Professional Write; Lotus 1-2-3 and Quattro Pro; Paradox; PKZIP; Symantex Q&A and Quicken.[8]

Eric Thompson, president of AccessData, reported that they had a recovery rate of 80–85 per cent with the encryption in large-scale commercial commodity software applications. He also noted that 90 per cent of the systems are broken somewhere other than at the crypto engine level, for example in the way the text is pre-processed (CSI 1997). A passphrase or key might be found in the swap space on disk.

In those cases where there is no shortcut attack, the key might be determined by brute force search, that is, by trying all possible keys until one is found that yields known plaintext or, if that is not available, meaningful data. Keys are represented as strings of 0s and 1s (bits), so this means trying every possible bit combination. This is relatively easy if the keys are no more than 40 bits, and somewhat longer keys can be broken given enough horsepower. In July 1998, John Gilmore, a computer privacy and civil liberties activist, and Paul Kocher, president of Cryptography Research in California, won $10,000 for designing a supercomputer that broke a 56-bit DES challenge cipher in record time, in their case fifty-six hours or less than three days. The EFF DES Cracker was built by a team of about a dozen computer researchers with funds from the Electronic Frontier Foundation. It took less than a year to build and cost less than $250,000. It tested keys at a rate of almost 100 billion per second (EFF 1998; Markoff 1998).

Unfortunately, criminals can protect against such searches by using methods that take longer keys, say 128 bits with the RC4, RC5, or IDEA encryption algorithm or 168 bits with Triple DES. Because each additional bit doubles the number of candidates to try, a brute force search quickly becomes intractable. To crack a 64-bit key, it would take 10 EFF DES Crackers operating for an entire year. At 128 bits, it is totally infeasible to break a key by brute force, even if all the computers in the world are put to the task. To break one in a year would require, say, 1 trillion computers (more than 100 computers for every person on the globe), each running 10 billion times faster than the EFF DES Cracker. Put another way, it would require the equivalent of 10 billion trillion DES Crackers! Many products, including PGP, use 128-bit keys or longer.

With many encryption systems, for example PGP, a user's private key (which unlocks message keys) is computed from or protected by a passphrase chosen by the user. In that case, it may be easier to brute force the password than the key because it will be limited to ASCII characters and be less random than an arbitrary stream of bits. Eric Thompson reports that the odds are about even of successfully guessing a password. They use a variety of techniques including

Markov chains, phonetic generation algorithms, and concatenation of small words (CIS 1997).

Often, investigators will find multiple encryption systems on a subject's computer. For example, PGP might be used for e-mail, while an application's built-in encryption might be used to protect documents within the application. In those cases, the subject might use the same password with all systems. If investigators can break one because the overall system is weak, they might be able to break the other, more difficult system by trying the same password.

To help law enforcement develop the capability to stay abreast of new technologies, including encryption, the Federal Bureau of Investigation proposes to establish a technical support centre. The centre would maintain a close working relationship with the encryption vendors. The Clinton Administration announced support for the center in its September 1998 update on encryption policy (White House 1998a).

One issue raised by the development and use of tools for breaking codes is how law enforcement can protect its sources and methods. If investigators must reveal in court the exact methods used to decipher a message, future use of such methods could be jeopardized.

Finding an access point

Another strategy for acquiring plaintext is to find an access point that provides direct access to the plaintext before encryption or after decryption. In the area of communications, a router or switch might offer such access to communications that traverse the switch. If the communications are encrypted on links coming into and going out of the switch, but in the clear as they pass through the switch, then a wiretap placed in the switch will give access to the plaintext communications. We noted earlier how digital cellular communications could be intercepted in this manner, while at the same time offering users considerably greater security and privacy than offered by analogue phones that do not use encryption.

Network encryption systems which offer access points of this nature were given an export advantage over those that do not (ibid.). The approach was initially called a 'private doorbell' approach to distinguish it from one that uses key recovery agents (Corcoran 1998; Cisco Systems Inc. 1998). New products are readily exported without a recovery capability, as noted earlier.

For stored data, Codex Data Systems of Bardonia, New York, advertises a product called Data Interception by Remote Transmission

(DIRT) which is designed to allow remote monitoring of a subject's personal computer by law enforcement and other intelligence gathering agencies. Once DIRT is installed on the subject's machine, the software will surreptitiously log keystrokes and transmit captured data to a pre-determined Internet address that is monitored and decoded by DIRT Command Center Software. DIRT add-ons include remote file access, real-time capture of keystrokes, remote screen capture, and remote audio and video capture. The software could be used to capture a password and read encrypted e-mail traffic and files.

When all else fails

The inability to break through encryption does not always spell doom. Investigators may find printed copies of encrypted documents. They may find the original plaintext version of an encrypted file, for example, if the subject forgot to delete the original file or if it was not thoroughly erased from the disk. They may obtain incriminating information from unencrypted conversations, witnesses, informants and hidden microphones. They may conduct an undercover or sting operation to catch the subject. These other methods do not guarantee success, however.

If there is sufficient evidence of some crime, but not the one believed to be concealed by encryption, a conviction may be possible on lesser charges. This happened in Maryland when police encountered an encrypted file in a drug case. Allegations were raised that the subject had been involved in document counterfeiting and file names were consistent with formal documents. Efforts to decrypt the files failed, however, so the conviction was on the drug charges only.[9]

In another case, a 15-year-old boy came to the child abuse bureau of the Sacramento County Sheriff's Department with his mother, who desired to file a complaint against an adult who had met her son in person, befriending the boy and his friends and buying them pizza. The man had sold her son $500–$1,000 worth of hardware and software for $1.00 and given him lewd pictures on floppy disks. The man subsequently mailed her son pornographic material on floppy disk and sent her son pornographic files over the Internet using America Online. After three months of investigation, a search warrant was issued against a man in Campbell, California and the adoption process of a 9-year-old boy was stopped. Eventually, the subject was arrested, but by this time he had purchased another computer system and travelled to England to visit another boy. Within ten days of acquiring the system, he had started experimenting with different encryption systems, eventually settling on PGP. He had encrypted a directory on the system. There was information indicating that the subject was engaged in serious corporate espionage, and it was thought that the encrypted files might have contained evidence of that activity. They were never able to decrypt the files, however, and after the subject tried unsuccessfully to put a contract out on the victim from jail, he pleaded no contest to multiple counts of distribution of harmful material to a juvenile and the attempt to influence, dissuade, or harm a victim/witness.[10]

If encryption precludes access to all evidence of wrongdoing, then a case is dropped (assuming other methods of investigation have failed as well). Several cases that had been aborted or put on hold because of encryption were noted earlier.

Other technologies for hiding evidence

The modern day criminal has access to a variety of tools for concealing information besides encryption.

Passwords

Criminals, like law abiding persons, often password protect their machines to keep others out. In one gambling operation with connections to New York's Gambino, Genovese and Colombo crime families, bookies had password-protected a computer used to cover bets at the rate of $65 million a year (Ramo 1996). After discovering that the password was one of the henchmen's mother's name, the cops found 10,000 digital betting slips worth $10 million.

Another gambling enterprise operated multiple sites linked by a computer system, with drop-offs and pick-ups spanning three California counties. The ring leader managed his records with a commercial accounting program, using a password to control access to his files. Although the software manufacturer refused to assist law enforcement, police investigators were able to gain access by zeroing out the passwords in the data files. They found the daily take on bets, payoffs, persons involved, amounts due and paid or owed, and so forth. The printed files showed the results of four years of bookmaking, and resulted in a plea of guilty to the original charges and a sizeable payment of back taxes, both state and federal.[11]

Passwords are encountered much more often than encryption in computer forensics cases. Of the 299 computer examination reports received by the FBI's CART between April and December 1998, sixty (20 per cent) indicated use of passwords. This was five times as many as had indicated use of encryption.[12]

Digital compression

Digital compression is normally used to reduce the size of a file or communication without losing information content, or at least significant content. The greatest reductions are normally achieved with audio, image and video data; however, substantial savings are possible even with text data. Compression can benefit the criminal trying to hide information in two ways. First, it makes the task of identifying and accessing information more difficult for the police conducting a wiretap or seizing files. Second, when used prior to encryption, it can make cracking an otherwise weak cipher difficult. This is because the compressed data are more random in appearance than the original data, making them less susceptible to techniques that exploit the redundancy in languages and multimedia formats.

Steganography

Steganography refers to methods of hiding secret data in other data such that their existence is even concealed. One class of methods encodes the secret data in the low-order bit positions of image, sound or video files. There are several tools for doing this, many of which can be downloaded for free off the Internet. With S-tools, for example, the user hides a file of secret data in an image by dragging the file over the image. The software will optionally encrypt the data before hiding it for an extra layer of security. S-tools will also hide data in sound files or in the unallocated sectors of a disk. Figure 6.2 shows the effect of using S-tools to hide a 17-page book chapter inside an image file that is less than four times the size; that is, about a quarter of the file contains a hidden document. The difference between the before and after images is barely noticeable.

There have been a few reported cases of criminals using steganography to facilitate their crimes. One credit card thief, for example, used it to hide stolen card numbers on a hacked web page. He replaced bullets on the page with images that looked the same but contained the credit card numbers, which he then offered to associates. This case illustrates the potential of using web images as 'digital dead drops' for information brokering. Only a handful of people need even know the drop exists.

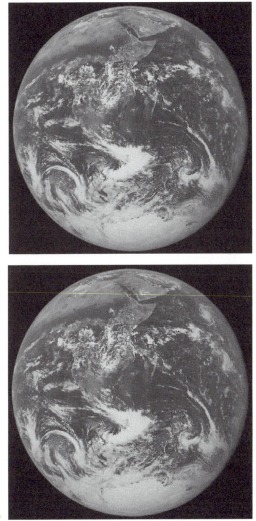

Figure 6.2   Image of earth taken from Apollo 17 on 7 December 1972 before (a) and after (b) hiding a 74 kilobyte chapter in the image. Both files are 281 kilobytes

Source: NASA (photograph AS17-148-22727)

Steganography can be used to hide the existence of files on a computer's hard disk. Ross Anderson, Roger Needham and Adi Shamir propose a steganographic file system that would make a file invisible to anyone who does not know the file name and a password. An attacker who does not know this information gains no knowledge about whether the file exists, even given complete access to all the hardware and software. One simple approach creates cover files so that the user's hidden files are the exclusive or (XOR) of a subset of the cover files. The subset is chosen by the user's password (Anderson *et al.* 1998).

Remote storage

Criminals can hide data by storing them on remote hosts, for example, a file server at their Internet Service Provider (ISP). Jim McMahon, former head of the High Technology Crimes Detail of the San Jose Police Department, reported that he had personally seen suspects hiding criminal data on non-local disks, often at ISP locations, but sometimes on the systems of innocent third parties with poor security, leaving them open to intrusions and subsequent abuse. Eugene Schultz, former manager of the Department of Energy's Computer Incident Advisory Capability, said that a group of hackers from the Netherlands had taken so much information from Defense Department computers that they could not store it all on their own disks. So they broke into systems at Bowling Green University and the University of Chicago and downloaded the information to these sites, figuring they could transfer it somewhere else later.[13] Software pirates have been known to stash their pilfered files in hidden directories on systems they have hacked.

Data can be hidden on removable disks and kept in a physical location away from the computers. Don Delaney, a detective with the New York State Police, told us in early 1997 that in one Russian organized crime case involving more than $100 million in state sales tax evasion, money laundering, gasoline bootlegging, and enterprise corruption, they had to obtain amendments to their search warrants in order to seize disks and records from handbags and locked briefcases in the offices at two locations. After an exhaustive six-month review of all computer evidence, they determined that the largest amount of the most damaging evidence was on the diskettes. The crooks did their work in Excel and then saved it on floppies. The lesson they learned from this was to execute the search warrant with everyone present and look for disks in areas where personal property is kept. As storage technologies continue to get smaller, criminals will have even more options for hiding data.

Audit disabling

Most systems keep a log of activity on the system. Perpetrators of computer crimes have, in many cases, disabled the auditing or deleted the audit records pertaining to their activity. The hacking tool RootKit, for example, contains Trojan horse system utilities which conceal the presence of the hacker and disable auditing. ZAP is another tool for erasing audit records. Both of these can be downloaded for free on the Internet.

Concealing crimes through anonymity

Crimes can be concealed by hiding behind a cloak of anonymity. A variety of technologies are available.

Anonymous remailers

An anonymous remailer is a service that allows someone to send an electronic mail message without the receiver knowing the sender's identity. The remailer may keep enough information about the sender to enable the receiver to reply to the message by way of the remailer. To illustrate, suppose Alice wishes to send an anonymous e-mail message to Bob. Instead of e-mailing Bob directly, Alice sends the message to a remailer (an e-mail server), which strips off the headers and forwards the contents to Bob. When Bob gets the message, he sees that it came via the remailer, but he cannot tell who the sender was. Some remailers give users pseudonyms so that recipients can reply to messages by way of the remailer. The remailer forwards the replies to the owners of the pseudonyms. These pseudo anonymous remailers do not provide total anonymity because the remailer knows who the parties are. Other remailers offer full anonymity, but they cannot support replies. All they do is act as a mail forwarder.

A remailer can accumulate batches of messages before forwarding them to their destinations. That way, if someone is intercepting encrypted Internet messages for the purpose of traffic analysis, the eavesdropper would not be able to deduce who is talking to whom.

There are numerous anonymous and pseudo anonymous remailers on the Internet. Some provide encryption services (typically using PGP) in addition to mail forwarding so that messages transmitted to and from the remailer can be encrypted. Users who don't trust the remailers can forward their messages through multiple remailers.

Anonymous remailers allow persons to engage in criminal activity while concealing their identities. President Clinton, for example, has received e-mail death threats that were routed through anonymous remailers. In one case involving remailers, an extortionist threatened to fly a model airplane into the jet engine of an airplane during takeoff at a German airport, the objective being to cause the plane to crash. The threats were sent as e-mail through an anonymous remailer in the United States. The messages were traced to introductory accounts on America Online, but the person had provided bogus names and credit card numbers. He was caught, however, before carrying out his threat.[14]

Anonymous digital cash

Digital cash enables users to buy and sell information goods and services. It is particularly useful with small transactions, serving the role of hard currency. Some methods allow users to make transactions with complete anonymity; others allow traceability under exigent circumstances, for example, a court order.

Total anonymity affords criminals the ability to launder money and engage in other illegal activity in ways that circumvent law enforcement. Combined with encryption or steganography and anonymous remailers, digital cash could be used to traffic in stolen intellectual property on the web or to extort money from victims.

In May 1993, Timothy May wrote an essay about a hypothetical organization, BlackNet, which would buy and sell information using a combination of public-key cryptography, anonymous remailers and anonymous digital cash.

> BlackNet can make anonymous deposits to the bank account of your choice, where local banking laws permit, can mail cash directly ... or can credit you in 'CryptoCredits,' the internal currency of BlackNet ... If you are interested, do *not* attempt to contact us directly (you'll be wasting your time), and do *not* post anything that contains your name, your e-mail address, etc. Rather, compose your message, encrypt it with the public key of BlackNet (included below), and use an anonymous remailer chain of one or more links to post this encrypted, anonymized message on one of the locations listed ...
>
> (May 1996a)

Although May said he wrote the essay to point out the difficulty of 'bottling up' new technologies (May 1996b), rumours spread shortly after May's essay appeared on the Internet of actual BlackNets being used for the purpose of selling stolen trade secrets.

In an essay called 'Assassination Politics', James Dalton Bell suggested using cyber betting pools to kill off Internal Revenue Service (IRS) agents and other 'hated government employees and officeholders'.[15] The idea was simple: using the Internet, encryption and untraceable digital cash, anyone could contribute anonymously to a pool of digital cash. The person, presumably the assassin, correctly guessing the victim's time of death wins. After spending nearly two years peddling his ideas on Internet discussion groups and mailing lists, Bell was arrested and pleaded guilty to two felony charges: obstructing and impeding the IRS and falsely using a social security number with the intent to deceive. In his plea agreement, he admitted to conducting a 'stink bomb' attack on an IRS office in Vancouver (McCullah 1997).[16] He also disclosed the passphrase required to decrypt e-mail messages that had been sent to Bell by his associates encrypted under PGP.

Although Bell did not implement any betting pools, an anonymous message was posted to the Cypherpunks Internet mailing list announcing an Assassination Politics Bot (program) called Dead Lucky that did. The message also listed four potential targets. A related message pointed to an interactive web page titled Dead Lucky, which contained the statement 'If you can correctly predict the date and time of death of others then you can win large prizes payable in untaxable, untraceable eca$h.' The page also stated 'Contest will officially begin after Posting of Rules and Announcement of Official Starting Date (Until then it is for Entertainment Purposes Only).' Another anonymous message posted to Cypherpunks had the subject 'Encrypted InterNet DEATH THREAT!!! / ATTN: Ninth District Judges / PASSWORD: sog'. The PGP encrypted message, when decrypted with 'sog,' contained death threats and a claim to authorship of the Assassination Bot. Investigators linked the messages and Bot to an individual by the name of Carl Edward Johnson. In August 1998, a warrant was issued charging Johnson with threatening 'to kill certain law enforcement officers and judges of the United States, with intent to impede, intimidate, or interfere with said officers and judges on account of their official duties'.[17]

Computer penetrations and looping

By breaking into someone's computer account and issuing commands from that account, a criminal can hide behind the account holder's identity. In one such case, two hackers allegedly penetrated the computers of Strong Capital Management and sent out 250,000 ads with fraudulent headers that bore the company's name. The ads were for online striptease services ('cyber stripping'), computer equipment and sports betting. SCM filed a $125 million lawsuit against the hackers, demanding penalties of $5,000 per message (Kabay 1997).

Hackers can make it difficult for investigators to discover their true identity by using a technique called 'looping'. Instead of penetrating a particular system directly, they can enter one system and use that as a springboard to penetrate another, use the second system to penetrate a third, and so forth, eventually reaching their target system. The effect is to conceal the intruder's location and complicate an investigation. In order to trace the connection, investigators need the help of systems administrators along the path. If the path crosses several national borders, getting that cooperation may be impossible.

Cellular phones and cloning

Drug lords, gangsters, and other criminals regularly use 'cloned' cell phones to evade the police. Typically, they buy the phones in bulk and discard them after use. A top Cali cartel manager might use as many as thirty-five different cell phones a day (Ramo 1996). In one case involving the Colombia cartel, DEA officials discovered an unusual number of calls to Colombia on their phone bills. It turned out that cartel operatives had cloned the DEA's own number! Some cloned phones, called 'lifetime phones', hold up to ninety-nine stolen numbers. New numbers can be programmed into the phone from a keypad, allowing the user to switch to a different cloned number for each and every call. With cloning, whether cellular communications are encrypted may have little impact on law enforcement, as they do not even know which numbers to tap.

Digital cellular phones use stronger methods of authentication that protect against cloning. As this technology replaces analogue cell phones, cloning may be less of a problem for law enforcement.

Cellular phone cards

A similar problem occurs with cellular phone cards. These pre-paid cards, which are inserted into a mobile phone, specify a telephone number and amount of air time. In Sweden, phone cards can be purchased anonymously, which has made wiretapping impossible. The narcotics police have asked that purchasers be required to register in a database that would be accessible to the police (Minow 1997). A similar card is used in France, however buyers must show an identification card at the time of purchase. In Italy, a pre-paid card must be linked to an identity, which must be linked to an owner.

Conclusions

Criminals and terrorists are using encryption and other advanced technologies to hide their activities. Indications are that use of these technologies will continue and expand, with a growing impact on law enforcement. Although the majority of investigations we heard about were not stopped by encryption, we heard about a few cases that were effectively derailed or put on hold by encryption. Even when the encryption was broken, however, it delayed investigations, sometimes by months or years, and added to their cost, in a few cases costing agencies hundreds of thousands of dollars to crack open encrypted files.

Efforts to decrypt data for law enforcement agencies or corporations in need of recovering from lost keys have been largely successful because of weaknesses in the systems as a whole. That success rate is likely to drop, however, as vendors integrate stronger encryption into their products and get smarter about security. It is not possible to break well-designed cryptosystems that use key lengths of 128 bits or more. It is not just a matter of paying enough money or getting enough people on the Internet to help out. The resources simply do not exist – anywhere.

Most of the investigators we talked to said that they had not yet detected substantial use of encryption by large organized crime groups. This can be attributed to several factors, including the difficulty and overhead of using encryption (particularly the personnel time involved) and a general sense that their environments are already reasonably isolated and protected from law enforcement.

Maria Christina Ascents, who runs the Italian state police's crime and technology centre, said that the Italian Mafia is increasingly looking to use encryption to help protect it from the government. She cited encryption as their greatest limit on investigations, and noted that instead of hiring cryptographers to create their codes, mobsters download copies of Pretty Good Privacy (PGP) off the Internet (Ramo 1996).

As the population becomes better educated about technology and encryption, more and more criminals will have the knowledge and skills needed to evade law enforcement, particularly given the ease with which unbreakable, user-friendly software encryption can be distributed and obtained on the Internet. We recommend ongoing collection of data on the use of encryption and other advanced technologies in crime. We need to know how encryption is impacting cases – whether it is broken or circumvented, whether cases are successfully investigated and prosecuted despite encryption, and costs to investigators.

Encryption is a critical international issue with severe impact and benefits to business and order. National policy must recognize not only the threat to law enforcement and intelligence operations, but also the need to protect the intellectual property and economic competitiveness of industry. Encryption policy must also respect consumer needs for encryption and basic human rights, including privacy and freedom of expression. Addressing all of these interests is enormously challenging.

Notes

1 The chapter is an update of a study we conducted in 1997 at the invitation of the US Working Group on Organized Crime, National Strategy Information Center, Washington, DC.
2 Additional information was provided by Detective R. J. Montemayor in the Dallas Police Department.
3 The key used by Ames was disclosed to us by Robert Reynard on 18 February 1998.
4 Data provided by CART on 9 December 1998.
5 United States District Court, Northern District of Illinois, Eastern Division, Search Warrant, Case Number 97–157M, 8 May 1997; *United States of America v. Adam Quinn Pletcher*, United States District Court, Western District of Washington at Seattle, Magistrate's Docket No. Case No. 97–179M, 9 May 1997.
6 Byron W. Thompson, presentation at HTCIA/FBI Training Seminar, Perspectives on Computer Crime, 12–13 November 1998.
7 Information on this case was provided by Fred B. Cotton of SEARCH Group, Inc. Cotton was the investigator who activated the PGP program on the defendant's computer.
8 http://www.hiwaay.net/boklr/bsw_crak.html as of February 1997.
9 This case was reported to us by Howard Schmidt.
10 This case was reported by Brian Kennedy of the Sacramento County Sheriff's Department.
11 This case was first reported to us on 22 February 1997 by Jim McMahon, former head of the High Technology Crimes Detail of the San Jose Police Department. We received additional information from Robert Reynard on 10 June 1998.
12 Data provided by CART on 9 December 1998.
13 Communication from Eugene Schultz, 15 May 1998.
14 Presentation by Christoph Fischer at Georgetown University, 22 July 1998.
15 A version of Bell's essay on Assassination Politics is in Winn Schwartau, *Information Warfare*, 2nd edn, Thunder's Mouth Press, 1996, pp. 420–425.
16 http://jya.com/jimbell3.htm.

17 *United States of America v. Carl Edward Johnson*, Warrant for Arrest, Case No. 98–430M, United States District Court, Western District of Washington, 19 August 1998.

7 Encryption, anonymity and markets

Law enforcement and technology in a free market virtual world

Philip R. Reitinger[1]

Introduction

The ongoing debate over the regulation of encryption, and the developing concern over the regulation of anonymity, present complex issues regarding government regulation of and adjustment to technology in free societies. These parallel issues place in sharp contrast our emerging views of privacy and law enforcement activity, including surveillance, on communications networks. Encryption – the scrambling of information to prevent unauthorized persons from reading it – can provide nearly perfect protection for the privacy of our communications and our stored data. Anonymity also protects our privacy by preventing others from determining what *we* (virtually) do or say on networks – with the emphasis on the '*we*' because a watcher might determine *what* is being done or said, but not *who* is doing it. Both encryption and anonymity are, therefore, closely tied to our developing notions of privacy, but each poses severe difficulties for law enforcement in its efforts to protect public safety because law enforcement must prove identity and criminal conduct in every criminal case.

Privacy is clearly important, but so too is public safety. Who would want, for example, a child predator to remain anonymous? Who would want a kidnapper to be able to converse freely with his confederates without fear of being overheard? Assuming, then, that there is a balance to be drawn among several sometimes conflicting values, societies have to decide how to draw that balance. For example, should the market draw the balance responding to market needs, or should the government regulate to achieve the best result, or should there be a combination of the two? This is the essential question and focus of this chapter.

The risks posed by encryption and anonymity, and the needs of public safety

Confidentiality and anonymity on computer networks present parallel issues affecting privacy and public safety. As noted above, both are closely tied to privacy – confidentiality is privacy of content, while anonymity is privacy of identity.[2] In addition, a person's ability to obtain confidentiality or anonymity is greatly enhanced on computer networks; as is explained below, computer networks permit near-perfect anonymity and confidentiality. And near-perfect anonymity and confidentiality pose considerable and related risks to law enforcement, because they impair its ability to prove identity (the opposite of anonymity) and criminal conduct which often depends on documentary evidence (which is unusable if it remains unreadable) in criminal cases.

This chapter, however, addresses encryption and anonymity, and not confidentiality and anonymity. Encryption is, of course, different from confidentiality and anonymity, because it is a process (that protects confidentiality) and not a goal like confidentiality and anonymity. Nevertheless, it is useful to compare the dilemmas posed by anonymity and encryption, rather than anonymity and confidentiality, because in practice, encryption is the best way to provide near-perfect confidentiality on computer networks. There are others, but none so effective or convenient,[3] and so there is little reason to consider regulating other forms of confidentiality to permit law enforcement to function. In contrast, there are multiple ways that near perfect anonymity can arise on computer networks, and each of these ways can prevent the effective functioning of law enforcement. Thus, it is anonymity and encryption, not anonymity and confidentiality, that pose dilemmas for law enforcement on computer networks.

Encryption

The difficulties encryption and anonymity pose for public safety deserve some further explanation. Let us start with encryption, because the debate over encryption is more hoary than that over anonymity. 'Encryption' is the process of scrambling data using a mathematical algorithm so that content of the data is obscured. In fact, cryptographers or mathematicians will tell you, the content of the data can be obscured so effectively that, using present technology, the data could not be made readable (decrypted) for billions of years. However, if one has the 'key' – some secret number known to the person intended to be able to decrypt the data – then the data can be quickly and easily decrypted into 'plaintext' (readable) form. Using this process, data can be protected so that only the person who knows the key can read the data.

Of course, encryption brings considerable benefits. Encryption protects the security of all types of information, including businesses' trade secrets, proprietary information and financial information. Encryption can protect the privacy of personal data, including medical records. This is especially important as we begin to store more and more data with entities such as Internet service providers. And encryption may be the only effective way of protecting the privacy of communications over public communications channels, like the Internet or the airwaves. For example, encryption is by far the best way of protecting the confidentiality of electronic mail and cellular phone conversations. Finally, encryption is essential for electronic commerce, such as for encryption of credit card information for online purchases.

But the difficulties that encryption can pose in the investigation and prosecution of criminal cases are also conspicuous. To prove criminal conduct, law enforcement needs the ability to obtain usable, plaintext evidence when it has legal authorization to do so. Encryption can, however, stymie the efforts of law enforcement to obtain usable evidence.

Criminals can encrypt data and be assured that law enforcement will not be able to obtain the plaintext. So, for example, a drug dealer could encrypt his records, keeping a list of customers and quantities bought and sold, yet if law enforcement seized that data pursuant to a court-authorized search warrant, the data would not be readable. So far as law enforcement could discern, the records could be related to criminal activity, or could be a grocery list. Similarly, a child pornographer or paedophile could encrypt the illegal pictures he keeps on his computer. In such a case, even if law enforcement were able to convict the child abuser without the pictures, the encrypted material could easily have identified additional victims. Without access to the content of the pictures, law enforcement would be unable to identify and protect those victims.[4]

In the United States, the loss of the ability to effectuate search warrants for electronic data would be devastating to public safety. Search warrants are among the most common and useful techniques for investigating crime. Search warrants for documents are critical investigatory tools in large categories of cases, including fraud cases and child pornography cases. In addition, as our world becomes increasingly electronic, more and more records will be stored on computers rather than in paper form, compounding the difficulties encryption will pose for law enforcement.

Law enforcement in the United States faces similar difficulties with respect to communications. Using encryption, criminals, terrorists and drug dealers can communicate freely without fear that law enforcement, pursuant to a court order, will be able to intercept and read their communications. Because such court-ordered 'wiretaps' occur only in the most serious cases,[5] and only if other investigatory techniques have been tried and have failed, are unlikely to succeed, or are too dangerous,[6] the loss of the ability to conduct them would severely hamper some of the most important investigations undertaken by law enforcement, such as investigations of organized crime, terrorism and, most particularly, drug trafficking.[7]

To be sure, encryption is just one process for protecting the confidentiality of data, and there are other ways of protecting confidentiality. You can hide a document, lock it in a box, or memorize and destroy it. But none of those are nearly so secure or convenient as encryption. It is hard to memorize a large document and, if you hide it, someone else (including law enforcement) might find it. If you lock the document up, law enforcement can break the lock if a court issues a warrant. In contrast, encryption, properly implemented, can be nearly foolproof. The distinction, I think, is not merely one of degree, because encryption leaves law enforcement with no workable options to obtain plaintext.

The problem for law enforcement will increase over time. Encryption, as noted above, is an effective way of protecting the security of data and communications, and is critical for protecting data and communications transmitted over or stored on insecure networks where they can be accessed improperly. In addition, encryption can be readily implemented on personal computers and other intelligent devices. Thus, because of encryption's high value and low price, we can expect increasing market pressure to include encryption in software and devices. Encryption will become incorporated more and more in commercially available mass market software, and, therefore, its use will increase markedly, especially on the Internet and other networks. Finally, as the global information infrastructure develops, individuals and businesses will increasingly use computers and networks to communicate and store important records. Eventually nearly all important data and communications will be encrypted. This means that encryption can spell the end of searches for electronic information and of wiretaps. The loss will be catastrophic.

Anonymity

Like encryption, anonymity is of incontestable value in protecting privacy. Almost everyone has a reason to speak or act anonymously at some point. People such as political dissidents in repressive regimes, whistleblowers, victims of sexual or child abuse, and persons who have medical conditions that may subject them to discrimination, all have special reasons to speak or read anonymously. We vote anonymously. Finally, the right to engage in anonymous speech is constitutionally protected in many circumstances in the United States.[8]

As noted above, a variety of processes can provide anonymity. Indeed, anonymity on networks can arise at any point (intentionally or unintentionally) where there is no authentication of the source of a communication. For example, a person signs up for a free Internet access service using a false name, and no one verifies his identity. He has just achieved a certain level of anonymity, because his actions cannot readily be attributed to him. Anonymity can also be achieved technically. An anonymous web browsing service can, for example, strip all identifying information related to an individual and allow that person to 'surf' the web without the websites she visits being able to determine who she is, or keep records of her habits tied to her real identity. Anonymous remailers perform a similar function for electronic mail. Such remailers, for example, allow people who have a wish or need to remain anonymous, such as whistleblowers and sexual abuse victims, to share concerns with other people in similar situations. But anonymity, like confidentiality, can be abused. Both speech-related crime, such as threats and extortion, and crime that involves no speech at all, such as an unauthorized access to a computer system ('hacking'), are facilitated by anonymity. The problems this poses for law enforcement are immediately apparent. It is hard to put a pseudonym in jail. Law enforcement in criminal cases relies upon the ability to impose a sentence, frequently imprisonment, on someone as a punishment for criminal conduct. To accomplish that end, law enforcement needs to be able to arrest, indict, prosecute, convict and possibly imprison a specific, physical person. This is not possible if the criminal remains anonymous. Therefore, 'untraceable' anonymity means that crimes can be committed on networks with impunity.

To say that anonymity may be 'untraceable' identifies an important point about anonymity. On a superficial level, anonymity is a binary concept – either my identity is known or it is not. In a deeper sense, however, anonymity can vary in degree depending on how 'traceable' my real identity is. The more difficult it is to determine who I am – to trace my identity – the more anonymous I am.

In this regard, anonymity is different with respect to crime on networks – in the virtual world – than it is with respect to crime in the physical world. For a number of reasons, determining identity on networks can be far more difficult and complex than in the real world.

- First, networks enable crime at a distance. To rob a real bank, you have to be there. To rob a virtual bank, all you need is a computer connected to the Internet, and you can perform the theft from anywhere in the world. This means that the location of the victim tells you little, if anything, about the location of the suspect.
- Second, in the real world, it is difficult to commit a crime without providing some means of physical or other identification – a robber appears on a surveillance video – based on what is said or done during the crime. And with respect to many forms of communication, such as the telephone, there are means of identification based on what is said or how that information is communicated, such as by identifying the voice of the speaker. In contrast, on computer networks it is fairly easy to avoid such identification. An e-mail, for example, purportedly from me could in reality be from anyone, as the recipient cannot hear my voice or see my signature.[9]
- Third, because crime on networks is based on communications, attempting to determine the identity of network criminals involves tracing the relevant communications to their source, such as determining who sent a threatening message. However, on computer networks, and especially the Internet, the source information that exists may be false or may mean nothing. Electronic mail 'from' addresses are easily faked, and even source 'IP addresses', the source addresses for the packets of information passing across the Internet, can be faked. Moreover, even if you have the correct source address, it may not mean anything – discovering that a harassing e-mail came from an anonymous electronic mail service available over the World Wide Web is unlikely to tell you anything useful.

For example, assume I am a computer hacker. I want to break into a US military computer system. Instead of launching my attack directly from my home system, I engage in a process called 'looping' or 'weaving.' I first log on to a computer system that I compromised (obtained access to) long ago. Then I hop to, that is, log on to, another system that I have previously compromised, and access it using an account belonging to someone else. I repeat this activity many times, each time logging on to systems using accounts that are not registered to me. Finally, I reach the system from which I will launch the attack on the US military computer system, perhaps a university computer system in Europe, and launch the attack. Through this process I have achieved a very high level of anonymity, because (1) I can be physically far removed from the victim, (2) there may be no means of identifying me from the content of the communications I use to attack the victim computer system, and (3) to the final victim, I appear to be some student or faculty member in Europe.

To determine who I really am, law enforcement would have to follow back over each of my hops or connections. And unless each of those systems keeps very good records *and* I fail to alter those records, it is nearly impossible to trace back through these many hops unless done in real time. If a law enforcement agent wants to determine the source of the attack on the military computer system, he must first go to the European university system. Because that is not the true source, he must then determine the source of the prior hop – perhaps the attacker logged on to the university system from a corporate system in the United States. He must do this repeatedly until he finds the ultimate source; however, this assumes that each system in the chain keeps accurate 'audit logs' showing the incoming and outgoing connections, which is often not the case. Moreover, hackers quite frequently obtain complete control over a system, 'root' access, so they can delete the audit logs that are created. Thus, for tracing to be successful, it must often be done in real time, that is, while the hacker is connected, before he or she has a chance to delete the relevant information.

You might think, based on this example, that anonymity on networks is a small problem for law enforcement – computer hacking, despite growing public concern, is not yet viewed with the same concern as violent crime.[10] That conclusion would be incorrect. Anonymity is already a tremendous problem in whole categories of cases, including not just unauthorized access to computer systems (hacking), but also threats and harassment, and software piracy. And as our society moves to using networks for more and more of our basic activities, anonymity, like encryption, will grow in importance and as an impediment to effective law enforcement investigations. Finally, there are services available on Internet, like anonymous web browsing services and anonymous remailers, that provide untraceable anonymity to anyone with a computer and modem, so no special skill is required. We can expect that both low-tech and high-tech criminals will use the benefits provided by these services.

To respond to this threat, law enforcement needs traceability. Without traceability, entire categories of crime on computer networks can and will go unpunished.

The need for a balanced solution

There are obvious polar solutions to the encryption and anonymity debates. One solution is universal, perfect confidentiality and anonymity on networks. This is a rather unappealing solution – it would permit terrorists to conspire freely with one another secure in the knowledge that law enforcement could not either determine what they were saying or with whom they were communicating. In such a world, law enforcement simply would have no capability to investigate crimes on a network.

The other solution, under which confidentiality and anonymity would not exist at all on networks, is equally unappealing. You would be free to communicate with anyone, but, of course, not privately. You might want to 'blow the whistle' on fraud in your workplace, but you would face the risk of retaliation because your identity would be known. This is the world of the panopticon, a world without privacy.

Of course, both of these supposed solutions are extreme – and neither is very likely. Some sort of balance between privacy and public safety will be struck. The best solution would ensure that persons could obtain privacy and confidentiality, but that law enforcement could effectively operate by obtaining plaintext evidence and determining identity where society thought it appropriate. However, as is explained in more detail below, society cannot simply decide on the best solutions regarding encryption and anonymity and impose them, because imposition of solutions by regulation has its own costs which may exceed the benefits of regulation. Thus, the more fundamental question is *how* this balance should be drawn.[11] For example, the market can draw the balance responding solely to market needs (the 'market' model); the market can draw the balance responding to the market as modified by government incentives intended to encourage a favourable outcome from the perspective of public policy (the 'incentives' model); the government can draw the balance, imposing that favourable outcome by legislation, regulation or standards, with the market able to select among technologies (the 'regulatory' model); or the government can mandate a single solution and ignore the market (the 'mandatory' model). In short, the question is the extent to which the government should influence market decisions to achieve outcomes deemed favourable by public policy.

To explore the appropriate mix of market and government action, it is useful first to explore the interaction of privacy and technology, and of law enforcement, regulation and technology, to determine the possible costs and benefits of regulation.

Privacy and technology

In part, the difficulties we face in balancing privacy and public safety arise because as we conduct more of our activities (including our private activities) on computer networks, we lose the physical constraints and historical context that provided balance in the past. For the most part, privacy has depended on physical, and observable, facts, in combination with laws that enforce normative rules that are based in large part on those physical facts. For example, in the physical world, sometimes you can be seen and your actions recorded, and sometimes not – these factors, along with others, control how much anonymity you have. With respect to confidentiality, you can hide an item in a private place, and can choose between speaking to a friend or publishing your views. These facts are observable by you – you know when you have privacy and when you do not.[12]

Technology has changed this practical, and historical, balance, by providing means to obtain perfect privacy or no privacy. In many ways technology could be said to reduce privacy, for example, by increasing the amount of information that other persons may have about us, such as credit card charge information and bank records. Technology also provides new ways for government to intrude on privacy, such as specialized listening devices. But in other ways technology can increase our privacy. Pay phones, for example, and prepaid telephone calling cards, permit us to make anonymous phone calls. But whether technology is enhancing or reducing privacy, as a result of technology privacy has become further divorced from physical reality and physical limits; instead technology, and which technologies we as individuals choose to use, can determine the amount of privacy we have.

The technology/privacy connection has at least two important consequences. First, as privacy becomes disconnected from our everyday reality, the amount of privacy we have becomes less apparent. Many, if not most, people do not understand what information can be kept about them. Second, the amount of privacy we have can depend upon the sophistication with which we use technology, with more sophisticated users having a greater degree of privacy because, for example, they use technology to limit information in the hands of third parties, or do not use technologies that reduce privacy.

These consequences are most apparent in the virtual world, as it is based on technology. On the Internet, for example, an Internet service provider can watch almost everywhere we go, and can record with whom we communicate. At the same time, and on the other side of the issue, anonymous web browsing services permit maintaining privacy regarding our web browsing habits, anonymous remailers provide untraceable and anonymous communication, and encryption can provide complete confidentiality of content. Technology, in other words, can provide either no privacy or perfect privacy, with the result having little to do with what the best outcome is for society. Moreover, sophisticated users can have near-perfect privacy, where common citizens have little unless they are aware of the consequences of their actions and act accordingly. Together, these possibilities suggest that regulation may be necessary to avoid the extreme outcomes of total privacy, which means ineffective law enforcement, and no privacy, which also has unacceptable costs,[13] and to ensure that policy, and not the vagaries of technology, determine what the balance is.[14] However, the regulation of technology has its own inherent costs.

Technology, regulation and law enforcement

Technology and law enforcement have a mixed relationship. Sometimes technology provides benefits to law enforcement, at other times it provides benefits to criminals, and most often it does some of both. Fingerprinting, for example, is a technology that is usable by law enforcement but not by criminals. But in most cases technology will be usable both by criminals to commit crime and by either law enforcement or private citizens to fight crime, and so will offer mixed benefits. For example, automobiles can be used as get-away cars for bank robberies and by police to chase criminals. Moreover, technology normally offers independent, and comparatively overwhelming, benefits to private citizens that have nothing to do with crime – automobiles are extremely useful for both business and personal transportation.

In part for these reasons, law enforcement is generally at the mercy of technology. Society does not prohibit the use of automobiles simply because they can be used for criminal purposes. Indeed, it is somewhat uncommon to regulate the use of technology solely based on concerns over law enforcement's ability to *investigate* crimes – the benefits of technology are too great to restrict it in most cases. Instead, law enforcement often depends upon regulation imposed for multiple purposes, such as the requirement that cars be licensed. Although automobiles must bear licence tags for many purposes, including for tax reasons, automobile licence tags also have manifest benefits for law enforcement investigations. Regulation is often unnecessary also because protections brought about by business requirements are sufficient for law enforcement purposes. For example, telephone companies keep long distance toll records for billing purposes, and even though this is done for business purposes, it benefits law enforcement.

Another consideration is that regulation of technology, for law enforcement purposes or otherwise, quite frequently does not work well. Technology moves very quickly in our modern world, and it is difficult for regulation to keep pace. Moreover, even light-handed regulation imposes costs on a technology that can decrease its development, and these costs increase if the regulation lags behind technology. For example, the US government avoids regulating the Internet – it wants the Internet to develop as quickly as possible because of its manifest benefits for business and consumers through electronic commerce, for quality of life through entertainment and other applications, and for education.

Regulation can be especially ineffective in the virtual world. The Internet spans the globe, and regulation by a single country, or even a group of nations, is often less effective because there are alternative geographic channels for information and technology. For example, the US can and does restrict online gambling, but that regulation is made less effective by the ready availability of gambling on the Internet in other countries. Moreover, even if there are not alternative geographic channels, there are generally alternative technical channels, so that if a government prohibits the use of a particular technology, an alternative technology appears that avoids the regulation – and to avoid this, regulations must be broadly drawn, which increases the scope and the possible cost of the regulations.

These considerations lead me to draw several conclusions with respect to regulation of activities on computer networks. First, there should always be an initial resort to technological and market-based solutions as opposed to regulatory ones. If the market achieves or can be influenced to achieve the desired end, much of the cost of regulation can be avoided. Second, any regulation should be necessary to meet essential needs and should be tailored to address those needs – and, if at all possible, regulation should parallel business require-ments so that there will fewer incentives to work around the regulation.

Drawing the balance

Encryption

The question of the appropriate level of government influence on the market for encryption can be simply framed. The question is, in order to provide law enforcement with the ability to obtain plaintext evidence, should the government mandate access by the government to plaintext, encourage such access, or leave the market completely alone?

For example, the government could require that law enforcement be given the capability to decrypt data and communications, by insisting that everyone use a specific encryption technology that allows for government access – because the government would require use of a specific technology, this is the mandatory model. Most probably this would be imposed through a key escrow system, in which all users of encryption would be required to store their decryption key with a key escrow agent or trusted third party from whom law enforcement could obtain it with appropriate authorization. This would balance privacy and public safety by providing individuals and businesses with strong encryption that also meets the needs of public safety, supporting the ability of law enforcement to access plaintext. Alternatively, the government could, under the regulatory model, also impose limits through regulation, but allow more freedom to choose among technologies. For example, a government could require that all encryption products manufactured, sold or used in the country provide a usable mechanism for law enforcement to obtain readable data, that is, that all encryption products be 'recoverable'. 'Recoverable' encryption is encryption that provides its user with both very strong encryption and the ability to 'recover' plaintext even if the decryption key is lost,[15] an ability which law enforcement can also use to obtain plaintext. In an incentives regime, the government would encourage the use of encryption that allowed law enforcement to access plaintext. Finally, in a market regime, public safety costs, which do not necessarily survive a traditional cost/benefit analysis, might be deemed unsupportable by the marketplace.[16]

Currently the mandatory and regulatory models are out of favour in most industrialized nations – most governments have, as suggested above, resorted initially to market-based solutions to see if they meet the needs of public safety. The US and the United Kingdom[17] have indicated they are not seeking to impose such a system at this time, and France has recently abandoned its mandatory policy.[18] The initial costs of a mandatory key escrow system are quite high, because it requires the creation of a new key storage infrastructure. In addition, the costs of operation could also be high,[19] because the key storage facilities would be targets for criminals, and the costs of compromise of a single key could be extremely high. A regulatory system imposes fewer costs, but they still exist. The benefits of encryption for privacy and the security of information have been deemed too important to restrict its growth and availability through imposition of such regulatory costs.[20]

Conversely, a market-oriented system probably provides greater benefits for privacy and the security of information, because it supports faster growth of the use of encryption due to fewer costs. And what are the costs of a market-oriented system? In terms of public safety, they differ for data as opposed to communications. There are already inherent incentives to use recoverable encryption for data, because of the risk that a decryption key will be lost. And so we can expect that most businesses, at least, and many individuals,[21] will use recoverable encryption to ensure that if a key is lost, they can, for example, recover the plaintext of important commercial or financial information.

That said, there is little incentive for businesses to use recoverable encryption for communications – only those businesses that have a need to monitor their employees' communications, such as to prevent fraud, will have an incentive to use recoverable encryption for communications,[22] and individuals will not have any incentive to use recoverable encryption for communications. In addition, there is little incentive to use forms of recoverable encryption that support law enforcement's needs. For example, I may use recoverable encryption because I want to be able to recover data; however, I have little incentive to use an encryption product that specifies where my key is stored, so that law enforcement can find it if it wants to.[23] Therefore, assuming the use of encryption continues to rise over time, a market-based approach to encryption means that law enforcement will lose much of its ability to wiretap electronic communications, and some or most of its ability to obtain stored data.[24]

There is an important caveat here – it is impossible to predict at this time the effect of other incentives that may arise. For example, how will tort law, and more specifically products liability law, handle the case of encryption that is not recoverable and that is used to commit a crime? At present, it seems unlikely that a manufacturer of a non-recoverable product would face a successful liability suit – along with other obvious problems, it would very hard to prove causation (that the harm would not have occurred but for the use of non-recoverable encryption). Perhaps suits by heirs who discover the amount and location of the family's assets, or perhaps the family's electronic cash itself, are encrypted, are more likely.

With the public safety risks from the widespread use of non-recoverable encryption in mind, the US has in the past supported the use of incentives to encourage the use of recoverable products. For example, the US has permitted easier exports of recoverable products to encourage their worldwide use. The US has also indicated its intent to purchase recoverable products, providing a further incentive for their development. Such incentives support public safety needs without impairing privacy of US persons, because the domestic use of encryption is not restricted.

However, it is important to recognize that there is a significant weakness of any market approach. Detractors of the US government policy often argue, even if recoverable encryption is the norm, criminals will not use recoverable encryption if non-recoverable encryption is available. There is an important degree of truth in this criticism, because some criminals will never use recoverable encryption – the risk that law enforcement can obtain the plaintext of the criminals' data outweighs any other risks.[25] However, law enforcement long ago accepted that there would be no 100 per cent solution to the problems posed by encryption, and sufficiently strong incentives could ensure that most encryption (especially encryption provided by the infrastructure) is recoverable, which would result in some or most criminals using that type of encryption. For example, criminals today use unencrypted telephones, even though they can be wiretapped, because that is what is readily available and easy to use. But if non-recoverable encryption is also readily available, then at least some and probably many criminals will not use recoverable encryption, limiting the effectiveness of any non-regulatory policy.

The above considerations, and applying the principles laid out in the last section regarding how regulation of technology for the benefit of law enforcement/public safety should be addressed, suggest that if regulations regarding the use of encryption are under consideration, regulation of encryption of stored data is more likely to be successful than the regulation of encryption of communications. There is already an incentive to use recoverable encryption for stored data, so regulations would parallel business requirements. Furthermore, requiring the use of recoverable encryption for stored data would increase considerably the use of recoverable encryption by criminals, because recoverable encryption would, by necessity, become a standard and more readily available. Of course, the principles of the prior section also suggest that regulation should be adopted only if less intrusive policies, including incentives, fail to address or will fail to address overwhelming public safety needs.[26]

Given the manifest costs of regulation, and the uncertainty at this point with respect to what the market will provide in the future, a mandatory or heavily regulatory approach to encryption may not be justified at this time. But given the manifest risks from the use of encryption by criminals, an unfettered market-based approach is also not justified, at least if you believe that law enforcement should have the ability to obtain electronic evidence. While this result may change as the costs and benefits of encryption become clearer, an incentives model appears to be the best approach for the immediate future.

Anonymity

In some senses, drawing the privacy/public safety balance for anonymity is far more complex than for encryption. Anonymity is an end or goal, not a technique, and so there are manifold ways to regulate it. Remember also that anonymity or a lack of traceability can arise anywhere on a network where there is no strong authentication. Thus, a government could regulate anonymity by requiring improved authentication at any point where it was concerned that anonymity or a lack of traceability posed a real problem. For example, anonymity could be restricted at the 'infrastructure' level in computer networks by requiring that machine-to-machine communications be strongly authenticated (that each machine must know for certain with what other machine it is communicating), or by requiring that information concerning past network communications, such as sources and destinations, be kept for a certain period. Anonymity could be restricted at the 'application' level of networks by requiring that specific high level applications, or all applications, contain identification information, such as that any e-mail sent be signed using a 'digital signature' that strongly identifies the sender. Finally, anonymity could be reduced at the network border by requiring that, for example, Internet service providers or other telecommunications companies identify and keep records on their customers' identities.

In some cases such restrictions could be placed on one or more of the different persons or entities involved. For example, an application-specific identification requirement, such as for e-mail, could be imposed on providers (all e-mail sent from an Internet service provider must be signed), on users (no person may send an e-mail without signing it),[27] or on manufacturers of products (no person may manufacture or sell an e-mail application if it does not require that communications be signed).

Because of this diversity of possibilities, it is hard to generalize about whether a mandatory, regulatory, incentives or market-based approach is appropriate to meet the public safety need of traceability. Some types of regulation would be very expensive, such as requiring that all machine-to-machine communications be strongly authenticated. This would require a fundamental change in the way the Internet operates (a change in Internet 'protocols'), and, therefore, would probably be justified only as based on business requirements (including fraud prevention), not as a law enforcement tool. But other types of regulation might be far less intrusive and still permit law enforcement to trace communications on computer networks.

Let us start with the incentives and market approaches – remember that, in considering whether to regulate, because the first resort should be to market-based solutions, we should look for areas where the market is not supporting or will not support the needs of public safety. In the case of anonymity, I think there is little difference between the incentives and market models because there are already a number of incentives that support traceability on networks, although, of course, the government could always provide additional incentives. The existing incentives arise from business needs. As the Internet becomes more commercial, companies are increasingly looking to market products based on the known preferences of Internet users, which requires that companies know what those preferences are, and so the companies need to know who is doing what on the Internet. Telecommunications companies and Internet 'host' computer systems also need to protect their own networks and systems from abuse and to bill their customers, and so they may keep records for these purposes that allow the tracing of communications. Finally, civil liability may provide an incentive to support traceability. For example, if the victims of computer crime start to sue 'upstream victims' (i.e., computer systems or networks that have been previously attacked by the same criminal and which are then used to attack the victim) on the theory that the upstream computer operator failed to take precautions to prevent the attack or to keep records to trace the attacker, we will see an increase in incentives both to secure computers and to support traceability.

In fact, one could argue that these incentives are sufficient to address the traceability problem.[28] However, we must also recognize that the above incentives apply unequally to different parts of the network infrastructure. For example, some Internet hosts, such as universities, do not normally record or keep marketing data, and may in practice be less concerned about security than commercial businesses. Other infrastructure members actually sell anonymity as a service, such as anonymous e-mail and web browsing services. It is unlikely that any 'incentive' would encourage such companies to provide traceability. If a government wants to support traceability despite the market conditions these entities face, then it would need to bring powerful incentives to bear, or use regulation.

Moving back to the regulatory or mandatory models mentioned above, we should first consider, under the regulatory maxims discussed above, whether we have actually reached the point where we can say with confidence that the market is not providing a solution. Anecdotally, as explained above, it appears that a lack of traceability is causing considerable problems in tracking computer criminals and that the problem will continue to grow. But the area of anonymity, and in particular traceability, on computer networks clearly deserves further research. More data on the lack of traceability, its impact, and feasible solutions would assist policy-makers in determining whether and how to ensure that law enforcement can function on computer networks.

If a lack of traceability is a problem severe enough to require a regulatory solution, under the regulatory maxims discussed above, we must look for minimally intrusive regulations that parallel business needs, and are tailored to the specific harm. Regulations requiring strong authentication of all communications are out of the question on the first ground, as they would require redesign of the Internet. Similarly, regulations requiring communicators to identify themselves are intrusive, possibly unconstitutional in the United States, and not well tailored to address the problem. The law enforcement problem is specifically traceability, and so a solution for law enforcement should be designed to make tracing communications possible.

At this point we must return to the incentives model, because, as discussed above, many companies already have an incentive to keep some records that assist tracing. The problem for law enforcement is that some relevant companies do not keep records that assist tracing, or do not retain those records, perhaps because of expense of perhaps as a service (as explained above, some companies offer as a service the removal of identifying information from communication). A regulatory regime could, therefore, supplement existing incentives (and parallel business requirements) by requiring computer communications providers and others to keep records about incoming and outgoing communications, for a specific period. For example, Internet 'host' computer systems could be required to log particular incoming or outgoing communications. This would permit in many cases law enforcement to trace criminal communications based on historical records,[29] at least in cases in which the criminal being traced lacked the ability to illegally alter the very records that could be used to trace his activity. Intrusive regulation of individuals, and burdens on speech, could also be avoided.

Accordingly, required record-keeping for certain entities on computer networks appears to be the most likely possibility for regulation of anonymity and traceability on computer networks.[30]

Conclusion

Debates concerning regulation of computer networks, particularly the Internet, tend towards the extreme because communications on these networks eliminate physical limits to the activities of both individuals and the police. Individuals can obtain near-perfect privacy and near-perfect anonymity through technology, but technology can also eliminate privacy. Mechanisms created for policing the Internet, such as for obtaining access to encrypted material and tracing communications, can appear to overreach acceptable law enforcement because of a lack of public understanding of the threat, and because they raise the spectre of the surveillance society.

Thus we see the Internet often portrayed as either a freewheeling marketplace of ideas and information in which the best inherently excel, or a 'wild west' overrun and effectively controlled by technologically sophisticated villains of all sorts. To proponents of the former view, proposals for government regulation conjure notions of censorship and *1984*, while law enforcement asserts that a failure to address the need to protect public safety on computer networks will lead to increasingly ineffective enforcement of the law as our communications, business and other activity increasingly occur on computer networks. While there is truth in both viewpoints, we must all do our best to achieve a reasoned dialogue among citizens, industry, privacy advocates and governments about how to ensure the protection of both privacy and public safety as our society becomes increasingly virtual.

Notes

1 Senior Counsel, Computer Crime and Intellectual Property Section, Criminal Division, Department of Justice. The opinions expressed in this article are those of the author, and do not necessarily reflect the opinions of the Department of Justice or the United States Government. There is no claim of copyright on US Government works.

2 It is possible to distinguish between anonymity and pseudonymity, depending on whether the person at issue identifies himself in some, generally fictitious, way. See generally: A. Michael Froomkin, *Anonymity and its Enmities*, 1995 Journal of Online Law, accessible at http://www.wm.edu/law/publications/jol. However, in this article I will use anonymity to refer to any person whose identity is unknown, whether or not a pseudonym is used.

3 The best competitor to encryption may be steganography, the process of hiding data in noise. However, for routine storage of data, steganography is not nearly as convenient, and, unless encryption is used also, not nearly so secure. If one knows that steganography (without encryption) has been used, one can extract the data if one knows or can guess the algorithm used to perform the steganography, which is a much more simple process than guessing the key necessary to decrypt data. And if a key is used in the extraction process, then we are in effect actually talking about encryption.

4 As is explained in n. 16, law enforcement's need for access to plaintext would not be met by imposing a legal requirement that suspects turn over decryption keys pursuant to a warrant or subpoena, because (1) the privilege against self-incrimination (in the US) makes such a course constitutionally difficult, (2) it is not covert, and (3) the suspect will simply assert a lack of memory.

5 In 1998, only 1,329 wiretap orders were issued in criminal cases in the United States, and, of that total, only 566 were issued by federal judges, with the remainder being issued by state and local judges. See 1998 Wiretap Report, Administrative Office of the United States Courts, at 7.

6 See 18 USC. § 2518(3)(c).

7 Narcotics investigations accounted for 72 per cent of the total wiretap orders issued in 1998. 1998 Wiretap Report, at 9.

8 See e.g., *McIntyre v. Ohio Elections Comm'n*, 115 S. Ct. 1511 (1995) (a ban on distribution of anonymous campaign literature violates the Free Speech Clause of the First Amendment to the US Constitution); *Talley v. California*, 362 US 60 (1960) (anonymous hand-billing advocating an economic boycott is constitutionally protected).

9 Notably, even a digitally signed document, unlike a physically signed document, normally provides no biometric form of identification. A 'digital signature' proves, through a cryptographic process, that a document was signed and that it has not been altered. But the digital signature only shows that someone who knows the right key signed the document – it does not prove conclusively who that person is – unless the key is somehow tied to a personal characteristic of the key owner.

10 The threat to public safety from computer crime and cyber-terrorism is higher than many people believe. The 1999 Computer Crime and Security Survey completed by the Computer Security Institute, available at http://www.gocsi.com/prelea990301.htm, indicates that, according to the responding institutions, system penetration by outsiders increased for the third year in a row, with 30 per cent of respondents reporting intrusions, and unauthorized access by insiders also rose for the third straight year, with 55 per cent of respondents reporting incidents. Moreover, single incidents of computer crime can pose considerable risks. In one case,

charges were brought in 1998 against a juvenile for disabling in 1997 vital telephone services to the Federal Aviation Administration control tower at the Worcester airport in the state of Massachusetts in the United States. See http://www.usdoj.gov/criminal /cybercrime/juvenilepld.htm.

11 At the same time, differences in how one views the relative benefits of privacy and law enforcement activity can affect considerably the resolution of the 'how' question. For example, a person who believes that law enforcement should not have the ability to wiretap will not be troubled by the fact that law enforcement may lose its ability to wiretap communications if the market alone determines what types of encryption are available.

12 Expectations based on this physical reality are enforced through appropriate legal rules. For example, the state cannot freely enter your house without your consent; in the United States, for example, the government generally must obtain a search warrant before entering a private home. Notably, the legal test for what is protected from arbitrary government searches and seizures is based on such expectations. To be protected, the person whose property is searched or seized must have a subjective expectation of privacy that society is prepared to recognize as reasonable. *Smith v. Maryland*, 442 US 735 (1979).

13 This is particularly true with respect to data held by third parties. Technology encourages us, for purposes of convenience and economic advantage, to put increasing amounts of information about ourselves in the hands of other entities, including both content which we may store with third parties like Internet service providers, and transactional information about our online activities. In the hands of third parties this information is outside our control, making legal rules regarding privacy more important.

14 'Technology should not dictate public policy, and it should promote, rather than defeat, public safety.' Letter from the Attorney General of the United States and other law enforcement officials to Members of Congress, 18 July 1997, available at http://www.usdoj.gov/criminal /cybercrime/aglet.htm.

15 Key recovery and key escrow are forms of recoverable encryption.

16 It is important to recognize that providing law enforcement with *ex post* remedies to address the problems posed by encryption is unlikely to meet the needs of public safety in many cases. For example, one method of attempting to meet public safety needs is to require that a person using encryption turn over his decryption key to law enforcement when he receives an appropriate demand, such as a court order. However, this type of regulation is, to begin with, of little use for wiretaps, because wiretaps must be covert and asking for the key reveals the investigation. Moreover, and setting aside the legal difficulties that would arise from compelling a person to produce his key in response to a government demand, see Philip Reitinger, *Compelled Production of Plaintext and Keys*, 1996 U. Chicago Legal Forum 171, no savvy criminal would produce a key in response to a government demand (the appropriate answer being 'I forgot it') unless the penalties for forgetting one's key were sufficiently draconian to deter possibly legitimate users from using encryption.

17 See *Encryption and Law Enforcement*, a Report of the Performance

and Innovation Unit, available at http://www.cabinet-office.gov.uk/innovation/1999/encryption/index.htm.

18 See *Interministerial Committee on the Information Society (CISI)*, 19 January 1999, Decisions Taken, available at http://www.premier-ministre.gouv.fr/GB/INFO /FINCHE1GB.HTM.

19 See generally: Hal Abelson, *et al.*, *The Risks of Key Recovery, Key Escrow, and Trusted Third Party Encryption*, available at http://www.cdt.org/crypt/risks98/index.html; *Encryption and Law Enforcement*, see n. 17.

20 See *Encryption and Law Enforcement*, see n. 17.

21 Many criminals, however, may be unaffected by 'business' incentives to use encryption, because they face a different set of costs than traditional business persons. The risk of a loss of a key, for example, may be out-weighed by the risk of imprisonment if law enforcement is able to obtain the plaintext of the criminal's data. See above.

22 In addition, despite whatever incentive exist, employers can monitor employee communications only in those jurisdictions where this is legal.

23 Nevertheless, we can expect that law enforcement will be able to find the key in an indeterminable number of cases. If an individual wants his data to be readable after his death, for example, he may provide sufficient clues to find his decryption key, and law enforcement may be able to locate these clues.

24 As suggested above, this outcome may not be troublesome to those who believe that law enforcement should not be able to wiretap communications or obtain 'private' papers.

25 See n. 21.

26 There is also a risk in waiting too long to regulate, because if an infrastructure is built that does not support the needs of public safety, it will be difficult, and expensive, to alter that infrastructure later.

27 Imposing an identification requirement on users would raise substantial free speech concerns, at least in the United States. See *McIntyre*, 514 US at 357.

28 An alternative and equally interesting question is whether existing incentives are sufficient to support privacy needs. While there clearly is an incentive to offer privacy services to those willing to pay, for the reasons expressed in the section above on Privacy and Technology, it is possible that some form of regulation may be required in order to protect privacy. See 47 USC § 222, prohibiting disclosure of certain information relating to customers of telecommunications carriers. Of course, the first resort should be to market-based solutions.

29 As noted above, further data on the extent to which a lack of record keeping by service providers, anonymity providers, etc., are impairing investigations, and also on what types of regulation are feasible, would be useful. For example, a regulation requiring Internet computer systems to keep a particular record would be unlikely to be feasible unless all the relevant operating systems supported logging the appropriate event.

30 To be most effective, given the international nature of computer networks, required record-keeping would need to be international in scope. Otherwise, computer criminals could still hide their tracks by moving through foreign computer systems that do not keep records.

8 Keeping secrets

International developments to protect undisclosed business information and trade secrets

Margaret Jackson

Introduction

Before 1994, there was no common international approach to the protection of undisclosed business information and trade secrets. In a number of countries, particularly in Asia, there had not even been a recognition or concept of a legal protection of information. However, despite these factors, three different approaches to the protection of business information had evolved – in the British Commonwealth, in continental Europe and in the United States – and these approaches had influenced the development of laws in a number of other countries. Unfortunately, such legal protection operated only at a national, rather than an international, level. As the internationalization of business and the growth in transborder flows of data meant that information had become an international commodity, an international solution to its increasing vulnerability was needed.

This chapter identifies and analyses how international developments are leading to changes to the traditional ways in which business information has been protected by the law and examines what these changes may be. We are concerned with those areas of law which enable an organization to restrict *access* to, and *use* and *disclosure* of, business information, rather than with areas of law which permit others to use the information with the consent of the originator of the information, such as patent, design, and trade mark law. Copyright law falls between these two legal approaches to protection of information because, although it is primarily concerned with publicly available works, in some circumstances it will offer protection to confidential information contained in a literary work or software package.

Since 1988, international developments concerned with the protection of business information and business data have moved in two directions, one direction advocating the introduction of national laws which meet minimum international standards, and the other advocating national implementation of technical guidelines and solutions to keep information secure from unauthorized access and use.

Three international agreements, all of which have the potential to affect how business information can be protected, are examined. They are the 1994 Uruguay Round Agreement on Trade-Related Aspects of Intellectual Property Rights (TRIPs), a part of the General Agreement on Tariffs and Trade (GATT); the 1992 OECD Guidelines on Security of Information Systems, and the 1997 OECD Guidelines for Cryptography Policy. Of these three, the TRIPs Agreement is a legally binding treaty, while the OECD Guidelines fall into the category of soft international law.

Existing approaches to the protection of undisclosed business information

Before 1994, trade secrets and other types of confidential business information and ways to protect them had not been the subject of international treaty. The multilateral treaty most relevant to the protection of business information was the Paris Convention for the Protection of Industrial Property (the Paris Convention) which was first signed on 20 March 1883. While the Paris Convention deals primarily with industrial property in the form of patents, trade marks, trade names and designs, it is also concerned with the suppression of unfair competition. Generally, acts of unfair competition include false or misleading allegations or acts which might create confusion about goods, industrial or commercial activities, or about competitors. However, the misuse of trade secrets and other confidential information is not expressly referred to in the Convention, although such misuse has been interpreted by courts as being an act of unfair competition (WIPO 1994). The lack of a specific international treaty covering business information has meant that the provision of legal protection against its misuse has been dealt with at a national level.

Three main legal approaches by which an organization can protect its information from unauthorized access, use and disclosure have evolved in the British Commonwealth, in continental Europe and in the United States. In Commonwealth countries, like Australia, the United Kingdom and Canada, criminal law, contract, equity and copyright are the main areas of law which provide measures by which a business organization can protect its information from others. Also, in many cases, government officers and those working in particular fields, like health and telecommunications, are prohibited from disclosing information by numerous secrecy and confidentiality clauses contained in statutes. The area of law used by an organization will depend on the type of information which is to be protected and the circumstances of its possible unauthorized access, use or disclosure.

In the Commonwealth, both contract law and the equitable breach of confidence action offer protection to an organization against the unauthorized access to, use or disclosure of confidential information by employees and, to a lesser extent, by ex-employees, and those under an obligation of confidence. Where no contractual relations exist, the breach of confidence action is the only means available to protect information. The action allows one party who has imparted information in confidence to another to obtain relief if the other party without authority either uses the information or imparts it to a third party (Ricketson 1984). The action may be used to protect confidential information of any type, not just business information. It exists outside any contractual relationship which may also impose an obligation of confidence either expressly or by implication.

The breach of confidence action is designed to protect the relationship of confidence between the confider and the confidee, rather than to protect the information itself. It can be used to stop a person from breaking a promise or breaching a duty but does not confer a right to keep information private. Protection of the information itself is an outcome but is not the main object of the action. A third party who receives confidential information in breach of an obligation of confidence will only be placed under the same obligation of confidence as the person to whom it was originally confided if the third party is aware, or subsequently becomes aware, of it having been imparted under a duty of confidentiality. The action overcomes the limitations of privity of contract which provides that only the parties to a contract can sue in cases of breach of contract. In such cases, the injured party to a contract is able to seek recovery from a third party who is aware that information received is subject to a confidentiality clause in a contract (Ricketson 1984). It should be noted, however, that a person affected by the unauthorized misuse or disclosure of the information, perhaps the subject of the information who is neither the confider nor the confidee, has no right to sue for breach of confidence (ibid.).

The protection available under the breach of confidence action is unclear in situations where there is no obligation of confidence owed by one party to another and where the information is obtained surreptitiously by one party. There is particular uncertainty about the extent of protection which may be available where the person accessing, using or disclosing the information without authority may not be under an obligation of confidence to the organization, or where an innocent third party receives the information (Jackson 1998).

In most continental European countries, the access, use and disclosure of trade secrets and other categories of business information have been governed by unfair competition rules, that is, the unauthorized acquisition, use or disclosure of business information is treated as an act of unfair competition. The emphasis is placed on the unfair act of the defendant, rather than on any special relationship between plaintiff and defendant. The undisclosed information must have been kept secret, must have been kept reasonably secure, and must have economic value because it has been kept secret. Personal information is not protected with this approach. Historically, the way in which European countries protect business information differs, although all countries which protect information do so by treating its unauthorized use as an act of unfair competition. Countries such as Germany, Austria, Switzerland, Hungary and Spain have introduced specific unfair competition acts which contain sections covering unfair practices relating to trade secrets. On the other hand, countries like France, Belgium and Italy protect trade secrets under their general tort provisions, their penal codes, or both (Wise 1981).

The European approach to unauthorized use and disclosure of a trade secret or business information avoids the perceived difficulties of the breach of confidence action, with its requirement for information to have been imparted in confidence, and its uncertain applicability in cases of unauthorized access, use and disclosure by persons who have no relationship of confidence with the original holder of the business information. The approach also ensures that innocent third parties are excluded from the operation of the law.

A third approach to the protection of trade secrets and undisclosed business information evolved in the United States. Although it inherited the equitable action for breach of confidence from the United Kingdom as part of its common law heritage, American courts began in the nineteenth century to develop both the breach of confidence action and the tort of passing off into a general tort of unfair competition (Knight 1978). This development occurred unevenly at both state and federal level until 1938, when the case of *Erie Railroad v. Tompkins* (304 US 64 (1938)) determined that a federal court hearing any state case was required to follow the substantive law of the state in which it was sitting (Leistensnider 1987). This decision had the effect of stopping the development of a unified common law of unfair competition and relegating trade secret law, among other areas of the common law, to being solely a state concern (Price 1978).

In 1939, in an attempt to harmonize the developments in the common law at state level, including the law relating to confidentiality of business information, the American Law Institute produced a Restatement of the Law of Torts. This Restatement attempted to define the correct legal principles of a number of topics, often having to choose between conflicting principles, so that a uniform set of laws could be developed. The American Law Institute and its Restatements have no formal legislative standing but many parts of its Restatements have been approved by courts and become the accepted interpretation of the law (Coleman 1992).

Sections 757 and 759 of the Restatement describe the trade secret tort, treating it as being an improper trade practice. Generally, the trade secret tort occurs when a person or organization acquires a trade secret of another by improper means, either directly or indirectly. The Restatement was revised for the third time in January 1995.

In 1968, the National Conference of Commissioners on Uniform State Laws recommended the development of a Uniform Trade Secrets Act (UTSA). The purpose of such an Act was to provide a model law or a draft bill which could be adopted by individual states and amended if necessary to fit each state's particular circumstances. The UTSA was approved by the National Conference in 1979, and amended in 1985 (Keays 1991). By 1997, forty states had adopted the UTSA. There are differences in the various acts, however, not only as a result of which version of the Act was adopted, but also as a result of amendments made to the Act by different states. However, as the UTSA was based on the First Restatement and served as the model for the Third Restatement, it does mean that the approach to trade secret protection in the American states is generally consistent.

Despite being derived from the action for breach of confidence, the American law now operates purely within a commercial setting. The definitions of 'trade secret' in both the Third Restatement (§39) and the Uniform Trade Secret Act (§1 [definition] (4)(i)) contain the requirement that the information has actual or potential *economic* value, and in the case of the former, the information must be used in the business. This means that personal confidences are clearly excluded from the operation of the tort or Act.

Many American states have also made theft of a trade secret or business information a criminal offence, by amending their existing criminal laws, by enacting specific trade secret offences or by introducing new computer crime sections which incorporate theft of information (Bloombecker 1993). Also, on 11 October 1996, the Federal Economic Espionage Act of 1966 became law, making trade secret theft (including theft using the Internet) a federal criminal offence. The purpose of the Act is to 'protect the trade secrets of all business operations in the United States, foreign and domestic alike, from economic espionage and trade secret theft and deter and punish those who would intrude into, damage, or steal from computer networks' (Halligan 1996).

The main difference between the European and American approaches, and the approach taken under the breach of confidence action used in Commonwealth countries, is that the European approach is concerned only with the actions of the person who has acted unfairly in a business context. If a person acquires the trade secret innocently and is not negligent in knowing how the information was obtained from the original holder, then such an act of acquisition is not deemed to be unfair. The Commonwealth and American idea that an innocent party, who subsequently becomes aware that the information had been improperly or unfairly acquired, will be required to pay damages to the original owner does not exist in the European approach to business information protection. Parties who acquire and use a trade secret will only be liable if they, too, have acted unfairly.

One development over the last three decades which went some way to producing an international approach to the protection of information was the enactment of new criminal offences relating to the misuse of computers. This was a worldwide trend in the 1980s which recognized that the problems associated with the use of computers were international, rather than national, issues because of the international operation of computer networks and communication technology. Although the new computer misuse laws avoided dealing with the legal status of information *per se*, they did create the offence of unauthorized access to a computer, which, in most cases, implies unauthorized access to the data stored on that computer. A number of countries like Australia and the United Kingdom introduced legislation which makes unauthorized access either to a computer or to data stored on a computer a criminal offence. Usually, however, the offence of unauthorized access does not make the use or disclosure of the data an offence.

The trade-related aspects of intellectual property rights agreement (TRIPS)

In 1994, the subject of the legal protection of confidential business information was specifically included for the first time in an international treaty. The Uruguay Round Agreement on Trade-Related

Aspects of Intellectual Property Rights (TRIPs Agreement) is a part of the General Agreement on Tariffs and Trade (GATT) concluded on 5 April 1994. The TRIPs Agreement requires member states to comply with certain minimum standards of protection for the following forms of intellectual property: copyright and related rights; trademarks; geographical indications; industrial designs; patents; layout-designs of integrated circuits; and undisclosed information.

The United States was the main instigator of the inclusion of intellectual property, including trade secrets, in the Uruguay round of GATT negotiations which commenced in 1986. The United States was concerned that its previous attempts to protect its intellectual property rights, particularly against misuse by developing countries, were too time-consuming and created resentment. Furthermore, the lack of compatibility of existing national intellectual property laws, the lack of intellectual property laws in some countries, the gaps in the existing international framework, and the lack of measures to allow for enforcement of intellectual property rights were seen as major reasons for attempting a new intellectual property standard.

The purpose of the TRIPs Agreement is to reduce international trade barriers while at the same time promoting effective and adequate protection of intellectual property rights. It is set against an existing framework of international agreements protecting aspects of intellectual property and is designed to supplement the operation of such existing agreements.[1] The obligations in these agreements are taken as the starting point for the standards of protection in TRIPs, although where the existing standards are silent or considered inadequate, new or higher standards are introduced (WTO 1996). The Agreement in Section 8 also sets out standards for the control of anti-competitive practices in contractual licences. The TRIPs Agreement is a multilateral trade agreement binding on all members of World Trade Organization (Article II: 2, WTO Agreement).

Part I of the TRIPs Agreement sets out the basic principles guiding it as well as some general provisions. Article 1(1) states that 'Members shall give effect to the provisions of this Agreement' but they are free to determine how they will legally implement them. Article 1(3) states that 'Members shall accord the treatment provided for in this Agreement to the nationals of other Members'. In addition, Article 3(1) states that members 'shall accord to the nationals of other Members treatment no less favourable than it accords to its own nationals with respect to the protection of intellectual property'.

Article 39(1) of the TRIPs Agreement provides for the protection of undisclosed information in the 'course of ensuring effective protection against unfair competition as provided in Article 10bis of the Paris Convention (1967)'. The effect of this paragraph is to incorporate Article 10bis into the TRIPs Agreement so that it applies to members who are not a party to the Paris Convention. It also ensures that protection of business information is firmly embedded in the European approach to unfair competition and that the difficulties in the approach to protection adopted in Commonwealth countries, which often involves the issue of whether information is property, are avoided.

Paragraph 2 of Article 39 explains how individuals and legal persons may protect undisclosed information:

2   Natural and legal persons shall have the possibility of preventing information lawfully within their control from being disclosed to, acquired by, or used by others without their consent in a manner contrary to honest commercial practices so long as such information:

    (a)   is secret in the sense that it is not, as a body or in the precise configuration and assembly of its components, generally known among or readily accessible to persons within the circles that normally deal with the kind of information in question;

    (b)   has commercial value because it is secret; and

    (c)   has been subject to reasonable steps under the circumstances, by the person lawfully in control of the information, to keep it secret.

A footnote to this paragraph explains that the term 'a manner contrary to honest commercial practices' means:

at least practices such as the breach of contract, breach of confidence and inducement to breach, and includes the acquisition of undisclosed information by third parties who knew, or were grossly negligent in failing to know, that such practices were involved in the acquisition.

Article 39(2) is concerned, therefore, only with the unfair acts of people in acquiring undisclosed business information and would appear to cover the procurement of undisclosed business information. Third parties who acquire such undisclosed information in a manner which is *not* contrary to normal commercial practices are not affected by the Article. Nor would accidental disclosure of information to a third party lead to the right to take action against them.

Paragraph 3 specifies that data submitted to governments or governmental agencies for the purposes of patent and other approval procedures are to be protected.

3   Members, when requiring as a condition of approving the marketing of pharmaceutical or of agricultural chemical products which utilize new chemical entities, the submission of undisclosed test or other data, the origination of which involves a considerable effort, shall protect such data against unfair commercial use. In addition, Members shall protect such data against disclosure, except where necessary to protect the public, or unless steps are taken to ensure that the data are protected against unfair commercial use.

In this paragraph, the requirement to protect the information is imposed on governments, not on individuals or businesses. The paragraph makes it clear that the government concerned must offer more than the possibility of protection; it must protect the information from disclosure or take the necessary steps to ensure that adequate security precautions to protect the data have been installed.

Enforcement of intellectual property rights under the TRIPs Agreement is achieved by placing both general and specific obligations on members (Articles 41–61). The general obligation, contained in Article 41, is that:

Members shall ensure that enforcement procedures as specified in the Part are available under their law so as to permit effective action against any act of infringement of intellectual property rights covered by this Agreement, including expeditious remedies to prevent infringements and remedies which constitute a deterrent to further infringements. These procedures shall be applied in such a manner as to avoid the creation of barriers to legitimate trade and to provide for safeguards against their abuse.

In accordance with Article 68, a Council of Trade-Related Aspects of Intellectual Property Rights has been created to monitor the operation of and compliance with the Agreement. In 1997, the TRIPs Council commenced a review of the legislation of developed countries to determine if such legislation satisfies the provisions of Section 7 of the TRIPs Agreement.

Since the TRIPs Agreement took effect, there has been a clearly identifiable trend for countries without such laws to introduce, or to commence a process to introduce, legislative protection for undisclosed business information based primarily on Article 39(2) and, to a lesser extent, on Article 39(3) of the TRIPs Agreement. This trend has been particularly noticeable with developing and least developed countries even though they have up to five and ten years respectively to introduce such laws if they are members, or are seeking membership, of TRIPs. Most of these countries have not previously had intellectual property laws at all or have had only limited laws and they have chosen to introduce comprehensive intellectual property statutes to satisfy their existing or potential TRIPs commitments. In those cases where the content of the legislation is known, all of the requirements of Article 39 have been adopted into national law. In particular, Indonesia, Thailand, Vietnam, Myanmar and the Philippines are all in the process of creating new laws relating to the protection of business information, with such laws also expected to adopt the model for protection contained in Article 39. This trend is reflected in developing and least developed countries in Africa, South America and the Caribbean (Jackson 1998).

By way of contrast, the developed countries, not unexpectedly, have attempted to demonstrate that their existing laws satisfy the requirements of Article 39 without the need for amendment. In the Commonwealth countries, the breach of confidence action has been put forward as the main legal remedy in cases of unauthorized use of undisclosed business information. Countries like Australia, Canada, the United Kingdom, New Zealand and Ireland have argued in their Article 62(3) notifications to the WTO that the breach of confidence action completely satisfies the requirements of Article 39(2).

Technical international developments

A different approach to the protection of undisclosed business information has been adopted by the OECD. In the 1990s, it introduced two sets of non-binding guidelines concerned primarily with the technology which controls and handles the international flow of information. The first set of guidelines covers the measures to be implemented to keep information systems secure. The second set covers how governments should develop policies relating to security of information stored and processed in computer systems through the use of cryptography.

The OECD has taken a leading role in these developments because of its interest in the social and legal implications of new technology on economic development and because its members consist of all the technologically advanced countries in the world, including the United States, Japan and Germany. Its role began in 1969 with the creation of the Data Bank Panel to explore issues relating to transborder data flows. The Panel sponsored a Symposium in 1977 which recognized five guiding principles for its work – the need for uninterrupted flows of information between countries; the need for countries to protect their own national security; the economic value of information and the importance of protecting business information by accepted rules of fair competition; the need for security of computer systems to protect personal and business data from unauthorized access; and the need for a set of core principles for the protection of personal data (OECD Data Protection Guidelines 1980).

The OECD's first venture into the arena of protection of information was the 1980 Guidelines on the Protection of Privacy and Transborder Flows of Personal Data. The purpose was to ensure that economic barriers to international data flows in the form of personal data protection laws were not created by countries. The Guidelines were developed to be minimum standards which could be adopted into domestic law by member states. Despite their non-binding status, these Guidelines proved to be very influential internationally.

In 1985, the OECD adopted a Declaration of Transborder Data Flows which was to be its capstone for development activity in relation to business information over the next two decades. This Declaration stressed the need for common approaches to issues relating to transborder data flows, particularly harmonized solutions and transparency in regulations and policies.

OECD guidelines on security of information systems

The OECD recognized that computer technology was creating international challenges relating to control and security of information but that the mechanisms for dealing with these challenges, particularly legal systems, were nationally based and varied substantially in some countries.

The Data Bank Panel had already identified the area of security of computer systems as one which needed some guidelines. The 1980 OECD Data Protection Guidelines contained a requirement in paragraph 11 that information holders should implement reasonable security measures to protect the information stored on computer systems. Also, key reports examining computer crime-related issues at the international level which were released between 1986 and 1990 raised the need for greater computer security to be adopted by organizations and governments to protect international data flows (OECD 1988). In March 1990, the OECD established a Group of Experts to draft guidelines for the security of information systems.

In September 1992, the OECD Guidelines for the Security of Information Systems were released. These Guidelines apply to all information held on any type of information system and provide for the holder of information to be responsible for availability, confidentiality and integrity of the information. They offer a series of security principles for adoption in both the public and private sectors, designed to prevent unauthorized access to and use of information, which are expected to be complemented by domestic laws which can penalize those who violate the security of information.

The term 'information system' is defined in Article 5(c) of the Guidelines as involving:

> computers, communication facilities, computer and communication networks and data and information that may be stored, processed, retrieved or transmitted by them, including programs, specifications and procedures for their operation, use and maintenance.

The Explanatory Memorandum which accompanies the Guidelines noted that this definition was only an attempt to broadly define what an information system encompassed in 1992. Computer and communication technology was changing so rapidly that a future information system might be radically different (OECD 1992a). What the OECD considered to be certain, however, was that a global information society existed and that this society was now dependent upon the continued proper functioning of information systems (OECD 1992a). As this dependence grew, so did the vulnerability of information systems to attack, failure and misuse at all levels and across all boundaries.

The OECD believed that the answer to such vulnerabilities and the way to ensure the confidence of users in information systems was to ensure the security of information systems through the application of uniform, internationally accepted, national rules (OECD 1992b). Security of such systems involved the protection of three aspects — availability, confidentiality and integrity.[2] To achieve the objective of security, nine principles, contained in Articles 7 to 15, were developed as part of the Guidelines. The first principle, *accountability*, requires the owners, providers and users of information systems and other parties to be accountable for the security of the system. The second principle, *awareness*, states that, in order to foster confidence in the information systems, the owners, providers and users of information systems should be aware of and informed about the existence and extent of the security measures in place. The third principle, *ethics*, requires all persons and entities involved in information systems to act ethically and respect the rights of others. The fourth principle, *multidisciplinarity*, requires that the security procedures should be developed with input from all discipline areas involved in the information flow, including technical, legal, commercial, educational, administrative and political viewpoints. The fifth principle, *proportionality*, accepts that it is reasonable, when determining the security measures required, to balance the risks to be avoided against the cost of the security measures. The sixth, seventh and eight principles, which are *integration*, *timeliness* and *reassessment*, require governments, and the private and public sectors not only to act in a timely way to prevent security breaches and to ensure that the security measures are integrated and coordinated but to reassess the measures periodically. The final principle, *democracy*, requires that the security of information systems should be compatible with the legitimate information flows in a democratic society.

In brief, these principles require that the owners of information systems and other parties should be accountable for the security of the system and should make users aware that such security procedures are in place. All persons and entities involved in information systems should act ethically and respect the rights of others, and should deal in legitimate information flows. The security procedures should be developed with input from all discipline areas involved in the information flow, including technical, legal, commercial, educational, administrative and political viewpoints. It is reasonable, however, when determining the security measures required to balance the risks to be avoided against the cost of the security measures. Finally, not only should governments and the private and public sectors act in a timely way to prevent security breaches but the measures should be reassessed periodically.

The implementation procedures formed an important section of the Guidelines. In Article 16, national governments were urged to support the Guidelines through legal, administrative, self-regulatory and similar measures and to create awareness of them at all levels and in all sectors. The OECD anticipated that governments and international organizations would also collaborate so that worldwide technical standards on security protection could be developed. In particular, governments should work to overcome any legal problems related to electronic commerce and paperless contracts. Sanctions for unauthorized use of computer systems which might jeopardize the security of information should be introduced by nations, if they had not already done so. Finally, nations should cooperate internationally to ensure that the flows of data are not attacked in any way.

In early 1997, the OECD undertook a review to determine the extent to which the Guidelines have been adopted and implemented at a national level. The final report, *Review of the 1992 Guidelines for the Security of Information Systems*, was released in 1998 and summarized the sixteen responses to the OECD survey (OECD 1998a).[3] The main response to the Guidelines has come primarily from action by national standards bodies, like Standards Australia and the American National Institute of Standards in Technology, and from national and international professional bodies, like the Council of European Professional Informatics Societies and the British Computer Society. Few countries appear to have introduced legislation to enforce computer security as a result of the OECD Guidelines, although Germany had implemented the Guidelines through the legislative creation of the German Information Agency. Voluntary public sector procedures containing the Guidelines was also common. A number of countries apparently feel they do not have the constitutional power to legislate the implementation of the Guidelines, particularly in respect of the private sector (Orlowski 1997).

The OECD review of the Guidelines found that most of the respondents to its survey did not consider that the Guidelines needed changing. Some respondents suggested, however, that consideration should be given to including 'information security' in addition to security of information systems in the scope of the Guidelines, and that the Guidelines, together with the Data Protection and the Cryptography Guidelines, should attempt to cover all issues relating to security, privacy, electronic commerce, intellectual property, law enforcement and consumer issues, with particular emphasis on the use of the Internet (OECD 1998a).

OECD guidelines for cryptography policy

Encryption of information or data offers another way to protect business information from unauthorized access. The use of an encryption device allows organizations to protect proprietary information by protecting the privacy of telephone conversations and preventing unauthorized access to and release of electronically transmitted and stored data. It is assumed that readers of this article will have an understanding of what cryptography is and how it operates so that it is not proposed to provide an overview of cryptography.

Governments have been particularly sensitive about encryption and have sought to control the extent of it, primarily because it potentially threatens law enforcement and national security. This sensitivity is the main reason why the OECD developed Guidelines for Cryptography Policy, fearing that governments may impose bans on the use of encryption which might affect the international flow of information. Cryptography had been monopolized by governments until only a few decades ago but public awareness of public key cryptography and computer technological developments has made it impossible to restrict its use to the government sector. The use of encryption by individuals and the private sector means that access to computer and telephonic communications, both nationally and internationally, by law enforcement officers and national security agencies may not be possible.

Governments have responded to the spread of encryption to the non-government sector in a number of ways (Clarke 1996). The first way is to build an electronic 'trap-door' or backdoor into all encryption schemes, to allow approved government agencies access for law enforcement purposes and to ban the sale of encryption schemes without such backdoor devices. The second way is to restrict the availability of powerful encryption schemes to the government and to allow the commercial sale of only relatively weak encryption which the government can decipher. The fact that others outside the government may also be able to break a weak encryption scheme is an obvious defect of this alternative. The third way is that encryption schemes are only available from organizations approved by the government. The fourth way is that copies of all private keys are placed in escrow with an agency or with a trusted third party (TTP) who hands over the key to the government authorities on receipt of a court order (Clarke 1996; Pattison 1997; National Research Council 1996). As would be expected, arguments against these government responses to encryption have come from those concerned with civil liberties, manufacturers of encryption schemes and the private sector generally.

The United States government has been particularly active in its attempts to control the use of encryption by non-government users. It has adopted two main approaches, first, to restrict the export of cryptographic software, and, second, to enforce the use of encryption schemes which either provide a backdoor for government access through the use of the Clipper Chip or which involve private keys being held in some form of escrow, supervised or authorized in some way by the government.

While the attempts by the United States administration to control encryption technologies has received considerable criticism from both inside and outside America, other countries are still grappling with the encryption control issue. Most countries, however, are moving very cautiously (Koop 1999; OECD 1998b). Government attention is now focused on the use of cryptography for authentication and certification because of their importance in encouraging electronic commerce.

There is an international instrument dealing with export controls on cryptographic technologies, the Wassenaar Arrangement on Export Controls for Conventional Arms and Dual-Use Goods and Technologies. In July 1996, the Wassenaar Arrangement was formally approved by thirty-three countries, including twenty-seven of the twenty-nine OECD countries. As is clear from its name, the purpose of the Arrangement is to provide a set of guidelines covering armaments and sensitive dual-use goods and technologies such as cryptography (OECD 1998b). Members to the Arrangement agree to control the export of the goods and technologies specified through their national laws, regulations and policies. It is not designed to control software which is in the public domain or generally available to the public.

The other important international guidelines addressing cryptography were issued by the OECD in 1997. While the OECD first held meetings on the subject of cryptography technologies and policies in 1992, it was not until 1996 that it formed an *ad hoc* Group of Experts to draft guidelines for a cryptography policy. It met three times in 1996 and prepared draft guidelines which were released at the end of 1996.

On 27 March 1997, the OECD Council adopted non-binding Guidelines for Cryptography Policy, designed to provide principles for countries to adopt in developing their own policies and legislation relating to the use of cryptography. According to the OECD, the guidelines arose from 'the explosive world-wide growth of information and communications networks and technologies and the requirement for effective protection of data which is transmitted and stored on those systems' (OECD 1997a). The problem of data security, linked as it is to issues relating to data protection, confidentiality of business information, national security, technology developments and commerce, could only be dealt with on an international level and in a way which led to a co-ordinated approach to national laws and policies. The Guidelines are aimed primarily at governments but the OECD considers that businesses and individuals should be involved in development and co-ordination of national policies and laws (OECD 1997a).

The OECD saw cryptography as an important method to use in protecting business information and personal privacy. As it explained:

> failure to utilise cryptographic methods can adversely affect the protection of privacy, intellectual property, business and financial information, public safety and national security and the operation of electronic commerce because data and communications may be inadequately protected from unauthorised access, alteration, and improper use, and therefore, users may not trust information and communications systems, networks and infrastructures.
>
> (OECD 1997b: 1)

It further recognized that the use of cryptography to ensure integrity of data was different from its use to ensure confidentiality of data, and so both the issues arising from both aspects of the use of cryptography had to be addressed.

The Guidelines contain eight guiding principles for cryptography policy:

1 Cryptographic methods should be trustworthy in order to generate confidence in the use of information and communications systems.
2 Users should have a right to choose any cryptographic method, subject to applicable law.
3 Cryptographic methods should be developed in response to the needs, demands and responsibilities of individuals, businesses and governments.
4 Technical standards, criteria and protocols for cryptographic methods should be developed and promulgated at the national and international level.
5 The fundamental rights of individuals to privacy, including secrecy of communications and protection of personal data, should be respected in national cryptography policies and in the implementation and use of cryptographic methods.
6 National cryptography policies may allow lawful access to plaintext, or cryptographic keys, of encrypted data. These policies must respect the other principles contained in the guidelines to the greatest extent possible.
7 Whether established by contract or legislation, the liability of

individuals and entities that offer cryptographic services or hold or access cryptographic keys should be clearly stated.

8   Governments should co-operate to co-ordinate cryptography policies. As part of this effort, governments should remove, or avoid creating in the name of cryptography policy, unjustified obstacles to trade.

(OECD 1997c)

The OECD also stated that any national controls on cryptography should be clear and publicly available. The Guidelines will be reviewed at least every five years to determine progress with implementation and whether amendments are needed (OECD 1997b).

It is not possible at this stage to attempt an assessment of the likely effect of these Guidelines or to determine whether member states will adopt them. The OECD Guidelines require member states to be open about the types of law enforcement controls they are seeking, not to restrict the use of encryption in the private sector as far as possible, and to not introduce encryption policies which will impede the international flow of encrypted data. To date, there are certainly differences in the way countries have responded to, or are handling, encryption issues. The United States has made constant attempts to control access to encryption keys. Other countries appear to be taking the middle ground and trying to achieve a workable compromise between the security needs of users and the needs of law enforcement agencies.

Conclusion

The three international developments examined in this chapter have led, or are in the process of leading, to consistent international approaches, both legal and technical, to the protection of business information.

They have led to the creation of new international standards relating to the protection of business information. The most influential of these is contained in Article 39 of the TRIPs Agreement and it has led to international acceptance of a minimum standard for the legal protection of undisclosed information. The approach adopted for this international standard is that of continental Europe, namely, to treat the improper acquisition, use and disclosure of undisclosed information as a type of unfair competition. The undisclosed information must have been kept secret, must have been kept reasonably secure, and must have economic value because it has been kept secret. Confidential business information has now been formally recognized as a form of intellectual property which needs specific legal protection in situations where it is acquired or disclosed without the consent of the holder of the information. The TRIPs Agreement requires member states to ensure that a legal remedy is available to an individual or organization who has experienced an act of unfair competition in respect of undisclosed business information. How a member state provides that legal remedy is left up to each state but minimum standards of how the law should work, contained in Section 7 of the Agreement, must be met.

Both of the OECD Guidelines address another aspect of the protection of business information. The OECD Guidelines on Security for Computer Systems are standards aimed at ensuring that a computer system is managed in such a way so as to offer security of information stored in it. They encourage, *inter alia*, the development of technical standards operating at both a national and, increasingly, at an international level. The OECD Guidelines for Cryptography Policy provide businesses and individuals with a means of keeping information confidential so that unauthorized access to it, or to the computer system if it is stored on a computer, becomes impossible or at least extremely difficult. Some governments, however, believe they have certain rights, normally related to law enforcement and national security, to be able to access and read encrypted data and so wish to restrict in varying ways the use of encryption by users external to the government. The OECD Guidelines seek to provide a way to achieve a compromise between the rights of individuals and businesses to protect data and keep it private and the rights of governments to pursue law breakers so that barriers to the international flow of information are minimal. It is too early to determine whether the Guidelines will lead to a common legislative approach, as was the case with the 1980 OECD data protection guidelines, to common technical standards as appears to be occurring as a result of the OECD computer security guidelines, or a combination of both, or whether it will have only limited impact at all on either international or national policies.

Notes

1   The international conventions mentioned in the Agreement are: the Stockholm Act of the Paris Convention for the Protection of Industrial Property of 14 July 1967, the Paris Act of the Berne Convention for the Protection of Literary and Artistic Works of 24 July 1971, the International Convention for the Protection of Performers, Producers of

Phonograms and Broadcasting Organizations, adopted at Rome on 26 October 1961, and the Treaty on Intellectual Property in Respect of Integrated Circuits, adopted at Washington on 26 May 1989.

2   These words were defined in Article 5 of the Guidelines as follows:

   (d)   'availability' means the characteristic of data, information and information systems being accessible and useable on a timely basis in the required manner;
   (e)   'confidentiality' means the characteristic of data and information being disclosed only to the authorized persons, entities and processes at authorized times and in the authorized manner;
   (f)   'integrity' means the characteristic of data and information being accurate and complete and the preservation of accuracy and completeness.

3   Responses had been received from Australia, Austria, Finland, France, Germany, Ireland, Italy, Japan, Korea, Norway, Portugal, Sweden, Switzerland, the United Kingdom, the United States and Interpol/ Helsinki.

9 Privacy and security at risk in the global information society

Simone Fischer-Hübner

Introduction

Since the Clinton government in the United States has started the National Information Infrastructure Programme (US Government 1993) most other technologically developed countries have issued information infrastructure programmes for the further development of information highways and to strengthen information and communication industry. A group of representatives, mainly from industry, under the chair of the vice-president of the European Union (EU) Commission, Martin Bangemann, has elaborated a report and an action plan for the EU to carry Europe forward into the global information society (Bangemann 1994).

The various national and global information infrastructure programmes promote different initiatives such as teleworking, distance teaching, health networks and network access to all households with applications such as telebanking. They are motivated mainly by economic interests and hold great promise, such as the generation of new jobs, economic growth, better chances for people constrained by geography or disability, possibilities to overcome structural problems such as in traffic or in health care. On the other hand, the new information infrastructure will change our lives completely, and it bears different risks for society.

The Internet as a contemporary data highway on which the global information society may be built is known for many security risks. Thus, the vast development of new information infrastructures will increase our dependency and might lead us to a vulnerable information society which is based on insecure technologies.

Besides, individual privacy is seriously endangered and this is becoming increasingly an international problem. More and more sensitive personal data can be quickly transferred around the world. Moreover, an increasing amount of transactional data for network services will be available and can be collected at different sites around the world. These data can be used to generate consumer and communication profiles. Privacy as a fundamental civil right has to be protected in a democratic society.

The EU Directive is aimed at enforcing a relatively high standard of data protection. It will probably not only be an instrument for harmonization within Europe but it can also have a coercive effect on countries outside Europe to enact efficient data protection laws based on the EU Directive. Nevertheless, a global international harmonization of privacy legislation in addition to the EU Directive on data protection is hardly achievable due to cultural, political and historical differences. Thus, more privacy-enhancing technologies which can technically enforce legal privacy requirements have to be designed, implemented and used.

This chapter discusses privacy and security risks in the global information society. It also compares and critically analyses the approaches to privacy protection of different information infrastructure programmes. The difficulties for a common harmonized legal approach to privacy protection, due to cultural differences, are analysed. Furthermore, privacy-enhancing technologies are discussed.

Privacy

> Privacy is the claim of individuals, groups and institutions to determine for themselves, when, how and to what extent information about them is communicated to others.
>
> (Westin 1967)

In general, the concept of privacy has three aspects (Rosenberg 1992; Holvast 1993):

- *territorial privacy* (by protecting the close physical area surrounding a person);
- *privacy of the person* (by protecting a person against undue interferences, such as physical searches or information violating his moral sense); and
- *informational privacy* (by controlling whether and how personal data can be gathered, stored, processed or selectively disseminated).

Data protection is the protection of personal data in order to guarantee privacy and is only a part of the concept of privacy.

The emphasis of this chapter is on the discussion of informational privacy of individuals. Individual informational privacy has also been defined by the German Constitutional Court in its Census Decision of 1983 as the term *right of informational self-determination*, meaning the right of an individual to determine the disclosure and use of his personal data on principle at his discretion. In order to protect the right of informational self-determination, national privacy laws of many Western states, codes of ethics of different computer societies as well as international privacy guidelines or directives (such as the EU Directive on Data Protection (EU Directive 1995)), require basic privacy principles to be guaranteed when personal data are collected or processed. These include:

- *purpose specification and purpose binding* (personal data must be obtained for specified and legitimate purposes and should not be used for other purposes) (see Article 6 EU Directive);
- *necessity of data collection and processing* (the collection and processing of personal data shall only be allowed, if it is necessary for the tasks falling within the responsibility of the data processing agency) (see Article 7 EU Directive);
- *the data subject's right to information and the right to correction, erasure or blocking of incorrect or illegally stored data* (see Article 10-14 EU Directive);
- *control by an independent data protection authority* (also called supervisory authority, data protection commissioner, or ombudsman) (see Article 28 EU Directive); and
- *requirement of adequate technical and organizational security mechanisms* to guarantee the confidentiality, integrity, and availability of personal data (see Article 6, 17 EU Directive).

The privacy-enhancing security criteria of *anonymity or pseudonymity* of a user is derived from the necessity principle. The privacy principle of necessity of data collecting and processing means that personal data should not be collected or used for identification purposes when not really necessary. Consequently, information systems should guarantee that, if possible, users can act anonymously. The best design strategy to enforce this requirement is the *avoidance of personal data*.

In general, privacy protection can be undertaken by

- privacy and data protection laws promoted by government
- self-regulation for fair information practices by codes of conduct promoted by businesses

- privacy-enhancing technologies adopted by individuals
- privacy education of consumers and IT professionals.

Threats to privacy in the global networked society

In the global information society, privacy is seriously endangered. A key problem is that the traffic on a global network (for example on the Internet) crosses international boundaries and is not centrally managed. On the Internet, there is no overall responsibility assigned to a certain entity, and there is no international oversight mechanism to enforce legal obligations (especially data protection legislation), as far as they exist (Budapest Draft 1996). There are severe privacy risks, because personal data about the users or other data subjects are available and can be intercepted or traced at different sites around the world. Major risks are discussed in the following sub-sections.

Privacy threats at application level

The Bangemann report (Bangemann 1994) and most other Information Infrastructure Programmes promote initiatives such as teleworking, distance teaching, research networks, telematic services for enterprises, road and air traffic management systems, health care networks, public administration networks, network accesses for all households through applications such as telebanking and video on demand. Meanwhile, the global information society is evolving rapidly and many new information highways and applications for the health sector, public administration, research, electronic commerce and private life are being developed. For these applications, there is a growing amount of personal data, such as sensitive medical data, business data and private data that are collected, processed and communicated through networks across state borders.

For example, according to the Bangemann report, European health-care networks for less costly and more effective health care systems for Europe's citizens are planned. A direct communication 'network of networks' based on common standards (e.g., standardized electronic patient case files) linking general practitioners, hospitals and social centres on a European scale shall be developed. These heath care networks shall improve diagnosis through online access to European specialists, online reservation of analysis and hospital services by practitioners extended on European scale, transplant matching, etc. A complete electronic medical patient case file which can be shared between specialists and can be interchanged between hospitals and with GPs can help to diagnose diseases correctly, to avoid repeating risky and expensive tests, and to design effective treatment plans.

Due to the development of new health care networks at the national level and on a global scale and the growing use of telemedicine and telecare, more and more sensitive medical data will be collected, electronically stored, shared among different health care professionals and transferred to different sites in the world. However, medical patient case files may contain some sensitive information about topics such as abortions, emotional and psychiatric care, sexual behaviours, sexually transmitted diseases, HIV status, genetic predisposition to diseases. The privacy of medical data which is endangered has thus to be especially safeguarded.

Furthermore, there are severe privacy risks, since more and more sensitive personal data can easily be communicated to and are often routed via different countries, which do not necessarily have an appropriate privacy level. Messages transmitted in plaintext could be intercepted or modified at each site of the communication path.

Privacy threats at communication level

A side effect of global communication is that connection data are available at different sites around the world revealing details about communication partners, time of communication, services used, connections, and so on. These transactional data may reveal who communicated with whom, when, for how long, and who bought what for what price. Users leave an electronic trace which can be used to create consumer or communication profiles.

Every electronic message contains a header with information about the sender and recipient, as well as the routeing and subject of the message. This information could be intercepted at each site passed. There is normally no anonymity of communication, because the recipient of an electronic mail (even if the e-mail is encrypted) can determine the sender's identity through the sender's e-mail address which normally contains information about the user's name, background (for example, university or company), and location.

Besides, communication profiles could be created by the service provider to whom the user is connected (like Internet or mailbox providers). Service providers are storing personal user data about their subscribers (such as user name, login name, address, bank connection, and status). Users are normally identified and authenticated by the service providers, and their communication behaviour (for example, accesses to news or world wide web (WWW) sites) could be easily traced and supervised by the providers. Normally, service providers are recording the use of services to create accounting data for billing purposes. Besides, the service provider has to collect connection data for operation of the cache.

Also, personal data about users can be recorded at remote servers. A recent study by the Electronic Privacy Information Center (EPIC) showed that none of the most frequently visited web sites on the internet meet basic standards for privacy protection (EPIC 1997). A WWW server can only record the Internet Protocol (IP) addresses of requesting users, which normally do not reveal the user's identity. Nevertheless, techniques, such as so-called 'cookies' or the proposed Open Profiling Standard (OPS), could be used by the remote WWW servers to monitor and track the user's accesses to web pages. Furthermore, a requesting user may be reidentified by the identd-protocol, which operates by looking up specific TCP/IP connections and returning the user name of the process owning the connection.

Cookies are blocks of ASCII text that a server can store and later retrieve from the local WWW browser of the user. Cookies, which were introduced by Netscape to allow user-side customization of Web information, are a mechanism that allows a Web site to record the user's comings and going, usually without his knowledge or consent. If a user is identified by the server as having ordered goods or registered for software, the cookies of this user revealing his interests in particular web pages can be related to his name or e-mail address by the server. Netscape soon modified its browsers so that cookies from one site could not be given to another site. However, web developers and Internet advertising companies (namely Double Click Network) soon found a way to use cookies to correlate user's activities between many different web sites to track the user's usage history and preferences. This could be done by adding cookies to GIF images that were served off third-party sites (see Garfinkel and Spafford 1997).

The current cookie usage is violating the provisions of the EU Directive on data protection and of other national data protection legislation (see also Mayer-Schönberger 1996): First of all, because of their expiration date option, cookies may violate the 'accuracy' and 'timeliness' principles of Article 6 of the Directive. Furthermore, the average user is unaware of cookie storage and access. However, to meet Article 7 of the Directive, a user has to give his informed consent to a cookie transfer, since the other alternative conditions of Article 7 (a legal obligation, vital interests and/or contractual arrangements) cannot be assumed. Browsers need to be specifically configured to disallow cookies or to display a cryptic warning that a cookie is going to be stored. The average user has not the technical knowledge to configure his system accordingly or to view or delete the cookie file and he can hardly make an informed decision based on such cryptic warnings. Consequently, there is no informed consent by the user and cookie technology is therefore violating Article 7 of the Directive. Besides, the extensive information and access rights granted to the user by Articles 10–12 of the EU Data Protection Directive is violated.

In May 1997, the American companies Netscape, Firefly Networks and Verisign announced the 'Open Profiling Standard' (OPS) which is defined by Netscape as 'a standard that enables personalisation of Internet services while protecting users' privacy' (Netscape 1997). In contrast to cookies, OPS specifies the structure of personal profiles, so that the same information can be used by many different websites. To enhance individuals' privacy, OPS shall give users control over their personal profiles and the ability to manage which information gets disclosed or withheld from a particular web site. Personal profiles can contain information of any sort, such as a unique identifier for the profile, unique identifiers to each service visited, demographic information (e.g., country, zip code, age, gender), contract information (e.g., name, address, phone and fax number, e-mail address), commercial information (e.g., credit card number) or side specific information (e.g., detailed personal preferences: favourite books or magazines).

Although, OPS can enforce the principle of informed consent by giving the users the ability to selectively release or withhold information in their profiles, OPS could severely endanger the individual's privacy. In contrast to cookies, OPS uses standardized personal profiles, which can be shared by different sites and can contain user identifying data and many more personal attributes. Even if the user has to give his consent for the disclosure of information in his profile, he could be forced in practice to do so. This could for example be the case if a user is relying on access to a service or to resources, and the access is only permitted to him if he is providing access to information in his personal profile (Brunnstein *et al.* 1998).

According to the German multimedia legislation the provider may not make the use of services conditional upon the consent of the user to the effect that his data may be processed or used for other purposes, if other access to these services is not or not reasonably provided to the user. However, since the internet has no national boundaries and personal data used for multimedia services often crosses national borders, corresponding international privacy regulations for multimedia services are needed as well.

Transactional data can reveal sensitive information about the user's communication behaviour and interests. For example, the choice of a news group or access to Web sites of a political magazine could reveal information about the political opinions of a user.

Marketing companies usually have a strong interest in such transactional data revealing the user's preferences. Users have reasons to be concerned over the distribution of their transactional data for financial gains, and the (mis)use for purposes other than the purposes for which it was collected: a noted case in the USA is the recent example of America Online (AOL) selling its subscriber contact information, financial information and Internet activities.

Security risks

A further problem of the global information society is whether the requirements of appropriate technical and organizational security mechanisms to protect the personal data on the information highways and to provide network reliability can be guaranteed sufficiently.

Important security and safety aspects that have to be guaranteed are:

- *confidentiality* (prevention of unauthorized or improper disclosure of data)
- *integrity* (goal of ensuring that data continues to be a proper physical and semantic representation of information, and that information processing resources continue to perform correct processing operations)
- *availability* (prevention of unauthorized withholding of data or resources)
- *functionality* (the system performs its functions always 'as required')
- *reliability* (all functions performed on a system are always equally performed under equal constraints).

The Internet, an important contemporary information highway that consists of several thousand computer networks with several million users, is known for many critical security holes and is missing essential security features of reliability, functionality, confidentiality, integrity and availability (see Brunnstein and Schier 1997). Various security attack techniques have demonstrated the insecurity of Internet technology and of contemporary information infrastructures:

- *manual* (such as the KGB hack) or *automated hacking attacks* (there are various Internet sites which offer hacking tools and introductory or assistant material on hacking techniques)

- *sniffing* attacks which monitor and store others' electronic traffic
- *spoofing* attacks which forge and misuse electronic addresses
- *malicious agents* which can exploit features or weaknesses of internet services. An agent can either be started by the user or automatically and may distribute itself through the network. Agents work in a hidden manner, and it will be difficult or even impossible to control activities or consequences of such agents. Examples of early malicious agent technologies are *worms* (the Internet worm experiment by Robert Morris has resulted in the break-down of several thousand Unix systems and has caused severe damage) or *chain letter attacks* (such as crismas.exe).
- *malicious documents/macro-viruses* which can import malicious side-effects into local Internet stations. Macro-viruses are computer viruses written in the macro or formula language of word processing and spreadsheet application programs. Macro-viruses spread when infected documents are transferred. Macro-viruses are a significant threat because they are platform independent, easier to write than 'traditional' file viruses written, for the most part, in assembly code, and because data files are exchanged far more frequently than executable files. Due to the increased use of electronic mail with the ability to attach file and mass access to the Internet and on-line services like AOL, macro-viruses are currently regarded as the most serious malicious code threat.
- *malicious web contents* such as hostile Java applets or Active-X controls. A Java applet is a Java program that is loaded over the Web and run from inside a web browser. In general, Java applets are restricted to a 'sandbox' and are prevented from reading and writing files on the client file system, and from making network connections except to the originating host. However, these restrictions have not prevented hostile applets (such as 'Noisy.Bear' or 'Killer-java') to misuse system resources to perform denial service attacks and to exploit various implementation flaws (bugs) in the Java run time system. In contrast to Sun Microsystem's Java, Microsoft's Active-X does not take the sandbox approach. Active-X programs have full access to the user's file system and can cause severe damage. The user's privacy is especially endangered by technologies that uses downloaded code, such as Active-X controls or Plug-Ins. Malicious downloaded programs can, through security holes, scan the end user's hard disk or network for important information and then smuggle the data to the outside world using

the computer's network connection (see Garfinkel and Spafford 1997).

A major reason for Internet security problems is that security was not an important aspect when the Internet was initially designed, and consequently, it is now virtually impossible to fix many security holes. Security and safety are design-inherent features (i.e. they must be specified in design and enforced in implemented systems). Later security enhancements, such as Internet Protocol Version 6 (IP V.6) including authentication and encryption or protocols such as S-HHTP or SSL, can only reduce security risks, but cannot cure past design faults. A further problem is the missing overall responsibility for security on the Internet; each site is responsible for its own security.

Problems of an international harmonization of privacy legislation

In the Bangemann report it is written:

> Without the legal security of a Union-wide approach, lack of consumer confidence will certainly undermine the rapid development of the information society. Given the importance and sensitivity of the privacy issue, a fast decision from Member States is required on the Commission's proposed Directive setting out general principles of data protection.

In the EU, privacy protection will be enforced by the EU Data Protection Directive.

EU Directive on data protection

The EU Directive on the protection of individuals with regard to the processing of personal data and on the free movement of such data (EU Directive 1995) was formally adopted in October 1995 by the European Council. Member states of the EU were supposed to amend their respective national laws (where necessary) to conform with the directive by October 1998. The main objective of the Directive is the protecting of privacy as a fundamental right which is more and more endangered in the networked society. Besides the privacy protection of individuals, another objective of the EU Directive is to require a uniform minimum standard of privacy protection to prevent restrictions on free flow of personal data between EU member states for reasons of privacy protection. The EU Directive makes no differentiation between rules applied in the public and in the private sector. It sets out general rules on the lawfulness of data processing which should also enforce the basic privacy principles mentioned above. It could be used to enforce a relatively good level of data protection in Europe. However, it has also been criticized because some rules (especially the criteria for making data processing legitimate – Article 7) are very general and allow a variety of specific implementations in national laws. These differences in interpretation could hinder the goal of reducing divergences between national laws.

The Directive contains a combination of concepts, which are enforced by the data protection legislation of different member states. For example, the concept of registration of processing operations (Article 18) is enforced in the British, French and Scandinavian data protection legislation (among others). The concept of a data protection official inside an organization (Articles 18 and 20) was taken from the German federal data protection act and the concept of special protection of special categories of data (Article 8) was taken from the French, Irish and Scandinavian legislation. Rules for industrial self-regulation of personal data systems (Codes of conduct, Article 27) were taken from the Dutch system.

The EU Directive also contains provisions for the transfer of personal data to third countries outside the EU. According to Article 25, the export of personal data to third countries, which do not provide an adequate level of protection, is prohibited. However, in open and free networks, such as the Internet, with no central agency of control, it is technically difficult to enforce this requirement (Koch 1995). It has also been criticized that many rules of the EU Directive include exceptions that are mandatory and may hinder states in providing a stricter standard of privacy protection (Greenleaf 1995).

Even if the EU Directive can help to enforce a relatively high standard of data protection in Europe, it will not be able to protect privacy sufficiently in the global information society. As discussed above, personal data can easily be transferred or routed across state boundaries to countries without any data protection legislation, where its information content or communication data can be intercepted. Privacy is therefore an international problem, and an international harmonization of privacy regulations is needed. However, a hope is that the EU Directive will not only be an instrument for harmonization within Europe. It can also for the following reasons have a coercive effect on countries outside Europe to enact efficient data protection laws based on the EU Directive: the Directive represents the 'most modern international consensus on the desirable content of data protection rights' and 'it may be a valuable model for countries currently without data protection laws' (Greenleaf 1995). Besides, due to the restrictions of Article 25 for the data transfer to third countries, there is an economic pressure on non-EU countries to enact efficient data protection acts. For these reasons, some states have already issued new data protection acts: for example, the 1983 Quebec data protection law (the first North American legislation to enact private sector data protection) was based on the earlier EC Directive Draft and was drafted explicitly to protect business from the possible blockage of data transfer from Europe. Another example is Hungary, which is seeking EU membership, and which in 1996 passed data protection legislation and established a data protection commissioner. It was the first country in Eastern Europe to do so. Countries outside the EU will increasingly use the EU Data Protection Directive as a model in devising or updating their legislation (see also Bennett 1997).

Nevertheless, the critical question remains whether a common harmonized approach to privacy will be possible due to cultural, historical and political differences. Anthropologists have stated that, on a low level, privacy (especially privacy of the person and of the close surroundings) is a human physiological need. But, on higher organizational levels, privacy is basically a cultural construct and there are considerable cultural variations in privacy needs and interests (Lundheim and Sindre 1994). In addition, experiences from the Second World War, especially the practice of the Nazi government in amassing and misusing great amounts of personal details about the population, have caused a greater sensitivity to privacy in Western European states (Madsen 1992). Another problem can be seen in non-democratic societies, where individual privacy is normally not protected by legislation. On the contrary, in these countries privacy is often invaded by the state.

In the following sections, the privacy approaches of technologically developed states that have set up information infrastructure programmes are compared with the EU approach. Thereby, considerable distinctions in the different national approaches to privacy protection are shown. Furthermore, all the approaches are critically analysed to determine the insufficiencies of privacy legislation (see also Fischer-Hübner 1997).

Singapore

Singapore was one of the first countries in the world to issue a national information infrastructure programme. The information infrastructure plan *IT 2000 – A Vision Of An Intelligent Island* was formulated by the Singapore government in August 1991 (Singapore 1991). Singapore, the Intelligent Island, should now be among the first countries with an advanced information infrastructure that will link government, business and people. *Singapore ONE (One Network for Everyone)* is a national initiative to deliver a new level of interactive, multimedia applications and services to all homes, businesses and schools throughout Singapore. So far, Singapore has worldwide the highest rate of internet connections per household. However, Singapore, like most other Asian states, does not have any privacy protection laws so far. On the contrary, privacy does not seem to be a topic at all. Intensive surveillance by security services is justified by Singapore's Internal Security Act. While promoting the use of the SINGNET (Singapore's Internet sub-network), the government is trying to control the content of the information transmitted over the net at the same time (Madsen 1995).

Japan

In June 1993, the Information Industry Committee of the Industrial Council in Japan issued a report stating the need for the government to promote information technology. In May 1994, the Ministry of International Trade and Industry (MITI) published a *Programme for Advanced Information Infrastructure*. In this programme under the topic 'Improvement of Environment for Realising Advanced Information Society', only security measures, and not privacy issues, are discussed (Japan 1994).

Japan, on the other hand, is one of the very few Asian countries to have implemented a data protection act. The awareness of privacy in Japan has resulted more from economic self-interest than from any longstanding tradition of ensuring individual privacy (Madsen 1992). The Japanese Act for Protection of Computer Processed Personal Data was made official in December 1988. In addition, cities, towns and villages have also enacted local privacy regulations. However, the Japanese data protection act only applies to national government organizations. Moreover, it does not install an independent data protection authority to control data processing. In 1989, MITI issued formal guidelines entitled *Protection of Personal Data Processed by Computers in the Private Sector* to encourage self-regulation in the private sector on privacy, information integrity and information quality. However, these guidelines for privacy in the private sector as a means of self-regulation are not mandatory and can only be adopted internally by private companies.

United States of America

In 1993, the Clinton/Gore government presented the *National Information Infrastructure (NII) Program – Agenda for Action* (US Government 1993). So far, the US have been criticized for being the first in technology but the last in data protection (Madsen 1992). The US Privacy Act of 1974 only covers the federal public sector. Besides the Privacy Act, there is only a non-uniform patchwork of various privacy and computer security legislation. The US does not have a data protection authority to oversee privacy protection and to act if there are complaints from data subjects about unfair or illegal use of their personal data. Consequently, the only way for data subjects to fight against data misuse is through the courts. It has been realized that the NII does not only promise many benefits, but is also increasing risks to privacy. Therefore, the Information Infrastructure Task Forces (IITF) Working Group on Privacy has developed privacy principles with the goal of providing guidance to all participants in the National Information Infrastructure (IITF 1995). They are intended to be applied to governmental and private sectors, and are based on the idea that all participants (information providers, collectors, users and data subjects) of the NII have a shared responsibility for the proper use of personal information..

General Principles for All Participants require that all NII participants should ensure and respect information privacy, information integrity, and information quality. *Principles for Users of Personal Information* require information users to assess the impact on privacy of current or planned activities and to use personal information only for these activities or for compatible uses. Data subjects will be informed by the data collector about the reason and purpose of data collection and about their rights. Information users should use appropriate security mechanisms to protect the confidentiality and integrity of personal data. Information users should not use information in ways that are incompatible with an individual's understanding. Furthermore, they should educate themselves about how privacy can be maintained.

According to the *Principles for Individuals Who Provide Personal Information*, individuals should obtain information about what data are being collected and for what reason, and how they will be protected. Individuals will have a responsibility to understand the consequences of providing personal data to others and will make intelligent choices on whether to provide or not to provide their personal data. Individuals will be able to safeguard their own privacy by having the means to obtain their data, to correct them, to use appropriate technical safeguards (for example, encryption), and to remain anonymous when appropriate. Furthermore, data subjects will have means of redress, if harmed by an improper disclosure or use of personal data.

The IITF privacy principles could raise the level of data protection in the US, especially if applied in the private sector. Unfortunately, the principles only offer guidelines for those who are drafting laws and regulations but they do not have the force of law. Although the IITF privacy principles are intended to be consistent with international guidelines such as the Organization for Economic Cooperation and Development guidelines, they do not in some respect offer the same level of privacy protection as the EU Directive. In practice, the idea of shared responsibility of equal partners will not always work, because data subjects (such as employees) often depend on services provided by the data processing agencies (for example, employers), so that they hardly have the chance to enforce their rights themselves. Consequently, besides the right of redress, the control of an independent data protection authority is necessary to protect data subjects efficiently. In *Options for Promoting Privacy on the NII* it is argued that the establishment of a data protection authority could reduce the likelihood that unfair information practices are prosecuted (IITF 1997). However, in practice it is normally more cumbersome and risky for a citizen to go to court than to appeal to a data protection authority, which acts as the citizen's lawyer. Besides, with a data protection authority that monitors and checks the observance of data protection regulations, it is much more likely that personal data abuses are detected.

Currently, the US and EU are discussing how the EU Directive might affect transatlantic data flow, and whether Article 25 will restrict the data flow from the EU to the USA and will thus have consequences on transborder electronic commerce. A main question in the discussion is whether 'adequacy' will be judged against the principles of the Directive or also against the methods of enforcement and oversight. The European side tends to demand the enforcement of clear requirements of legitimacy (especially purpose specification and binding) as well as an independent oversight authority, which can act on complaints of the data subjects. Currently, the US American side is opposed to enacting a data protection legislation according to the European model and instead favours means of self-regulation for the private sector.

A recent comprehensive report *Privacy and Self-Regulation in the Information Age* by the US Department of Commerce (US Department of Commerce 1997) explores the benefits and challenges of self-regulatory privacy regimes. According to this report, effective self-regulation must involve substantive rules as well as means to ensure that consumers know the rules, that companies actually do what they promise to do, and that consumers can have their complaints heard and resolved fairly. The Department of Commerce also recently proposed 'International Safe Harbour Principles', which are self-regulatory privacy guidelines that will prevent US companies' data transfer from being cut off by the EU.

In the USA, voluntary privacy codes have generally been developed in conformity with the OECD Guidelines, whereby some of these codes embody external mechanisms for complaints and oversight and others are merely statements of good intention (Bennett 1997). However, although several hundred USA companies signed to the OECD Guidelines, few adopted their provisions in practice (Madsen 1992).

The United States argue that an omnibus privacy legislation is a feature of a continental legal system, and that the Anglo-American system based on common law dictates a less regulatory regime. According to the US tradition of self-help and judicial enforcement, more responsibility is placed on the individual to demonstrate damage and make a claim through the court. However, in contradiction to this argument, in the USA there are several application-specific acts regulating privacy aspects in the private sector, such as the Fair Credit Reporting Act or the Video Rental Act. Moreover, there are other states with an English common law tradition that enforce or plan to enforce an omnibus data-protection policy. For example, the United Kingdom, has passed its data protection act covering the public and private sectors in 1984, and Canada is currently planning to expand its data protection legislation also to the private sector.

Canada

In September 1995, the Canadian Information Highway Advisory Council presented the final report *Connection Community Content: The Challenge of the Information Highway* (Canada 1995). In contrast to most other information infrastructure programmes, which were mainly influenced by input from representatives of the IT industry, the advisory council also included members from artistic, creative and educational communities, and from consumer and labour organizations. It was chaired by David Johnston, professor of law at McGill University's Centre for Medicine, Ethics and Law.

The Canadian Privacy Act of 1982 which, in contrast to the US legislation, established the Office of Privacy Commissioner, only applies to federal government bodies and agencies. Only the province of Quebec has enacted privacy legislation for the private sector. Voluntary privacy codes and standards have generally been the preferred approach of Canadian business and industry associations. The diversity of codes of practice in Canada was one reason for the Canadian Standards Association (CSA) to negotiate a Model Code for the Protection of Personal Information in the private sector with business, government and consumer groups. Besides, the CSA was motivated by the EU Directive and by the fear of the possible blockage of personal data transfer from Europe.

Privacy protection and network security were one of five principles that were set up by the Information Highway Advisory Council. The council recommended that the government should continue to collaborate with the CSA, business and consumer organizations, and other levels of government, in order to implement the CSA code and develop effective independent oversight and enforcement mechanisms. This recommendation was accepted by the federal government in May 1996. The Canadian Justice Minister promised that such legislation would be in place by the year 2000.

Privacy-enhancing technologies

In a fully networked society, privacy is seriously endangered and cannot be sufficiently protected by privacy legislation or privacy codes of conduct alone. Data protection commissioners are therefore demanding that privacy requirements should also be technically enforced and that privacy should be a design criterion for information systems. The Dutch Data Protection Authority (the Registratiekamer) and the Information and Privacy Commissioner (IPC) for the Province of Ontario, Canada, have collaborated in the production of a report (Registratiekamer/IPC 1995) exploring privacy-enhancing technologies that safeguard personal privacy by minimizing or eliminating the collection of identifiable data. The report on privacy-enhancing technologies by the Registratiekamer and IPC, and a prior study of the Registratiekamer on how to design and model privacy technologies (Registratiekamer 1995) mainly focus on privacy technologies that permit transactions to be conducted anonymously.

Extended security criteria for systems with high privacy requirements should cover a diversity of privacy-enhancing security aspects such as:

- *Anonymity, pseudonymity, unlinkability, unobservability of users*: The privacy principle of necessity of data collecting means that personal data should not be collected or used for identification purposes when not really necessary. Consequently, information systems should guarantee that, if possible, users can act anonymously.

- *Anonymity and pseudonymity of data subjects*: if storage is needed, personal data of data subjects should be anonymized or pseudonymized as soon as possible.
- *Security mechanisms*, such as access control or encryption, are necessary to protect the confidentiality and integrity of personal data, if personal data have to be stored, processed or transmitted. Such security mechanisms can also be classified as data protection technologies. Especially the privacy requirements of purpose binding and necessity of data processing of personal data of users and data subjects can be technically enforced through an appropriate security policy and access control mechanisms (for example, see Fischer-Hübner 1994, for a formal privacy enforcing access control model).

None of the early security evaluation criteria, such as the American *DoD Trusted Computer Systems Evaluation Criteria* (TCSEC 1985) or the European *Information Technology Security Evaluation Criteria* (ITSEC 1991), really covers user and privacy friendly functionality, as their focus is biased on the protection of system owners instead of users and data subjects. The harmonized Common Criteria (CC 1999) are at least covering the functionality class *Privacy* for the evaluation of the functionalities *Anonymity*, *Pseudonymity*, *Unlinkability* and *Unobservability* of users.

Examples for privacy technologies which are protecting the user's anonymity at application level are electronic payment systems based on anonymous prepaid cards (such as telephone cards) or David Chaum's *ECash* which is based on blind signatures (Chaum 1992). Further examples for systems which can provide anonymity of communication are communication Mixes (Chaum 1981), such as the Anonymizer, for anonymous web accesses (Boyan 1997), anonymous remailers (see Cottrell 1997; Chaum 1981) or Onion Routing for anonymizing interactive Internet communication (Goldschlag *et al.* 1999).

Anonymous remailers should allow the anonymous use of electronic mail. Simple anonymous remailers are intermediary computers, which secretly pass messages to a recipient. However, such remailer cannot sufficiently protect privacy, because a mapping of anonymous identities to real addresses must be maintained by the remailer which, for that reason, can be a sensitive point of attack. The Finnish remailer service anon.penet.fi was recently closed down, after it had been raided by the Finnish police in cooperation with the FBI.

So-called cypherpunk remailers enable the chaining of encrypted messages through a series of remailers. The structure of messages is a nested set of encrypted messages, where each message is encrypted to a remailer. Cypherpunk remailers should ensure that only the first remailer in the chain knows the address of the sender, and only the last remailer knows the address of the receiver. However, cypherpunk remailers can be attacked as well (see Cottrell 1997). Messages could be traced if incoming messages to a remailer are directly forwarded. Even if incoming messages are delayed or reordered, an attacker could send a batch of messages after your message arrives, so that your message will flushed back out of the remailer's message pool. Besides, messages could be tracked by their size (which decreases) or by the use of active replay attacks.

A remailer, which can guarantee anonymity effectively is Mixmaster (Cottrell 1997) which is based on the concept of Mixes (Chaum 1981). Mixmaster uses constant-length messages, includes defences against replay attacks and offers improved message reordering code to stop passive correlation attacks based on timing coincidences. In 'Electronic Frontiers Georgia, Reliable Remailer List' a current list of remailer services for the internet with an estimation of their reliability is offered (EFGA).

Conclusions

In conclusion, the global information society is at risk. A key problem is that most of the information infrastructure programmes emphasize economic opportunities and neglect social impacts. Nevertheless, a democratic participation of the public in the design and development of the information infrastructure should be encouraged. Social and legal impacts of the different initiatives have to be assessed in advance and have to be periodically reviewed. High standards for security and network reliability have to be required.

In addition to international privacy protection should also be ensured by implementing and adapting privacy-enhancing technologies. The report of the Registratiekamer and IPC (Registratiekamer/IPC 1995) concludes that, if privacy technologies are to play a more significant role, it will be necessary to create more public awareness as well as consumer demand for them. If there is a demand, providers will probably try to respond to market forces.

Privacy education is important to raise the awareness of the users, the data subjects, the system designers, the IT professionals and of the management. Most privacy-enhancing technologies themselves are not necessarily an effective mean to technically enforce privacy aspects, unless users or customers have sufficient technical knowledge to apply them. Thus, users and customers need information and education about their rights, about the value of their personal data, about privacy risks and the possibilities of self-protection by the use of privacy-enhancing technologies.

10 Data protection of law offenders

Peter Blume

> Privacy is at the very soul of being human.
>
> (Diffie and Landau 1998: 126)

This chapter concerns the protection of data related to people who have been convicted, have been charged or suspected in connection with a crime. It considers the extent of such protection and how the different conflicting interests should be balanced. In the information society personal data are diffused much more than previously and access to and usage of this information are called for in many different respects. The question of how criminal data should be processed is accordingly difficult, taking into account the necessity of an expedient crime prevention policy. Throughout the chapter, the phrase 'criminal data' covers data concerning people convicted, charged or suspected of criminal offences.

Basic assumptions of data protection

Data protection can be seen as a modern kind of privacy protection. The term informational privacy has been coined[1] and the main purpose is to ensure that personal data are not misused, leading to invasions of privacy. In the information society this kind of privacy is of course particularly important. The object of protection is often not so much the information as such but the knowledge it provides with respect to some aspect of the private life of an individual. This linkage between information and life is important to keep in mind in the following discussion.[2]

A major difficulty concerns the concept of privacy.[3] There is no commonly acknowledged definition of what is private and it is not possible in general to determine which type of information should be viewed as private.[4] It is often the case that privacy is not known until it has been lost. Privacy is an immaterial value which is not normally considered in day-to-day life. In some sense the individual takes it for granted that he has a protected private life. This could seem to establish a rather weak foundation for a legal policy. However, it could also be assumed that privacy is seen as something natural and that there must be strong societal reasons for protecting it. This is the starting point taken in the following discussion. Another difficulty is that individuals perceive different kinds of information as private. It is in many ways a personal viewpoint that determines what is private. When drafting legal rules it is not possible to define private information in a way that corresponds to everybody's notion, but this is in practice not a major obstacle as it is normally possible for the individual to waive his privacy protection. When legal regulation makes it possible for the individual to consent to processing of his personal data, then the protection can be broad as it is possible to limit it. However, in some cases consent should perhaps not be a possibility. There are certain kinds of data which should always be viewed as private. This is the case with respect to so-called 'sensitive' data such as criminal data.

The attitude towards privacy as a moral and legal value differs historically and in different types of societies.[5] In classical Rome the private sphere was not thought highly of as everything of value occurred in the public sphere. Another example is socialist countries where privacy must not interfere with the interests of state and society, and is sometimes not acceptable at all. It is well known that in small indigenous communities it is seen as positive that all information is shared. In contrast the ability to be private and to control your own information is viewed as an important value in Western societies. Privacy is considered a human right, e.g. as outlined in Article 8 of the European Human Rights Convention. The development of the information society has not changed this fundamental attitude and there is little doubt that many citizens consider privacy a necessity.

With this background it must be considered which rights should be entailed by privacy. A traditional starting point is that privacy means a right to be let alone and a right to self-determination with respect to personal information.[6] There are areas of life into which others are allowed only with the consent of the individual, who also has the right to control use of his personal information. A more modern approach has determined four 'states' of privacy which are solitude, intimacy, anonymity and reserve. Rights of this nature are fundamental but they cannot be absolute. Societal reasons make modifications necessary. This is the case in both the private and public sector but within the framework of this chapter it is primarily, but not exclusively, the public sector which is of interest. The running of a modern state with its importance for society cannot be managed if processing of personal data can only take place with the consent of the individual citizen. Even the most rigorous privacy advocate must acknowledge that the individual cannot be solely his own private person. It is only romantics who think that personal data can be absolutely private in all situations. These assumptions do not in any way mean that privacy is rejected. On the contrary they indicate that a privacy-promoting policy regarding modern society must be balanced in order to be realistic.

Modern informational privacy is often founded on certain basic principles, sometimes referred to as fair information practices. They are recognized in many national statutes, etc., including the legal texts discussed in the subsequent sections. These principles concern openness, individual access and correction, collection limitation, use limitation, disclosure limitation and security.

It is well known that strong interests often try to limit privacy and give priority to other societal values. New risks for privacy are constantly emerging. These must be met but this can best be done with a balanced policy. Accordingly, the general idea is that privacy is the primary value when assessing information-handling, but if it in practice is to be ensured that personal information is not misused, then it must be accepted that it can be processed independently of the individual under certain conditions. The legal policy discourse considers what these conditions should be and whether there are types of data that ought not to be processed under any circumstances. It is with this background that this chapter is concerned.

Data subjects who break the law

Informational privacy protects the individual citizen – in legal documents referred to as the data subject. The actual rules and the general principles are drafted in his or her interest. There can be other reasons for such rules but there is no doubt that focus is on the individual. With this reference it must be considered whether all individuals should be viewed under the same standard or whether distinctions should be made. With respect to the general principles this is rarely discussed while actual rules sometimes make distinctions, e.g. with respect to children or the dead.

However, it seems appropriate to consider whether data subjects who have violated the law and committed a criminal offence should have the same privacy protection as other citizens. Does the fact that a person is charged or convicted imply that his privacy is limited? The answer is probably yes and no. From the outset it is generally recognized that human rights such as privacy apply to all people regardless of how they are situated in society. This assumption is enforced by the fact that human rights in particular protect weak citizens. Their primary intention is to protect the citizen against the state. At the general level there is no doubt that criminal data subjects are protected in the same way as everybody else. However, it is evident that when a person commits a crime, this act paves the way for a more limited private sphere. Both during investigation and sentencing, and after punishment, the citizen has actually lost some of his privacy and this must also to some extent be the case. In all data protection laws there are possibilities provided for police and prosecution to process a considerable amount of personal data, often including data which is not directly linked to the actual criminal offence. On the other hand, it should be recognized that this situation does not in principle differ from other social events. If a citizen applies for a social benefit this will also imply that certain forms of personal data must be made known to the state. This does not mean that the data can be freely accessed by everyone or can be processed for other purposes outside the criminal justice sector. It should also from the outset be maintained that these data should be processed in accordance with the general data protection principles.

Accordingly, the discussion in the following sections of the chapter concerns to what extent criminal data can be processed and whether the special circumstances surrounding such data can make it legitimate to make use of them in a more extensive way than is the case with respect to 'normal' data.

Data on criminal offences

In this section the general rules concerning processing of data on criminal offences and the practical problems in this respect are discussed. The text focuses on three levels: national law, the Council of Europe regulation and EU law. The starting point taken is national law, as it is here that the practical problems have mainly emerged. The special problems relating to Schengen and Europol are discussed separately below.

Danish law

In the following discussion Danish law is considered.[7] Denmark has had statutory regulation since 1978 when two Data Protection Acts were passed. Denmark is about to change its laws due to the implementation of the EU Data Protection Directive (see under heading 'The European Union')[8] but the practical issues will still be the same and it is these issues that are of general interest.

First, it must be considered whether criminal data ought to be viewed differently in the private and the public sector. This is the general assumption. As data processing must be sustained by a reasonable purpose, it is from the outset most likely that these data can be processed by public authorities. This is also the position in Danish law where such data can be processed by private corporations, but only in special circumstances.

Public sector

In the public sector, criminal data are viewed as sensitive, implying that they can only be registered when this is necessary for the performance of tasks by a certain authority (Public Data Protection Act, Section 9(2)). There is no doubt that the police, the public prosecution and the courts can process such data. With respect to these authorities it only remains to determine when such processing actually can take place. The attitude to other authorities has, on the other hand, been cautious. The Data Protection Agency (DPA) has generally been reluctant to endorse such authorities having their own files containing criminal data. This creates unwanted security risks, especially with respect to unauthorized disclosure of such data. However, it has not been possible to prevent the collection of such files entirely. The current position is that an authority can process criminal data in so far as there is authority in statute and it is clear that such processing is necessary with respect to supervising tasks, and so on. An example of this is the Ministry for Fishery, which is permitted to have a file of fishermen who have violated rules concerning the amounts of fish that can be landed.[9] Although such processing is legitimate, it is fortunately an exception. With respect to the public sector, the main demand is that criminal data are processed carefully and not disclosed to a greater extent than absolutely necessary. This is best ensured when the data are processed by specialized authorities who can be fairly easily supervised. The risk of uncontrolled disclosure increases when many different authorities are processing the data. However, the necessity of statutory authority means that it always will be a political decision whether such processing should take place regardless of the dangers.

Private sector

The situation is different with respect to the private sector. From the outset it could be argued that it should be forbidden to process criminal data in this sector which does not play a role in the criminal justice system. This is to some extent an unrealistic position. There are certain situations where processing is reasonable which will also be discussed below in connection with the question of access. However, there is no doubt that criminal data ought to be viewed as sensitive and that processing accordingly should only take place when strict conditions are met. This is the position in Denmark (Private Data Protection Act, Section 3(2)) as in most countries.

It is special factual circumstances that can make processing legitimate. In Danish law it is mainly data on shoplifters that have been discussed. Private shopowners have an interest in the registration of these persons and would also like to exchange such data between shops in order to prevent further theft. Viewed in isolation this is a legitimate purpose, but from the outset the DPA was opposed to both registration and disclosure. In several decisions the DPA has maintained that data can only be processed if the incident is reported to the police, and that data can only be stored as long as criminal proceedings are still pending.[10] The reason for acceptance of storage is that witnesses have a duty to refresh their memory (Administration of Justice Act, Section 180). Disclosure of the data for other purposes is not permitted. These decisions illustrate that even though processing takes place in order to protect legitimate interests, it is seen as more important to protect the offender against violations of privacy.

In some situations use of criminal data is forbidden. This is the case with respect to credit reporting. Regardless of whether a certain piece of criminal information is relevant with respect to credit assessment, it is illegal to process it. It is not acceptable that credit reporting agencies process such data, as from a societal point of view they should not be taken into account.

This rule can be seen as representative of an attitude concerning the possible consequences of a criminal conviction. There a long tradition in Denmark with respect to resocialization of people with criminal convictions. The purpose is to prevent new crimes being committed and to make it possible that such persons can play a satisfactory role in society again. They must have a real chance of achieving this goal. Widespread use and disclosure of criminal data can be viewed as counterproductive with respect to such a goal. As will be elaborated below, considerations of this kind are relevant with respect to many of the situations where usage of criminal data is considered. Data protection and criminal law should be viewed together and to the extent that data protection rules can sustain a reasonable crime prevention policy, they should be promoted. Such an assumption is in accordance with the fact that data protection primarily is in the interest of the individual.

Extent of storage

Generally it is important that only correct criminal data are processed. As is the case in other areas, data quality should be ensured. However, there are no special aspects which have to be considered. Much more interesting is the question of for how long such data ought to be stored. This is in many respects a very difficult problem which has to be considered carefully. There are many conflicting interests which have to be taken into account. According to general data protection principles, data should not be stored for longer than they are useful with respect to the purpose of registration. The actual time of storage will differ according to the type of data and the purpose of usage. It is important to notice that the sensitivity of the data does not mean that they can only be stored for a short period. It is well known, for example, that some medical data are kept even after the person has died. However, it is reasonable that particularly sensitive data be deleted as soon as possible. It must be recognized that general data protection considerations do not provide precise answers.

If the discussion is limited to police files, there are two main reasons for storage of criminal data. First, it provides a record of previous convictions which can have importance for future sentencing and, second, it can help the police in the investigation of new crimes. In this last respect the data do not only consist of hard facts but can also provide indications of certain kinds of behaviour, and so on. In Danish law, the Central Criminal Register is divided into one file for each purpose and the rules of deletion are only known with respect to the file on convictions.[11] Here there are set times of deletion which differ, depending on the seriousness of the crime.[12] Most convictions are deleted at some stage. This is important with respect to access to criminal records which is discussed below. The actual periods can of course always be discussed but in this context it is important that dates of deletion actually are fixed. With respect to the investigation file, whose official purpose is to store data of police relevance, the rules are not known and it seems doubtful whether data are deleted at all. It might even be a possibility that deleted convictions are transferred to this file. This is often supposed. This is in principle not an acceptable situation as secluded registration is unwanted. However, it is also reasonable that the file cannot be freely accessible as crime detection would suffer seriously from such a situation. In practice the Data Inspectorate has the power to supervise the file and to control whether data are deleted. The efficiency of this authority has to be trusted.

To these general considerations should be added that the police investigation file has been recently much debated in Denmark. This is due to an incident where information on a drunk-driving offence by a leading politician which took place thirty years ago emerged simultaneously with him being appointed chairman of his party. This of course highlighted the question of when data are deleted from the file as it is difficult to envisage a police purpose for storage of such old data concerning a fairly trivial offence. The incident was of course also due to a breach of security and this aspect will be discussed below. From the debate it emerged that only very minor data are deleted automatically within set time limits, while all other data are deleted only if a new offence makes it necessary to consider the data again. If this is not the case, the data are kept at least until the person becomes 70 years old. It follows from this practice that the database is huge and that no real control of data quality is possible. It also demonstrated a peculiar paradox in that the best way of having data deleted from the file is to commit a new offence. In a decision of 15 May 1998 the DPA severely criticized the situation. A special working group under the Ministry of Justice has considered whether this procedure should be amended and has recommended that exact deletion periods are stated. The current situation is unacceptable, seen from the point of general data protection.

Size

It is not sufficient that there are controlled deletion times; even the mere size of such a database containing sensitive data can constitute a threat to privacy. The database can be used for surveillance and generally creates a certain amount of insecurity in society. It can be seen as an independent goal that databases containing criminal data ought not be too large. It is difficult to determine precisely what this should mean in practice. It is of course not possible to indicate the amount of data which should be in such a database. It must be an aim that the size of the database should be under careful control and that it should be evident that the stored data are relevant and necessary for crime prevention and detection. This aim is mainly dependent on the attitude of the police and the public prosecution. It is desirable that they are aware of the problem and try to restrict the amount of data that are indexed in the database. It ought regularly be considered whether the database is of a satisfactory size.

Security

Security is one of the foundations of data protection. It is essential that only people who are authorized can access the data, and that data are only used for authorized purposes. It is well known that this goal can be very difficult to achieve. There are basically three kinds of security: physical (i.e. securing buildings, etc.), organizational (i.e. rules for personnel) and system-oriented measures. Experience seems to show that, even though all three kinds of security can be breached, it is often the organizational aspects that constitute the weak link.

Current developments in Denmark illustrate this very clearly. The investigation of the above-mentioned case concerning disclosure of information on the drunk-driving offence committed by a leading politician showed that the computer screens at the different police stations are constantly linked up to the criminal register, and that anybody in the computer room at any time can perform searches in the register. For this reason it was not possible to detect who had disclosed the information and at the same time it became clear that many police officers use this possibility to retrieve information on their neighbours, and so on. Seen from the traditional data protection perspective it is rather difficult to understand why such an insecure environment can exist in connection with sensitive data. It is even more interesting to observe that the situation has not been changed immediately. The DPA has criticized the low level of security, but the police have argued that it is necessary to have open screens as data have to be retrieved very quickly. If a password has to be used this would take too much time and thereby reduce the quality of police work. This argument does not seem very convincing and the current situation demonstrates that security is insufficient and that sensitive criminal data in practice are not well protected.

Perhaps this is an isolated Danish problem but I am inclined to doubt it. It is accordingly important in general to emphasize that a primary condition for processing of criminal data is that this takes place in a secure manner. The security requirements with respect to such sensitive data must be high and modifications should not be accepted unless it is absolutely evident that major societal interests favour these. In the Danish example this is not the case. It should be added that this conclusion also applies to the international police systems that are discussed below.

Disclosure and access

Probably the most complex problem concerns disclosure of criminal data. In Danish law – as in all countries with data protection rules – the data subject has a right of access. This right can be modified but it at least applies to data on convictions, etc. ('objective data').[13] This is normally conceived as an essential right as it maintains the individual's ability to control his own data and to ensure that processed data are correct. It is presupposed that the right of access is used voluntarily and for purposes that are in the interest of the data subject. However, it is also presupposed that the right can be used without formalities and in particular that the data subject does not have to explain why data are to be accessed. The authority in possession of the data will accordingly only in rare situations be able to assess whether access is required due to some kind of pressure.

This legal situation, which in general should be supported, leads to problems within the field of criminal data. There is a clear tendency for more and more employers to require the criminal record of job applicants and employees. In the rules on the Central Criminal Register certain public authorities are given the right to request such a record, while this can be obtained in the private sector only with the consent of the data subject or through the right of access. If a person applies for a job and wants to have the job, there is no alternative to giving consent or using the right of access to provide the employer with the desired information. In this way there exists a major risk of criminal data being disclosed on a wide scale.

This is an important legal policy issue which is quite difficult to solve. It would not be advisable to restrict the right of access. This is a fundamental right, emphasizing the right to self-determination with respect to information, which should not be modified in any way. It is accordingly the behaviour of the controllers that must be regulated, preferably in statutory law. In Danish law a parallel can be found with respect to health data. Here a special Act, no. 286 (24 April 1996), prohibits employers from asking job applicants questions concerning health and in other ways to require such data. Only very special job situations are exempted from this rule. It is accordingly unlawful to force somebody to use his right of access for this purpose. Such a model can also be applied with respect to criminal data. Under a special Act employers should be forbidden to require the criminal record of job applicants and employees. This rule should apply in most cases. There are undoubtedly jobs where it is relevant to know whether an applicant has committed certain kinds of crimes.[14] In the statute or perhaps better in a statutory instrument such jobs can be listed as exemptions from the general rule. In these cases it should be emphasized that it is only data on relevant types of crimes that can be requested. The applicant should in all cases be informed that such data are being provided. With such legislation criminal data will be better protected at the same time as actual processing will become more transparent for the data subject.

Until such legislation is passed it is desirable that applications for access to the Central Criminal Register are viewed with caution and if there are indications that a request is not voluntary, then it should be rejected.[15] At the same time employers should be convinced that it is unnecessary to require such information and that this practice should be discontinued.

DNA register

A special problem, well known in many countries, concerns the use of DNA profiles as a method of identification with respect to police investigation. These profiles are the result of an analysis of biological material such as blood, hair and semen. The profile in itself merely provides an identification. It is a more accurate method than fingerprinting, to which it has often been compared. Today there is no central DNA register in Denmark but this has been proposed[16] and will probably become a reality within the next few years. The proposal states that people who have been convicted or charged with serious crimes should be included in the file. The reason for inclusion of charged people, who are acquitted, is that they are statistically 44 per cent more likely than others to commit crimes in the future. However, this is unwarranted, seen from a data protection perspective, as innocent people will be registered. This goes against the principle of proportionality. It has even been suggested that the whole population should be registered[17] but this is not reasonable and luckily very expensive. It is proposed that data first be deleted when a person is 80, or two years after death. The DPA has in March 1999 recommended that the issue of an DNA register is regulated by statute and the

Minister of Justice has indicated that he will follow this advice. A bill was proposed in December 1999.

As indicated, the profile is just a means of identification, and as long as the file is very limited it can be reasonable. More disturbing is the basic biological material that can be used to develop a much more detailed and precise profile of the individual. There are indications that this material is not always deleted and if this is true, a dangerous police surveillance system could emerge. DNA profiles are part of a brave new world that must be watched carefully in order to prevent erosion of privacy.

Conclusion

Although the processing of criminal data in Danish law is not in all respects ideal, especially in practice, it can be concluded that there exists a developed data protection regime and that this forms a good starting point for improved regulation. However, it is also evident that there are still many legal policy battles to be fought before informational privacy is sufficiently protected.

The Council of Europe

The Council of Europe has for many years been the major player in international data protection. In 1981 the Convention for the Protection of Individuals with Regard to Automatic Processing of Personal Data was issued.[18] It came into force in 1985 and has since then been the fundamental text in European data protection.[19] The Convention states the different basic data protection principles which have been mentioned previously. In connection with the Convention several recommendations have been issued by the Committee of Ministers. These are not binding like the terms of the Convention but have none the less a major influence on the practices of the Convention states. They provide a sectoral regulation which is more specific than the Convention.

Police data recommendation

This is also the case with respect to Recommendation R(87)15, regulating the use of personal data in the police sector. This is in many ways the most important international regulation of processed criminal data and contains several basic principles and rules. First of all, in Section 1 it is stated that use of data by the police must be supervised by an independent authority outside the police. It is well known that data protection rules are often drafted broadly and can be interpreted in many ways. It is their use in practice which is decisive for the level of protection. An independent authority is a basic precondition for satisfactory protection.[20] In practice it is important that this authority is given the means to enable it to carry out its functions efficiently. In particular in this area the police are often a closed community which can be very difficult to supervise. The data protection authority must therefore be very aware of the special features of the authorities that act as controllers of data.

In Section 2.1 the reasons for collection of police data are regulated. It is stated that collection must be 'necessary for the prevention of a real danger or the suppression of a specific criminal offence'. Exemptions are allowed in statutory law. The basic rule is clear: there must be a relevant police cause that makes it legitimate to store personal data. Whether this is the case will depend on criminal law in the specific country, and the principle does not in itself limit the extent of data being collected. However, it connects collection closely to statutory law and provides a good basis for supervision by the independent authority. The data protection rules cannot in themselves determine whether a specific criminal law is good or acceptable but they can make a modest contribution to such an assessment. If a certain action is made a criminal offence with the consequence that several kinds of personal data have to be processed, this can constitute a valid argument against such a law. It is in general important that the data protection implications of proposed new legislation are made clear and taken into consideration in the legislative process.

It is a characteristic feature of police work that data sometimes are collected without the knowledge of the data subject. This must be accepted as necessary, but should of course only take place in situations when this is clearly indicated. In Section 2.2, it is stated that the data subject should be informed that data have been collected and stored 'as soon as the object of the police activities is no longer likely to be prejudiced'. Somewhat disturbingly, this does not apply if the data are deleted in which case the data subject should also be informed. It is extremely important that hidden data processing does not occur and when this is societally necessary it should be as limited as possible. It is an important task of the supervisory authority to ensure that this practice is not applied more than absolutely necessary.

Personal data can concern facts or they can be based on assumptions and so forth. With respect to data quality this is an important distinction, as it is much easier to ensure the correctness of factual data. This problem is recognized in Section 3.2, where it is stated that stored data should be distinguished with respect to accuracy or reliability and especially that 'data based on facts should be distinguished from data based on opinions or personal assessments'. In police work it is likely that there will be many people assessing data, and that it often will be uncertain whether such data are correct. This emphasizes the importance of constant scrutiny of police databases in order to ensure that such data are not kept longer than necessary and are rectified in situations where it becomes evident that they are not correct. It must be ensured that the police develop adequate routines in this respect. In this connection Section 7.1 should be mentioned. It states the basic principle that data should not be kept longer than necessary for the police purposes for which they were stored. It is an unwanted situation that police databases contain data just because they might be relevant in some future situation which is not related to the original purpose. Such storage can be tempting, but it should be maintained that it is not acceptable and that excessive police databases in themselves can be viewed as a threat to civil liberties. Sufficient discipline in this respect must be required.

A fundamental issue is how stored police data are used. In particular it is interesting to what degree such data are communicated. In Section 5 detailed rules concerning communication within the police sector, to other public bodies, to private parties and internationally are stated. These elaborate rules will not be described here, where it is sufficient to observe that it is reasonable to give this aspect high priority in data protection policy. There must always be a reasonable cause for communication and this should in any case only take place on a limited scale. It is obvious that there are major risks of infringements of privacy if disclosure of criminal data is not carefully controlled.

Conclusion

In general the Recommendation is an important document. In a balanced way it details many important principles relating to the use of police data. Although some of the rules, in particular the modifications, are open to discussion, the Recommendation in general provides sufficient protection of the data subject. It is interesting to observe that the Recommendation in some sense forms the basis for the international police systems discussed below. Both Schengen and Europol are based on the assumption that the participating states have developed their national law in accordance with the Recommendation. It is accordingly soft law turned into hard law.

The European Union

Directive 95/46 EC on the protection of individuals with regard to the processing of personal data and on the free movement of such data is now the primary data protection instrument in Europe.[21] The Directive should have been adopted as national law by 24 October 1998 and this deadline was met in the UK, Italy, Spain and Sweden. All member states are expected to have implemented the Directive during 2000. Although the Directive provides some freedom for the member states, the vast amount of rules and principles will probably be the same in all states.

The Directive does not cover all areas of law as it of course only applies to regulatory areas that are covered by EU law. Furthermore Article 3(2) exempts data processing relating to 'the activities of the State in areas of criminal law'. The member states are here only bound by the Council of Europe convention and they can freely choose whether they will apply the provisions of the Directive or have independent rules. It is likely that there will be differences, but it would be best if the Directive is applied. This is, for example, the case in Denmark, where only a few exemptions will be made.[22] Seen from the perspective of the data subject, and often also of the controller, it is best that the same rules apply to all processing of personal data as this makes it easier to understand the legal position. Regardless of how this question is solved, the Directive contains many rules of interest.

First of all it must be considered how criminal data are viewed. The Directive makes the traditional distinction between ordinary and sensitive data. The latter are regulated in Article 8, where they are listed in Subsection 1. This list is surprising because it omits criminal data.

This is not explained in the recitals and it is difficult to understand the reasons for this omission. As the list cannot be extended, the Directive in principle weakens the protection of such data. However, in Article 8(5) special rules on criminal data are stated. According to this rule, criminal data may only be processed under the control of an official authority or in accordance with national law, which must contain 'suitable specific safeguards'. A complete register of criminal data must only be kept by a public authority. This is a rather complex regulation which makes it fairly uncertain how national law will be drafted. The forthcoming Danish Act can here be used as an example. According to this, criminal data can be processed in the public sector in accordance with the rules that apply to ordinary data. In the private sector criminal data may be processed when this is necessary for the controller, and the interest of the data subject cannot be considered as more important. These rules should mean that current Danish law is upheld.[23] It is unlikely that the rules in the member states will be similar and it is unfortunate that the Directive has not taken a more firm position with respect to these data which clearly are sensitive. This is also disturbing because the rules of the Directive will influence the understanding of the Schengen Convention.

The Directive contains the traditional data protection principles and in doing so these are emphasized at the international level. In particular Article 6(1b) is important as it states the purpose specification principle. Collected data may not be processed for other purposes than those that supported the collection. This is a principle that promotes transparency which is a major goal of the Directive. Data subjects must be able to know how and why their data are being processed, which is emphasized by a right of information outlined in Articles 10 and 11. With respect to processed criminal data, this is of course very important as uncertainty with respect to the actual data processing is one of the primary problems within this area. However, in Article 13 it is made possible for member states to make exemptions from these rules, for example with respect to 'the prevention, investigation, detection and prosecution of criminal offences'. It is likely that this possibility will be used by many states although this can only be done when it is a necessary measure to safeguard this kind of data processing. In legal policy it should be an aim that the informational rights are restricted as little as possible. Also criminal data should be transparent and the necessity for secrecy cannot be overestimated.

Another interesting right is found in Article 15, concerning automated individual decisions. According to this rule the data subject has a right not to be subjected to decisions 'based solely on automated processing of data intended to evaluate certain personal aspects' relating, for example, to 'reliability'. This rule can be relevant in the workplace, where modern decision-making systems can be used to evaluate employees and job applicants and where it is likely that the occurrence of criminal data will be programmed to have negative consequences. It is difficult to determine the importance of this rule but in any case it seems important to be aware of this new right.

Conclusion

In general the Directive aims at providing a high level of protection for citizens. Its purpose is to demonstrate that the European Union cares about human rights. This aim should be employed in concrete legal policy. The protection of people who violate the law has clearly not been a priority for the Community but the general aims can be utilized to this end. It should be an intrinsic goal to demonstrate that only if these citizens are protected, will comprehensive and laudable data protection measures have been instituted. Even though the EU does not in general have competence within criminal law, a policy along these lines might be advantageous. In any case there is little doubt that decisions on data protection made by the Union will influence the legal regulation in all fields. Efforts to influence the policies and attitudes of the EU are accordingly extremely important.

International police cooperation

The two major societal tendencies are currently internationalization and the development of the information society. Both tendencies have many implications for the police and thereby also for the processing of criminal data. The aims of a more unified Europe and the recognition that crime increasingly is an international phenomenon have led to the development of new legal structures that supplement the traditional international police organization, Interpol, which was founded back in 1923.[24] These new structures will become even more important with respect to the legal protection of criminal data. They are accordingly considered in this section.

The Schengen Convention

The Schengen Convention of 1990 on the gradual abolition of checks at common borders has been ratified by all EU member states with the exception of the UK and Ireland.[25] Although it is in principle an international treaty, the Amsterdam Treaty makes it a more integrated part of ordinary EU law. The Convention provides authority for the processing of personal data at the same time as it instigates a huge information system, SIS, located in Strasburg. From the outset it is interesting to note that it is presupposed that the ratifying states have implemented the Council of Europe Police Data Recommendation and Section 134 states that if the EU institutes more data protection rules these will substitute for the rules of the Convention. As will be elaborated below, from the outset the rules of the Convention are satisfactory in many ways and there is no doubt that data protection aspects have been considered carefully in connection with the drafting of the Convention.

General observations

However, there are certain general aspects that call for caution with respect to a legal instrument of this nature. The following remarks also apply to the Europol Convention. The Convention is based on cooperation between public authorities in the different countries. These authorities are given the same powers and restrictions. The Convention presupposes – as do other international treaties – that the rules are used in the same way. It is doubtful whether this actually will be the case. The legal culture and the connected police culture are very divergent and it is a clear risk that personal data will be used and understood differently. It should also be observed that the understanding of the relationship between citizen and police (state), of the concept of crime and also the definition of police may differ quite substantially. In many ways internationalization of criminal data in itself poses a risk for the data subject. It becomes uncertain how data are processed and data usage will almost certainly not be transparent. These observations cannot support the conclusion that international exchange of data between police forces, etc. should not take place. This would not be realistic and would also to some extent be societally unfortunate. The conclusion is rather that such exchanges should be viewed with a great deal of caution, and especially that the regulating legal texts cannot in themselves ensure that sufficient protection is provided in practice. The assessment of the Convention should take this into account. Furthermore, the fairly uncertain practical circumstances make it necessary that the legal rules are especially strict and unambiguous. The legal draftsmen have a very difficult task. With this background selected rules from the Convention will be discussed in the following.

SIS

In Articles 95–9 it is stated who can be registered in SIS. Examples are:

1   persons wanted for arrest for extradition purposes – data can include the nature and legal classification of the offence, the circumstances in which it was committed and its consequences;
2   data on refused aliens;
3   data on witnesses, persons summoned in connection with criminal proceedings in order to account for prosecuted acts or who are summoned to serve a custodial sentence;
4   data to be used for the purposes of discreet surveillance (Article 99(4)).[26]

As it appears, SIS contains many different kinds of criminal data and has already become a huge database. New figures (1997) show that 782,477 persons are registered. Most of these are categorized as refused aliens. Only 7,123 are wanted criminals. However, the system, slowly started in 1988, is still fairly new and there is little doubt that its growth will be significant in the coming years.

For this reason it is extremely important how these sensitive data are protected and how misuse is prevented. There are several rules in the Convention for this purpose. In Article 101 it is stated that only certain authorities may use the data. In Subsection 3 it is indicated that these 'users may only search data which are necessary for the performance of their tasks'. This is supported by the provisions in Article 102. It is furthermore emphasized in Articles 126(3), 127 and 129 that authorities who receive searched data may only use these for legitimate purposes. These rules take into account the fact that probably all the processed data are sensitive and that they accordingly should only be processed for restricted and clearly defined purposes. The issue is, of course, whether or not this is also the case in practice.

SIS consists of a central database within French jurisdiction and national databases containing the data that has been reported. More than 30,000 computers are linked to SIS. In Article 104 it is emphasized that national law applies to these databases and it is accordingly the national authorities that have the primary responsibility for the accuracy and reliability of the data. According to Article 114 there must be a national supervisory authority and there is also according to Article 115 a joint supervisory authority[27] that is responsible for controlling the central database. As for searches in SIS, there must be appointed a special national authority (Article 108);[28] this is normally a special police unit. Although this is not evident in the Convention, these units also use so-called working files, the SIRENE system, which seem to contain more data than SIS. The rules on this part of the Schengen Convention have not been made public, which is unfortunate. However, they have been leaked, and demonstrate major divergences from the Convention. First of all, supplementary data connected to Articles 94, 95, 97, 98, 99 and 100 can be stored and communicated. It is in particular interesting that data can be transferred directly between the national units which accordingly become the main link in the actual police cooperation. SIS is the primary information system, but it is not the only one. As already indicated there are many fears about Schengen, and it is quite unfortunate that it is supplemented with a secret system. It should be added that it is difficult to understand why it is necessary to keep the SIRENE system a secret.

Returning to the Convention, it can be observed that several rules emphasize the importance of ensuring the accuracy of processed data. According to Article 105, it is the reporting state that has the responsibility of ensuring data quality, and according to Article 106 as a rule only this state has the power to make changes in the data. This is evidently important as it could easily have led to chaos if this were possible for all participating states. These rules are supplemented by provisions on deletion stated in Articles 112 and 113. It should furthermore be noted that the data subject has a right of correction (Article 110). This can be viewed in connection with the right of access which, as stated in Article 109, can be exercised in accordance with national law. However, in Subsection 2 it is indicated that access is limited and must not undermine the performance of the relevant tasks. It seems likely that this reservation combined with the exemptions to the right of access that can be found in national law will mean that the main rule in practice will be that access is refused. The right of access will not make SIS an open and transparent system.

A main and basic demand is that the system is secure. In Article 118 it is stated that it is a national responsibility to ensure that unauthorized access to and use of the system do not occur. In this connection it is interesting that Article 103 prescribes that on average every tenth transmission of data is recorded in order to check their admissibility. There is no doubt that security is essential and unfortunately there have already been incidents in connection with the central system where sensitive data have been disclosed in a manner that demonstrates that the security measures are not acceptable.[29] This is of course quite frightening. It was also demonstrated that the joint supervisory authority at that time had not been given sufficient opportunities to carry out its tasks.

Conclusion

Taken at face value, the rules of the Schengen Convention appear acceptable, providing adequate protection of the criminal data that are being processed. However, there are indications that the reality differs from the fine rules and in any case it is necessary to scrutinize the system very carefully in the future. The secret SIRENE system does not inspire confidence. Regardless of the precautions stated in the Convention, the vast information system constitutes a risk to the legal protection of criminal data subjects.

The Europol Convention

A similar observation is valid with respect to the Europol Convention of 26 July 1995 that came into force 1 October 1998. This is in many ways a much more complex regulation, at the same time as it more or less solely concerns criminal data. The purpose and the kind of criminal activities that can be processed are outlined in Article 2. These cover a broad spectrum including unlawful drug trafficking, illegal immigrant smuggling, trade in human beings and 'other forms of international crime where there are factual indications that an organized criminal structure is involved' including at least two member states. Illegal money-laundering is also included and, finally, so are terrorist activities, which as a political crime often can be difficult to define precisely. It is expected that the scope of criminal activities that can be investigated through the Europol system will be increased in the future.

To perform its tasks a central database has been established in The Hague. In each country a unit is set up with the responsibility of reporting data to the system, and liaison officers from these units are placed at Europol (Articles 4 and 5). At the same time national and joint supervisory authorities are established to ensure sufficient data protection (Articles 23 and 24). In Article 15 it is stated that the member states have the legal responsibility with respect to data protection concerning the data they have communicated, while Europol is responsible in other situations.

The main concern is of course connected with what data can be placed in the system. This is indicated in Article 8 which is in particular interesting as it allows storage of assessive data. People who are suspected of having committed or taken part in a criminal offence, and people for whom there are 'serious grounds' to believe they will commit a crime, can be registered. Many data can be processed in connection with these people, including previously committed and *alleged* crimes, together with previous convictions if these are relevant with respect to Article 2. In Article 9 it is stated that only the national units and other authorized authorities can process the data, but this is of course not in itself a guarantee of their accuracy.

Even more interesting is the fact that there are established work files for the purpose of analysis combined with an index system. The rules are stated in Articles 10 and 11. In Article 10(1) it is indicated who can be registered. They include people who might testify in investigations, victims and 'persons who can provide information on the criminal offences under consideration'. The last category has in Denmark provoked public debate, as it seems to include journalists etc., and could be used to restrict freedom of information. Regardless of how this is viewed, it seems clear that the number of people that can be covered by the working files can become very large.

Data can be retrieved by the national units and Europol according to Article 17, but what is more interesting is that, according to Article 18, data can also be disclosed to third countries.[30] Europol is not a closed system merely for the benefit of the member states, but stored data can be diffused anywhere. This makes it particularly necessary to control the system, as wrongful disclosure can have a very damaging effect on the data subject. Rules on correction and deletion are found in Articles 20, 21 and 22. They are connected to the right of access stated in Article 19; a right which is fairly limited. It is in practice the supervisory authorities that must ensure that the system does not infringe human rights. It must be recognized that this is a demanding task and it seems doubtful whether it can be performed satisfactorily. Among other things, security must be supervised. Article 25 states that Europol must ensure a high level of data security and in this connection Article 16, that prescribes logging of transactions, should be observed.

Conclusion

In general there is little doubt that Europol should be viewed with caution. It demonstrates the potential risks of international communication of criminal data. These risks are being increased by the use of modern information technology. Europol has to some degree a legitimate purpose, as some crimes are international and must be combated, but it is essential that these efforts do not impose major risks of infringement of human rights. It should be added that it is likely that at the end of the day Europol, Schengen and other European information systems such as Eurodac (asylum seekers) will be merged into one comprehensive system. If this becomes a reality, the European citizen will be substantially surveyed and another era of innocence will have ended.

Concluding remarks

The basic starting point has been that law offenders – using the term in a broad sense – have human rights and that these must be protected. This is a position that probably nobody will argue against, but the devil is hidden in all the implications. In the area discussed in this chapter protection means that data concerning a criminal person cannot be used freely but only after serious consideration about to what extent privacy and personal integrity can make such data processing acceptable.

From the outset the different legal rules are in accordance with (or at least pay lip service to) this position, but they have to be constantly scrutinized in order to ensure that they are used in accordance with their stated intentions. It is furthermore important to ensure that modern information technology is not utilized blindly in efforts to fight crime, but that these efforts are proportional to the actions of the affected persons. The basic message is that data protection should be taken seriously. It should be accepted that these rules in some sense restrict use of modern technology and also can be envisaged as a restriction on the efficiency of crime detection and prevention.

It is a recognized assumption that people who are suspected of, charged with and convicted for a crime have a right to legal protection. The rules of criminal procedure are the primary example of this line of thought. There is no reason why data protection rules should be viewed in another way. It should also be taken into account that such rules in particular have the purpose of protecting weak citizens. It is those citizens who do not have the resources to protect their own rights that must be defended by the legal regime.

As the chapter has demonstrated, there are many limitations on the privacy of criminals and several problematic ways of processing criminal data. This is the case both nationally and internationally, with the emergence of a major EU surveillance system. At the beginning of the new millennium, there are a multitude of challenges. Developments are rapid and complex. To finish optimistically, if the fundamental principles are constantly kept in mind, it will still be possible to uphold and sustain an acceptable protection of criminal data in the future.

Notes

1 See Michael (1994: 3) and Rodota (1992: 261–72).
2 Data and information are abstract concepts and it is accordingly important to take into account that they refer to aspects of real life.
3 See Blume (1997).
4 'Of all the human rights in the international catalogue, privacy is perhaps the most difficult to circumscribe and define' (Michael 1994: 1).
5 In an American context see Regan (1995: 24–41).
6 See Brandeis and Warren (1890–91).
7 Danish data protection law is only described in any detail in Danish. The leading commentary is Blume (1996). The two acts in English are printed in Madsen (1992: 272–291). As the main literature is in Danish and

accordingly is not readable for English-speakers only few notes will be used in the following.

8 The Danish transposition is based on Betænkning (White Paper) no. 1345/1997 and Bill no. 44 (8 October 1999). Along with several other member states Denmark had not implemented the Directive before it came into force on 24 October 1998.

9 See *DPA Annual Report* 1990: 42–46. In the 1993 report (p. 52) the postal office is not permitted to register persons who have used bounced cheques.

10 Most recent decisions are found in *DPA Annual Report* (1992: 86) and (1993: 83–5).

11 The rules are stated in Statutory Instrument 13 (December 1991). It is not acceptable that the rules on the investigation file are secret; it is difficult to understand why this should be necessary for the police.

12 In Section 15 of the Statutory Instrument the time limit is set to ten years, but starting at various times, e.g. release from prison.

13 Section 32 of the Statutory Instrument of the Central Criminal Register provides this right to all data subjects. If under the age of 18 access presupposes consent from the custodian.

14 Examples can be security jobs and employment in child-care institutions.

15 It must be accepted that this will sometimes not be in the interest of the data subject, who might lose a job.

16 See *Rapport om etablering af et DNA register* (Report on the establishment of a DNA register) (1996). On the legal issues in general, see Council of Europe Recommendation R(92)1 on the use of analysis of DNA within the framework of the criminal justice system – Denmark has not adopted this Recommendation.

17 This idea has been promoted by the chairman of the legal committee in Parliament.

18 The Convention is printed in Madsen (1992: 962–973). It is described by Michael (1994: 35–40).

19 Denmark ratified the Convention in 1990.

20 This is emphasized in Flaherty (1989: 11–16, 381–385).

21 On the Directive in general, see Bainbridge (1996).

22 Exemptions will mainly concern rights to information and access (Articles 10–12) where rules in the Administration of Justice Act will apply.

23 The practice described above (under the heading 'Danish law') is upheld in the preparatory remarks to the Bill.

24 On Interpol and its Criminal Information System (CIS), located in Lyon, see Benyon *et al.* (1993: 121–133, 222–228). It is observed that the new European systems are given priority because Interpol is a worldwide organization which in 1993 had 174 member countries.

25 A general analysis of the Schengen Convention is given in Joubert and Bevers (1996).

26 In connection with these rules it is interesting to notice that the secret services play an active role in the exchange of data. This is clear in the SIRENE system (described above) while it is not evident in the text of the Convention.

27 *L'Autorité de contrôle commune* consists of two members from each state. The authority is fairly weak with no powers of sanction.

28 It is likely that Europol will gain access to SIS in the future.
29 Sensitive documents were found on a Belgian train station (Ghent) and in the home of an employee in 1997.
30 It is currently being considered how data from non-EU sources can be inserted in the system. This is reported in *Statewatch* 8 (2): 24–25 – this journal is a main source of information concerning both Schengen and Europol.

Part III

Information warfare, critical national infrastructure and security

Themes and issues identified

This part addresses some of the most important and enveloping issues of cybercrime, those of politics, national security and ICTs. In doing so, these essays examine how ICTs are fundamentally transforming the landscape of political expression and national security. As the twenty-first century begins, the role of information and ICTs in governmental and political infrastructures has provided an opportunity for a new category of cybercrime, that of extreme forms of political expression and information warfare.

While information and disinformation have always been a part of political strategy, statecraft and military action, the emergence of ICTs as central to the state's functioning has produced both increased capacities as well as new vulnerabilities. In the case of cyberwarfare, the reliance on command, control, communication and intelligence has provided the ability to orchestrate and coordinate military action with a level of precision previously unknown. ICTs have played a significant role in surveillance, reconnaissance and intelligence gathering and the amount of sensitive information and the need to protect government and military secrets are increasing in proportion to the technological advancements that make such information gathering possible.

The incorporation of ICTs into military strategy and planning has made ICTs a target for the most recent kind of cybercrime, information warfare. Information warfare targets ICTs and information infrastructures in an effort to disable or interfere with communications, to steal information, or to disable the technology itself. These essays explore the implications of information warfare, stressing the relationship of information and ICTs to national security and information infrastructures. Throughout, these essays provide a critical assessment of the role that ICTs play in national security as well as the vulnerabilities that new technologies present for new forms of warfare, sabotage, espionage and information gathering.

A second, related theme explored in this part is the use of ICTs by extremist groups. Like many of the themes explored throughout this volume, the use of ICTs for political expression creates new issues, particularly in terms of balance. Extreme forms of political expression, such as hate speech on the World Wide Web, force us to examine issues of balance in terms of freedom of expression and responsibility. ICTs provide the means to rapidly disseminate large amounts of information inexpensively, anonymously and without consequence. Information which may be otherwise controlled in terms of access, restricted, or deemed indecent or illegal is freely distributed in electronic forums, such as the World Wide Web, e-mail, bulletin boards and electronic news groups. The ease with which information traverses regional and national boundaries also presents problems for political expression. What may be considered harmful or illegal in one state, country or region, may be immune from restriction or prosecution if it originates from an area without such restrictions. Further complicating the problem is the power of ICTs to provide networks of communication and organization for political extremists, allowing the groups to organize and build their movements.

Like many of the questions raised by ICTs, extreme political expression forces us to balance the right to individual political expression with community standards and issues of hate speech, violence and the harmful effects of some forms of speech.

As these essays demonstrate, ICTs are forcing us to rethink issues of national security, public and political expression, and the ability to balance issues of access to information with the need for the state to protect its citizenry. Inherent in these assessments is an understanding that ICTs are not merely changing the rate at which information travels or the manner in which it is disseminated, but that ICTs are fundamentally changing the role and function of information in terms of our political economy.

11 Information warfare and sub-state actors

An organizational approach

Andrew Rathmell

Introduction

Although the Gulf War was subsequently labelled the first information war, at the time few had heard of the term information warfare (IW). With remarkable speed thereafter, however, the term became a central concept in American strategic thought. By the mid-1990s, the American armed forces were investing billions of dollars in acquiring IW capabilities and in developing doctrine. Meanwhile, thanks to the efforts of notorious hackers and popularization of the topic by IW 'gurus,' the entertainment industry and the media, the concept has entered the public consciousness.[1] In the USA, since 1996 the issue has been addressed at the highest levels and in the spring of 1998 President Clinton himself devoted a major speech to the problem (Clinton 1998). In Europe and other parts of the post-industrial world, governments are also beginning to pay serious attention to the topic.

The rapid adoption of the concept of IW has inevitably meant that there is still uncertainty over the exact meaning of the concept. In particular, there is considerable confusion over how all-encompassing to make the term. Very broad definitions count IW as being synonymous with conflict in the 'information age', an approach which expands the scope of the term beyond all utility. A more moderate approach is to argue that IW is about managing the perceptions of one's opponents and is therefore a strategy that embraces many policy instruments, from armed force through cyber-attack to diplomacy and propaganda. A narrower approach still is to focus on the vulnerabilities of digital information infrastructures and to posit that IW is about efforts to disrupt or exploit these infrastructures (Kuehl 1997).

This latter approach may, at the tactical level, consist merely of Command and Control Warfare (C2W) while at the strategic level it may encompass attacks on the entirety of the national information infrastructure (NII). It is this approach on which Western governments are beginning to focus their efforts, both defensive and offensive. The argument is that, as traditional critical national infrastructures, such as power generation and transport, merge with critical information infrastructures, such as telecommunications and remote control systems, then national governmental, military and economic activities become much more vulnerable to disruption of these infrastructures. These control networks may be disrupted by cyber-attacks but just as important is their vulnerability to physical or psychological attacks. Whereas it took the US Air Force weeks of sustained bombardment to shut down the Iraqi national power, communications and logistics infrastructure in the spring of 1991, similar results could, theoretically, be achieved with much more limited application of cyber and physical attacks today.

The reasons for the rise to prominence of IW in the mid-1990s are a fascinating study in themselves. In all countries it has been defence ministries or departments who have led the way. Following the US lead, they have become ever more aware of the ways in which they can exploit the vulnerabilities of digital infrastructures to decapitate and paralyse their opponents. At the same time, it has dawned on them that they are, if anything, even more vulnerable than their potential opponents. The US armed forces have moved most rapidly to embrace a digital battlespace and so are acutely aware of how vulnerable their smaller and more dispersed armed forces are to information attacks. Moreover, since they have come to rely heavily on civilian telecommunications and logistics systems, they have pushed for initiatives to protect these infrastructures. Although no other nation's armed forces are as connected and digitized as the Americans', most recognize that they have to follow the American lead in an era of revolutionary military change. They therefore also need to place greater emphasis on information assurance at national levels (Molander *et al.* 1996).

The upshot of this concern has been embryonic efforts, again led by the USA, to put in place structures and systems to provide national information assurance. In May 1998, President Clinton issued Presidential Decision Directives 62 and 63 which established the office of a Coordinator for Counterterrorism and Infrastructure Protection, working to the National Security Council (White House 1998b). The Presidential Commission on Critical Infrastructure Protection (PCCIP) was transformed into a Critical Infrastructure Assurance Office (CIAO) and the FBI's National Infrastructure Protection Center (NIPC) was put onto a formal footing. The PDDs followed from the PCCIP's study that had pointed out that the US NII was extremely vulnerable to IW attack. The PCCIP had recommended a number of measures to improve information assurance and urged immediate action (PCCIP 1997). PDD 63 mandated this rapid action and ordered government departments to formulate defensive plans. It also tasked government departments with coordinating defensive measures in the private sector.

The US initiatives are being followed closely in allied countries. Sweden, Norway, Finland and Switzerland have conducted studies along similar lines to the PCCIP and are formulating their defensive plans (FOA 1997; Ahvenainen 1998). Germany, France and the UK are likewise considering how to adopt their existing organizations and procedures to deal with the threat (Emmett *et al.* 1997; Campbell 1998). Further afield, Israel and Singapore, not to mention Canada and Australia, are investing in studies of defensive measures and approaches. Russia and China, which are often seen by America and its allies as more of a potential threat than as potential partners, are going their own way but undeniably see this as a serious threat. They however tend to regard the US as their main potential IW threat (Pillsbury 1997; Fitzgerald 1997).

The frantic defensive activity by governments on this issue however tends to founder on an underlying methodological problem. Quite simply, they do not really know the extent of the threat (Evers 1997). Due to the poor reporting systems and technologies they have in place, they have very little idea of what is actually going on in their own information infrastructures. They have even less idea what is going on in the private sector's information infrastructures (Swinburne 1998). There is therefore an inadequate baseline against which to determine if anomalous or malicious behaviour is taking place. Furthermore, they are finding it very hard to determine from whence the threat may come or how serious this threat may be.

Of course, there are efforts to assess the magnitude of the threat. In the US, the Defence Intelligence Agency (DIA) has made public an assessment of the seriousness and likelihood of IW attacks from a variety of groups (Office of the Undersecretary of Defense 1996: A-12). In the UK, the Defence Evaluation and Research Agency (DERA) has made public a similar analysis (DERA 1998). These studies assess the capabilities of potentially hostile states and groups. They conclude that the threat of strategic IW attack is low for now but is likely to increase in coming years.

However, relying on methodological approaches developed in the Cold War, when intelligence services focused on the armed forces of the Soviet Union, is inadequate when dealing with this problem. First, IW is a far more complex threat to quantify, since it involves many more fluid components than a traditional military threat. Second, the threat from sub-state groups, sometimes labelled empowered small agents (ESA), is in many respects more serious than that posed by states (Emmett *et al.* 1997: 25). This notion has been emphasized by the US presidential initiatives that have framed defensive IW as mainly a counter-terrorism issue.

In light of the inadequacy of existing methods for assessing the IW threat, especially from sub-state groups, researchers are beginning to turn their attention to more sophisticated approaches that may provide better models of a more complex reality and provide more holistic sets of indicators for governments concerned with predictive intelligence.

The ability to predict the likelihood or seriousness of an IW threat is not just of importance to national security agencies seeking to allocate intelligence resources or install protective measures. Given the porousness of the actual and conceptual boundary between IW and cybercrime, threat assessment is just as important for police and criminal intelligence agencies to enable them to prioritize resources and to plan for emerging criminal threats. Similarly, for the private sector, which after all owns and operates most of the information infrastructures of concern, there is a pressing need to develop more informed risk assessment mechanisms. However sophisticated the risk assessment procedure adopted by a corporation, without accurate predictive input from a systematic threat assessment, the output is of limited worth.

Capabilities and organization

Existing methods of assessing the threat from a particular group tend to focus on capabilities. Defence and national security intelligence threat assessments have tended to quantify capabilities by reference to hard factors such as size of armed forces, numbers and quality of equipment and economic strength. Sub-state groups, such as terrorist organizations, have likewise been assessed in terms of numbers of personnel, quantities of weaponry, support networks and logistical networks and targeting doctrine.

Capabilities assessment clearly has a central place in IW threat assessment. Some existing approaches that have been made public have provided quite sophisticated capabilities assessment. An excellent model is that produced by Canadian government researchers Norbert Gass and Tiit Romet (Gass and Romet 1998). Gass and Romet provide a carefully selected and weighted list of ICT capabilities that covers hardware, software and wetware – the human factor.

However, these methods do not go far enough. The focus on capabilities, even though it may incorporate predictive indicators of change, is essentially a steady state perspective. All the method does is to indicate what a group's capabilities are now and what they could be if there was change in certain elements. While this approach may make for the sort of presentational clarity preferred by consumers of intelligence, it ignores one of the key lessons of the information revolution. The essence of the ongoing information revolution is change and fluidity. The increasing interest in chaos and complexity theories to help explain international political developments reinforces this point (Alberts and Czerwinski 1997; Czerwinski 1998). The information revolution, combined with the ongoing international political revolution, means that we are operating in a fluid environment in which static, linear methods of predicting threat are, by themselves, inadequate (Freedman 1998).

In practical terms, the problem for predictive methods is to find ways of coping with rapid and non-linear change. One approach is to focus on organizational factors. This indeed is one of the lessons to be drawn from the literature on the information revolution. Commentaries on the impact of this revolution in the business world or the military world, the so-called Revolution in Military Affairs (RMA), stress that the key element in implementing this revolution is not technological but rather organizational. It is commonly, and convincingly, argued that it is not the entry into service of new technologies or skilled personnel that transforms an armed force. Rather, it is the organizational and doctrinal innovations that incorporate this hardware, software and personnel into new patterns that lead to truly revolutionary change (Blank 1997). A commonly cited example is the change in the *Wehrmacht* before the Second World War. New systems such as tanks, radios and aircraft by themselves made little difference. Indeed, these were available to all armed forces. Rather, it was the willingness of the Germans to innovate and the invention of new organizational structures and doctrines that led to the *Blitzkrieg* approach that swept aside Germany's opponents in 1939 and 1940 (Arquilla and Ronfeldt 1997b).

A focus on the organizational approach is also encouraged by the theoretical literature on the role of sub-state groups in future conflict. A theme of this literature, which has been picked up by governments with their focus on cyber-terrorism and ESAs, is that sub-state groups will be better placed to exploit ICTs since they already have networked rather than hierarchical organizations. The argument, familiar to the commercial world which has emphasized 'delayering', 'networked organizations' and similar concepts for several years, is that network forms of organization or, even better, 'organizational networks' will be better able to leverage ICTs in a conflict situation (Ronfeldt 1996: 35).

Culture and structure

A consideration of organizational culture and of organizational structure therefore seems logical in constructing methodologies designed to analyse threats in a dynamic environment. The former focuses the attention of the analyst on the propensity of a particular organization for change and innovation. The main interest is to determine the likelihood that the group may adopt new technological or doctrinal solutions that may result in enhanced IW-fighting abilities. The latter, organizational structure, encourages the analyst to focus on the internal dynamics of an organization and to identify those factors in its organizational make-up that may help or hinder exploitation of ICT and of IW techniques.

In adopting an organizational approach, the model builder can draw on a rich literature on organizational culture and organizational structure, as applied both to military organizations and more broadly to commercial organizations and indeed to societies in the round. Although the organizational literature on sub-state groups is limited there are encouraging beginnings. For instance, criminologists have paid attention to the organizational structures of organized criminal groups and to inner city gangs. Meanwhile, considerable attention has been paid to the dynamics of networks of computer hackers (Sterling 1992; Taylor 1997).

Culture

In applying concepts of organizational culture to this problem, one can draw on a particular interest of the literature – military innovation. The adoption of IW is a form of military innovation, whether it is adopted by sub-state groups already engaged in 'traditional' forms of warfare or by new groups who use only IW. We are therefore asking precisely those questions posed by scholars of military innovation who have examined the successes, and failures, of military organizations in adopting new technologies and doctrines (Farrell 1996).

This literature focuses our attention on the type of system that a particular organization represents and characterizes the system, in part, by its proclivity to change. Commonly, three types of system are identified: natural systems, rational systems and open systems. The natural systems approach characterizes organizations as fighting for survival in a hostile environment. They are not however driven by a rational vision of self-interest but are rather subject to the vagaries of internal 'bureaucratic politics'.

The rational systems approach proposes that organizations act to achieve designated goals. In response to environmental changes, they adapt their procedures, processes and structures to ensure more efficient achievement of their goal. An example of this type of system was the US Army in the Second World War which re-engineered itself during its drive across Europe.

The open systems approach argues that organizations are susceptible to pressure for change from external factors (environmental) and internal factors (institutionalism). This approach focuses on institutional rules and strategic culture that condition organizational behaviour (Gray 1986; Powell and DiMaggio 1991).

These models give some guidance to the propensity, or lack of it, of an organization to embrace change. For instance, in peacetime or after a victory, there is a distinct tendency among military organizations for institutionalism to prevail, as described in the open systems model. Although military innovators will sometimes make their views heard, it is often only as a result of a severe external shock that change will be embraced and the organization will be re-engineered. This is just as true of commercial organizations. The business management literature is replete with case studies and theoretical works detailing how companies can be reinvigorated through business process re-engineering (Miles 1996).

A particularly relevant branch of the organizational culture literature is that dealing with organizational learning. Business gurus now argue that success will belong to 'learning organizations'. These they define as 'organizations with an ingrained philosophy for anticipating, reacting and responding to change, complexity and uncertainty' (Malhotra 1996).

The lessons for organizational analysis of sub-state groups are self-evident. The question is, which sub-state groups are the most likely to embrace IW techniques and technologies? The answer is those that are learning organizations, those that are more open to environmental factors and those that are least bound by institutionalism and strategic culture that may be antipathetic to change and to technological, structural and military innovation. This level of analysis also usefully directs our attention to a crucial question. Why should a group want to adopt this new mode of warfare? As with corporations or militaries, a sub-state group is less likely to innovate if it is successful or insulated from external pressures. On the contrary, if the group has been defeated or is under severe external pressure then it is more likely to innovate.

Structure

Organizational structure and organizational culture are interrelated. The synergies and interconnections need to be recognized. None the less, it is useful to separate them out for analytical purposes. As with culture, the literature on structure draws on both military and commercial case studies. In relation to military examples it is however less mature, with most conclusions being drawn from the commercial world. In particular, attention has focused on the high tech sector.

For our purposes, the essence of the discussion of structure concerns the relative effectiveness of network or hierarchical forms of organization for operating in the 'information age'. Initial conclusions from the business world and from the non-governmental sector are that networked organizations and, even more, organizational networks, are better placed to exploit ICTs.

Political scientists and sociologists have begun to generalize from these conclusions. Ronfeldt, for instance, posits a progression in civilizations from tribe to network (Ronfeldt 1996: 11–20). He argues that the post-industrial era is witnessing the emergence of organizational networks. While these consist mainly of social actors, sometimes known as SPINs (segmented, polycentric, ideologically integrated networks), the model has been diffusing into the business sector. These multi-organizational networks are made possible, and effectively exploit, multi-channel and dense information flows.

The debate over organizational structure and warfare has only recently been joined. In principle, the US armed forces are adopting many of the concepts of networking and the Joint Chiefs of Staff have adopted the concept of 'network-centric warfare'. This emphasizes connectivity between all levels of the organization, a flattening of hierarchies and the free flow of information around the organization. The argument is that this form of organization makes for more efficient application of new military technologies and doctrines, not least of which are those relating to IW. However, there is considerable resistance to the notion of transforming armed forces from the rigid, bureaucratic hierarchies they have been since the advent of modern warfare into loose networks. While some of this resistance is due to institutional conservatism, there is also a genuine debate over the degree of centralization versus the degree of decentralization that makes for more efficient warfighting.

Precisely the same issues over warfighting efficiency in the information age need to be considered for sub-state groups. Although few sub-state groups are as hierarchical as the armed forces of a state, there are clear differences in the organizational structures of such groups. At one extreme could be an organization such as the Palestine Liberation Organization (PLO) in the late 1970s and 1980s. Based in Lebanon, the PLO deliberately sought to build a formal, hierarchical armed force. At the other extreme could be informal alliances of computer hackers or single issue pressure groups in the 1990s. These organizational networks have a flat structure.

The initial work that has been done on organizational structure and IW has tended towards the conclusion that, the more networked an organization, the more able it is to, first, confound a hierarchical organization and, second, the more adept it is at exploiting ICTs. Evidence for both views abounds but more thorough analytical work needs to done to isolate organizational structure as an independent variable in assessing success and adoption of ICTs. For instance, it is sometimes argued that highly networked insurgents, such as the Viet Cong, have invariably triumphed over inflexible, hierarchical armed forces (Arquilla and Ronfeldt 1997a: 38–39). While not without substance, this claim ignores a number of counter-examples, such as the British defeat of Communist insurgents in Malaya.[2] It may also place too much emphasis on organizational structure as compared to other factors.

As another example, it is often observed that this decade's organizational networks, who range from environmental and human rights pressure groups to political opposition movements, have been more effective than their state or corporate opponents in harnessing ICT and IW techniques to their causes. Again, this is a tempting conclusion but the evidence needs to be more rigorously and systematically assessed than it has been at present.

These caveats notwithstanding, the basic point made by the organizational structure literature is valid. There are, in general, benefits to be gained in the digital age from having a more networked and less hierarchical organizational structure. Networked organizations and organizational networks do seem to be better able to exploit ICTs. Therefore, assessing the organizational structure of a sub-state group will provide an indicator of its IW ability. Exactly how to measure the degree of 'networkedness' of a group or how to measure the warfight-ing implications of this 'networkedness' are pressing research questions.

Application

Analysts seeking to apply an organizational approach to threat assessment are faced with two methodological problems. First, how to translate the theoretical importance of organizational culture and structure into measurable indicators of IW proclivity. Second, how to construct metrics that will allow real world sub-state groups to be assessed (Rathmell 1998).

The first question can only be answered by conducting considerable case study work. Since few organizations, whether state or non-state, have actually engaged in IW, as yet there is a limited number of case studies one can draw upon. This will doubtless change, however, and the coming years should provide an ever richer data set from which to work. Initially, though, a cursory survey of contemporary sub-state groups suggests that there are causal links between organizational culture and organizational structure on the one hand and the adoption of ICTs and of IW approaches on the other.

Perhaps the most remarked upon users of ICT have been right-wing militias in the USA, Islamist opposition movements originating in the Middle East and single-issue pressure groups such as environmental activists or human rights campaigners. However they may differ in aims, membership or ideology, all of these groups have been quick to exploit ICTs for propaganda and psychological operations. These groups also tend to resemble organizational networks in their structure. They are also, in some ways, learning organizations. This may seem odd since the former two types of movement epitomize fundamentalist obscurantism in their world views. None the less, in their selection of tactics and methods, these groups have proved to be innovative and open to their environment (Rathmell 1997a; Junas 1995). The organizational theory literature reminds us that this is not surprising since they are representative of movements that have experienced catastrophic defeat and therefore have no status quo to defend.

Another set of users of ICT and of fairly sophisticated IW techniques have been organized criminal groups. Examples range from some Latin American drug cartels to Dutch criminal gangs. They have not been interested in propaganda but have concentrated on developing secure communication networks and on exploiting offensive IW to disrupt or monitor the information infrastructures of their opponents, whether these are the Amsterdam police force or the Drug Enforcement Administration (Kruyer 1997; ERRI 1997). Organizational analysis appears to have explanatory power here too. Such criminal groups are more hierarchical than the networks discussed above but they are more reminiscent of networked organizations than of hierarchies. At the same time, operating in a highly competitive environment with little time or space for dogmas to become institutionalized, they are very much learning organizations (Williams 1994; Bureau for International Narcotics and Law Enforcement Affairs 1998).

Turning to insurgent, guerrilla and terrorist movements, one finds interesting examples which illustrate the argument, if by providing a counter example. Many insurgents, from the Provisional IRA through Mexico's Zapatistas to Lebanon's *Hizbollah*, have incorporated ICT into their more traditional propaganda and fund-raising activities. They therefore have websites as well as newspapers (Reuters 1998). They do not appear, however, to have supplemented their kinetic attacks, using bullets and bombs, with cyber-attacks.[3] This is despite the fact that, in response to environmental pressures, groups such as the PIRA have shifted to attacking national infrastructures. It is even more striking given the publicity on the supposed advantages and cost-effectiveness of cyber-terrorism (Soo Hoo *et al.* 1997). The slowness to adopt offensive IW can in part be explained by organizational analysis. Many of the established insurgent organizations are as institutionalized as their state opponents. They do not often face existential threats and they are reluctant to embrace change. They may not have won their struggles but they have survived so there is little incentive to change. Moreover, they are comfortable with existing coercive methods which appear to work and which, often, form part of their organizational self-image (Rathmell 1997b).

At the same time, few of these groups are extensively networked. Whether they have adopted an urban guerrilla cell structure or a paramilitary rural insurgency structure, they are resolutely hierarchical. Indeed, given the vital importance of operational security and secrecy, they may less resemble learning organizations and organizational networks than many of their state opponents. This is not to say that such groups will not embrace IW in the future. These examples do however suggest that, all things being equal, they will do so less quickly and less comprehensively than will more open, flexible and networked groups.

In answer to the first question posed above, then, a cursory survey of existing sub-state groups does suggest a causal link between organizational factors and adoption of IW. This and the cases mentioned above, provides the basis on which to model this link and to categorize organizational elements in terms of their IW significance.

In response to the second question, how to construct metrics of predictive utility, one can draw upon two sources. First, the case studies and models discussed above. Second, the literature on business organization and change. Management consultants have generated a considerable body of work which seeks to measure organizational culture and structure. After all, such measurements form the baseline for any re-engineering of business processes. Military organizations have begun to adopt some of these techniques, seeking to model their business processes and to map their organizational knowledge (Tyrrell 1997). Similar methods could be applied to sub-state groups.

While analysing the business processes or information flows in a clandestine terrorist group may not be easy, this sort of analysis is being done by intelligence agencies. For instance, criminal analysts make use of link analysis to understand the dynamics of criminal organizations. Security services likewise apply this analysis to terrorist groups as they seek to understand who to target for recruitment, deception or elimination. Currently, this organizational analysis is carried out mainly for operational purposes. According to the argument here, it could usefully be adapted to provide predictive intelligence.

Conclusion

The problem of how to assess the IW threat posed by sub-state groups is one of the most urgent facing governments and corporations in advanced, networked societies. ICTs are empowering small actors and enable them to achieve strategic effect with limited resources. At the same time, the rush to digitize, connect and deregulate critical infrastructures is opening up a wide range of vulnerabilities. The nature of IW, especially in the unpredictable conflict environment which faces states since the end of the Cold War, makes it very hard to judge the direction from which threats will come, much less their seriousness.

While existing approaches to IW threat assessment are useful, there is a need for novel approaches that are better able to provide predictive indicators of emerging problems. This article has argued that, in a threat environment marked by dynamic and non-linear change, a steady state focus on capabilities is insufficient. One useful additional method is organizational analysis. By focusing on organizational culture and organizational structure, analysts will be better placed to predict the emergence of IW threats.

The argument has been made that sub-state groups are no different from armed forces or corporations. Armed forces and corporations vary in their ability to embrace change and to learn new modes of behaviour. They also vary in their organizational structures, with consequent impacts on their ability to exploit ICTs. Sub-state groups are as varied. They have specific organizational cultures and structures which, in part, will determine how they will react to the opportunities of the information revolution.

The notion of ESAs and organizational networks goes too far in proposing that sub-state groups will inevitably be the most effective and most rapid exploiters of ICT and adopters of IW. Some groups are clearly beginning to act as very dynamic and efficient ESAs. Others are not.

From the perspective of predictive intelligence, the crucial point is that the organizational level of analysis can provide an important set of indicators not captured by existing capability indices. Most importantly, in the dynamic and fluid postmodern security environment where non-linear change is a constant, a focus on organizational factors that may facilitate or inhibit change or adoption of ICTs and IW doctrines can provide warning signs that allow intelligence and information assurance resources to be better targeted.

Acknowledgment

I would like to thank Neil Robinson for his invaluable assistance in researching this chapter.

Notes

1   The gurus include Winn Schwartau (Schwartau 1996). Noted hacking incidents include Solar Sunrise (Kyl 1998). Films include *The Net* and *Wargames*.
2   Although it should be acknowledged that one of the factors for the British success was their adoption of guerrilla tactics in addition to their more rigidly structured methods.
3   Sri Lanka's LTTE guerrillas launched a Denial of Service attack on the e-mail servers of the Sri Lankan embassies in early 1998. Reportedly, this was in response to an attempt by the Sri Lankan government to disable an LTTE listserver.

12 Far right extremists on the Internet

Michael Whine

Introduction

Among the most dynamic of all the political extremes now is the far right. In the US, the growth of white supremacist groups, militias and so-called Christian fundamentalists has led to a belated recognition that domestic extremism poses great dangers. In Germany, neo-Nazi groups incite violence against foreign workers and asylum seekers, and official assessments suggest that they continue to pose a danger to the safety of citizens and the security of the state. As in the US, the trend in Germany since the 1980s has been for small groups to act out their campaigns on single issues, often coordinating their activities, but seldom seeking to come together to form larger groups with a political agenda.

British far right groups have achieved far less impact than elsewhere in Europe and America. Their support base, as expressed in votes at elections, is narrower and the size of the groups is very much smaller. However they too incite violence, and have even been responsible for acts of terrorism.

Common to many far right groups is a developing bond of ideological opposition to central government and its policies, to non-white residency and to the development of transnational contacts. In these respects the new Right differs from older, particularly wartime, models of fascism and neo-Nazism. New contacts and evolving ideologies are being facilitated and enhanced by information and communication technologies (ICTs).

Noted commentators have remarked on this employment of new cultural mechanisms and technologies to disseminate neo-Nazi ideas (Back, *et al.* 1996, 1998; Eatwell 1996). They suggest that what is being produced is a globalized racist and neo-fascist movement and culture that draws on international electronic networks, whilst simultaneously reinforcing old xenophobic ideas embodied in traditional racism and anti-semitism. They further suggest that a new virtual racism has evolved through the medium of the Internet, that the interpenetration of various nationalist movements is amplified within cyberspace, and that it is possible for far right groups of markedly different types to establish common networks and ideological alliances, particularly around a shared common enemy.

It is this tendency to use cyberspace as a means to communicate, and to a lesser extent to effect command and control, the dangers that arise therefrom and the legal sanctions used to combat these developments that are the subject of this chapter.

Current Internet usage

The militia movement in the USA is now deemed a potent threat to the authority of central government. According to Ken Stern (1998), the use of ICTs was one of the major reasons the militia movement expanded faster than any hate group in history. Its lack of an organized centre and its geographical spread across the whole country was more than made up for by the communication and rumour-mongering potential of the new medium. It meant that a militia member in a remote state such as Idaho or Montana could be part of an entire nationwide network.

The most important of the new technologies was the Internet, followed by fax networks and talk radio. Stern cites the short-wave radio stations WWCR in Nashville, WRNO in New Orleans, WHRI in South Bend Indiana and others that regularly broadcast racist and anti-government conspiracy theory programmes. It was on WWCR (World Wide Christian Radio) that a broadcaster gave instructions on how to build bombs with materials from local stores from 1994 onwards and which the Federal Communications Commission was subsequently reported to be investigating for a possible link with Timothy McVeigh and the Oklahoma City bombing (Stern 1998: 224)

Fax machines are useful for disseminating messages, but they are not interactive. Therefore it is the Internet which has been the main means of communication for the American far right. Stern noted that there were up to 300 such systems serving the far right in the USA in 1997, but since then other estimates have run much higher, including that of the Simon Wiesenthal Centre in Los Angeles, which now cites 600 'hate' sites. Among these it has identified 35, mostly US-based sites, run by militia groups advocating armed struggle, 94 sites that sought to establish a racial hierarchy, 87 neo-Nazi sites, 35 white supremacist sites, and 51 sites openly advocating terrorism. However it also found that some of the most extreme groups have placed their sites outside of the United States, in order to escape legal jurisdiction.[1]

Initially it was bulletin board services, including PatriotNet, LibertyNet, PaulRevereNet, which allowed the interconnectivity across great distances. Linda Thompson, a militia leader, stated that her bulletin board reaches 36,000 people.

> We are a news service. We use the computer as the end of the line, not the beginning. We get information in by Federal Express, faxes and phone, then we put it on the bulletin boards for the widest distribution.
>
> (Stern 1998: 226)

Thompson also stated that some of their messages were encrypted using Pretty Good Privacy: 'To confuse people who may be listening in … We send copies of the Constitution out encrypted, just to keep 'em (the CIA) busy' (ibid.).

Dan Gannon established the first far right hate site in Portland, Oregon, in December 1991, but from the mid-1990s onwards computers and computer services became cheaper, quicker and more readily available and these developments coincided with the birth of the militia movement. While bulletin boards had provided communication and a degree of control and security, the Internet news groups provide greater speed and audience. Newsgroups such as alt.conspiracy and talk.politics.guns allowed members of the militias to share information, advice and paranoia.

The militias owe much of their doctrine to the white supremacists and neo-Nazis. During the mid-1980s Louis Beam, a leader of the white supremacist group Aryan Nations, operated a computer network. He used it to issue a hit list which proposed the assassination of politicians, judges, FBI agents, federal marshals and even the President himself. In 1992 he published *Leaderless Resistance*, which defined the modern far right in America, and increasingly elsewhere. His particular doctrine downplays hierarchy in favour of a network of 'phantom cells'. Such cells communicate covertly in a networked format allowing offensive flexibility while protecting the security of the organization as a whole.

> Utilising the leaderless resistance concept, all individuals in groups operate independently of each other, and never report to a central headquarters or single leader for directional instruction … Participants in a programme of leaderless resistance through phan-

tom cell or individual action must know exactly what they are doing and exactly how to do it ... All members of phantom cells or individuals would tend to react to objective events in the same way through usual tactics of resistance. Organs of information distribution such as newsletters, leaflets, computers etc. which are widely available to all, keep each person informed of events allowing for a planned response that will take on many variations. No-one need issue an order to anyone.[2]

German neo-Nazis were the first to use the Internet in this way. They have been communicating with one another, and organizing their activities, via the *ThuleNetz* (Network) since the 1980s.

> Provided with passwords such as *'Germania'* or *'Endsieg'* (Final Victory) from a post office box, personal computer screens will display a calendar of forthcoming neo-Nazi events and list contact numbers of leading right-wingers ... On Remembrance Sunday, police saw in action for the first time, computer planned co-ordinated neo-Nazi action, involving the widespread use of secret codes and radio communication ... 'The advantage of electronic mailboxes is that they are free of censorship and bug proof' said Karl-Heinz Sendbuhler of the National Democratic Party.[3]

The German authorities express increasing concern about the Internet. They have noted the growth of far right home pages, from 30 in 1996 to 90 in 1997 and the manner in which football hooligans were mobilized during the 1998 football World Cup series by German Nazis via their websites.[4]

British neo-Nazis adopted the use of ICTs later than their counterparts in other countries. Although smaller in size, less sophisticated and certainly less violent, they are nevertheless now willing to take on new ideas and technologies. The writer of the National Front journal, *The Nationalist*, recently discussed the benefits that information and communication technologies were bringing to the group:

> All over the world anyone with access to the Internet can find a full range of information regarding the National Front at the touch of a button ... New friends from around the world have been made and important contacts have been established, particularly in the United States, where we regularly liaise via E-mail with a major nationalist organisation, with a possible view to

future long-term co-operation. The Internet will be the main political campaigning tool of the next decade and beyond.

(Ashcroft 1998)

The British National Party has also caught up with cyberspace and aims to use it extensively in the future. Its Internet Conference Weekend, held at the end of March 1999, was designed to help a small number of activists make their plans for a dedicated Euro-Campaign website, and to discuss electronic political outreach work. Also on the agenda were plans for the exchange of expertise, research and development for a Virtual Headquarters idea, and merchandising plans.[5] Even the much smaller National Revolutionary Faction, a descendant of the National Front, announced recently:

> The new homepage has put us in touch with an increasing number of National Revolutionary activists worldwide. If you have access to a computer, then why not check it out for yourself at: http//www.geocities.com/Athens/Troy/8854.[6]

A recent development has been the transnational cyberspace information bulletin, having no real national affiliation. The International Third Position's Final Conflict E-mail appears to be moving in this direction, with its increasing number of postings from far right groups around the world, but the Western Imperative Network (WIN) claims to be truly international. Its Mission Statement states that:

> The Western Imperative Network is a cyberspace organisation consisting of concerned White Men and Women who are dedicated to the essential urgent missions of educating our fellow Whites on racial issues and fighting anti-White attitudes, ideas and propaganda on the Internet ... WIN activists use the Internet to educate as to the problems and dangers we face as a people ... The second main directive of the Western Imperative Network is to actively oppose anti-White propagandists of whatever race operating on the Internet (typically on the usernet) ... if you are a White man or woman, have a computer and Internet account, a few hours per week, are ready to do your part in the White separatist struggle, have read the WINFAQ and agree with the goals and guidelines described therein, then contact us. WIN is always active fighting anti-White activities and attitudes on the Net.[7]

How threatening is the far right's Internet usage?

What particular dangers arise from the far right's use of ICTs, and are these dangers new or additional ones? Several reasons might suggest that they are. First, they allow interconnectivity, that is the power to communicate and network that previously were not available to them in such an easy manner and with such speed.

An example of this were the warnings given on the Internet to supporters after the simultaneous raids in America and Canada on the offices of Resistance Records, the leading producers of white supremacist and skinhead music and tapes, and the home of George Burdi, its founder.[8] A second example was when the killing, in Essex in February 1997, of Combat 18 member Christopher Castle by two of the group's leaders, was posted on the Internet site of the American National Socialist White People's Party within twelve hours.[9]

In early 1999, Final Conflict E-mail, the website of the International Third Position, a small British national revolutionary group, advertised an anti-European Union demonstration that was to have taken place in Rome in April. Few other adverts were seen for this in hard copy format, and it may therefore be assumed that the bulk of the advertising was carried out over the Net. (However they also subsequently published news of the demonstration's ban by the Italian police.)[10]

Second, the Internet allows covert communication and anonymity. Milton John Kleim Jnr, the former self-styled 'Net Nazi Number One' wrote of these powers, before he renounced his Nazi views:

> All my comrades and I, none of whom I have ever met face to face, share a unique camaraderie, feeling as though we have been friends for a long time. Self-less co-operation occurs regularly amongst my comrades for a variety of endeavours. This feeling of comradeship is irrespective of national identity or state borders.[11]

A third reason for using the Internet is that it is cheap. For the price of a computer and a modem an extremist can become a player in national and world events. ICTs lower the threshold for participating in illegal acts, and without state or other backing extremists will look for cost-effective instruments. A consequence of this is that presentation and quality may vary widely. At one end of the spectrum there are professional-quality sites such as Stormfront and RadioIslam, with coloured graphics, photographs and links to other similar sites, which are the equal of the best available produced by large organizations. At the other end of the spectrum are the poorly presented, often barely literate, hate sheets such as the Norwegian Julius Streiker's site or some of the messages on the bulletin boards and the news groups. The British National Party's Internet television site commenced transmission in early 1999, and represents the next generation and future direction for groups which seek to hide their hate messages in sophisticated packaging. What is common to all is the fact that they are produced with few resources, often by single persons, or very small teams, yet present a façade of authenticity to the innocent reader, despite their origins.

Four, ICTs act as a force-multiplier, enhancing power and enabling extremists to punch above their weight. They can now have a reach and influence that was previously denied them. Communication technology represents, in many respects, the 'death of distance' and the national borders that once separated the extremists from the objects of their hatred have ceased to exist. The British National Front summarized these opportunities in a recent issue of their journal *The Nationalist*:

> GREAT OPPORTUNITY ... The Internet will be the main political campaigning tool of the next decade and beyond. We have tested the technology with our audio broadcasts and it is entirely suitable for substantial investment, both in terms of time and money. Some people might think that the National Front Internet presence is not at all important and that funds should only be channelled into it after everything else has been paid for. Such a view represents a dangerous underestimation of the significance of the Internet and the great opportunities that it presents us with admittedly, many people do not own a computer with which to view our site at present, but all that will change with the advent of the digital revolution which will begin to sweep this country at the end of the year ... we have the opportunity to reach millions of people with our message over the next few months, but we must invest now and have the infrastructure in place in order to take full advantage of the opportunities that will present themselves in the near future.[12]

The Australian symposium on Holocaust denial organized by Frederick Toben's Adelaide Institute in the summer of 1998 was attended by a number of Nazi sympathizers and deniers. Some would-be participants however were precluded from attending by the distance and expense involved; others were banned from entering Australia by the authorities. However, those unable to attend were still able to participate by posting their presentations over the Internet or by the use of video links.

Fifth, ICTs enable extremists to reach their target audience when other outlets and media are denied them, and to reach new audiences, particularly the young and educated. In several European countries, their hate-filled postings would almost certainly be prosecuted if published in hard copy; the absence of specific sanctions, or protocols on the Internet have allowed the postings, so far. It has enabled the far right to reach across national boundaries and by-pass laws banning hate material, as in Britain, France, Germany and Scandinavia and has therefore become a priority from the point of view of their doctrine. Again it was Louis Beam who first pointed out these possibilities, as well as the barriers that law enforcement was likely to place in their way:

> The Internet, perhaps the last truly free means of information exchange in the Western world, may soon be choked by censorship and governmental controls. The circumscribing of the Net may cause the death of what has become the first people-to-people exchange of ideas and information on a worldwide basis ... at stake is nothing less than the regaining of information control which the Internet has shattered. Up for grabs is nothing more than the thinking and decision making abilities of informed men. Information has flowed from the top down for most of this century. Filtering of information by middlemen from government, newspapers, radio and then television has led most Americans depending upon Paul Harvey 'for the rest of the story'. Suddenly, almost without warning, the Internet mushroomed into popularity, connecting people all over the world together electronically and thereby threatening the power of those who can disseminate information.[13]

Some activists have sought to avoid legal proscription by moving their sites abroad to put them beyond their own countries' laws. Thus the British National Party now has a site registered in Tonga, the French Charlemagne Hammerskins moved their site to Canada following the termination of their service by America Online in September 1997 and Ernst Zundel, a German national residing in Canada, has his site registered in California. The Net strategy of Milton Kleim defined the far right's approach:

> The State cannot yet stop us from 'advertising' our ideas and

organisations on USERNET, but I can assure you this will not always be the case. NOW is the time to grasp the WEAPON which is the NET, and wield it skilfully and wisely while you may still do so freely ...

Crucial to our USERNET campaign is that our message is disseminated beyond 'our' groups: we MUST move out beyond our present domain and take up positions on 'mainstream groups' ...

Remember our overall USERNET strategy must be to repeat powerful themes OVER AND OVER AND OVER. We cannot compete with the Jews' media, of course, as our propaganda dissemination is but a very small fraction of the everywhere pervasive leftist propaganda. However, our ideas possess an energy that truth alone contains.[14]

Effective policing

Growing international concern is prompting governments to police the Net and to take legal action against those who post offensive and illegal hate material on the Internet. Two major issues arise however in their approach to these problems. They must balance the right of free expression with the protection of human dignity; and they must determine under whose jurisdiction any offence has been committed. However any national response will necessarily be based, in part, upon the main international legal instruments signed by governments.

In 1965 the United Nations adopted the International Convention on the Elimination of All Forms of Racial Discrimination. It is the oldest and most widely ratified UN human rights convention and defines racial discrimination as 'any distinction, exclusion, or restriction or preference based on race, colour, dissent or national or ethnic origin which has the purpose or effect of nullifying or impairing the recognition, enjoyment or exercise, on an equal footing of human rights and fundamental freedoms in the political, economic, social, cultural or any other field of public life'.

States ratifying the Convention are obliged to adopt legal measures for eliminating racial discrimination in all its forms and manifestations and preventing and combating racist doctrines and practices. They are expected to make all dissemination of such ideas based on racial superiority or hatred, and incitement to racial discrimination, an offence punishable by law, and are required to take effective measures to review policies in order to amend laws and regulations which might have the effect of creating or perpetuating racial discrimination wherever it exists. It is generally agreed that these requirements are applicable to hate-oriented groups using the Internet to disseminate their propaganda.

In August 1996 the Committee on the Elimination of Racial Discrimination, which was created to ensure that governments fulfil their obligations under the Convention, noted that there was a growing trend among racist organisations to use electronic mail or the Internet to spread racist or xenophobic propaganda, and that no national legislation had power over this worldwide network. A seminar on the Internet and Racial Discrimination held by the Committee in November 1997 noted with great concern that the Internet plays an increasing role in disseminating hate speech and racial discrimination worldwide. Although it failed to reach a consensus on a number of contentious issues it did recommend that member states continue in their efforts to establish international legal measures in compliance with their obligations under international law. More effective action has foundered however on the resistance of some countries, particularly the USA, to impose any barriers to free speech.

In Europe more concrete goals are possible through the European Union institutions, and there has been considerable effort to develop a regulatory framework, and the enactment of legal instruments, in recent years. In October 1996 the European Commission adopted the Communication On Harmful And Illegal Content on the Internet which set out proposals for immediate action against such material. The Communication concluded that it was the responsibility of the member states to ensure that existing laws apply to the Internet and that cooperation and coordination at a European and international level should assist the enforcement of the laws. It recommended a regulatory framework combining self-control by the service providers, the adoption of technical solutions such as rating and filtering software and the provision of monitoring intelligence by Internet users themselves. At the same time the Commission adopted a Green Paper on the Protection of Minors and Human Dignity in Audio-Visual and Information Services designed to engender debate on regulatory and legislative controls for particular types of illegal material, including anti-semitic and racist material. The Green Paper invited comment on three themes – strengthening legal protection, encouraging parental control systems, and improving international co-operation.

It is the consideration of these by the European Parliament and interested parties in member states that has led to a broad consensus on the problem of illegal racist material on the Internet. During 1997 the European Commission adopted a Proposal for a Recommendation of the Protection of Minors and Human Dignity, and an Action Plan promoting safe use of the Internet. The two documents are designed to be complementary. The Recommendation is legal in nature and aims to promote common guidelines for the implementation, at national level, of a framework for self-regulation and the Action Plan provides financial support for specific action on creating a safe environment, developing filtering and rating systems, education among users, and support action in the legal and economic spheres. In essence, the initiatives implemented thus far place responsibility for combating illegal content, at source, with law enforcement agencies whose activities would be governed by national laws and international agreement on judicial co-operation. It is expected that this will lead to the pooling of experience and information and the training of police officers and the judiciary, although the Internet industry is expected to play its part in reducing illegal content, particularly anti-semitic and racist material, through self-regulation, codes of conduct and the establishment of hotlines.

On another tack, the Working Party on Illegal and Harmful Content on the Internet was established following the 1996 Communication, and its area of research was extended when, in September 1996, the Telecommunications Council agreed to the addition of representatives of the ministers of telecommunications, service providers and others. The Working Party reported twice, in November 1996 and in June 1997. Their reports led to the adoption, in February 1997, of the Council Resolution on Illegal and Harmful Content on the Internet which invited EU states to adopt self-regulatory systems including representative bodies for service providers and users, effective codes of conduct, hotline reporting mechanisms for the public and the provision of filtering mechanisms and rating systems. The Resolution also requested the European Commission to follow up on previously suggested measures, which included faster coordination and exchange of information on best practice and research at a community level, and further consideration of the question of legal liability of Internet content.

In April 1997 the European Parliament adopted a resolution based on the Council Resolution and a report by Pierre Pradier, Chairman of the Committee on Civil Liberties and Internal Affairs. The Resolution *inter alia* called on member states to define common rules in their criminal laws, strengthen administrative co-operation on the basis of joint guidelines and, after consultation with the parliament, the establishment of a common framework for self-regulation, which would include objectives to be achieved in terms of the protection of minors and human dignity; principles governing representation of the industries concerned and the decision making procedures; measures to encourage the information and communications industry to develop message protection and filtering software, which should be made available to subscribers; and appropriate arrangements to ensure that all instances of child pornography be reported to the police and shared with Europol and Interpol. With respect to illegal and harmful content on the Internet the Resolution called on the Commission, and the member states, to encourage the development of a common international rating system compatible with the Platform for Internet Content Selection (PICS) protocol which would be sufficiently flexible to accommodate cultural differences.

An international ministerial conference (Global Information Networks: Realising the Potential), was held in Bonn in July 1997 as a consequence of the Council Resolution (of February 1997) and brought together all the players in the ICT industries, as well as representatives of users and other international organizations. A number of declarations followed the Conference which *inter alia* stressed the role which the private sector can play in protecting the interest of consumers and in protecting and respecting ethical standards through properly functioning systems of self-regulation.

At the police level the Justice and Home Affairs Council is sponsoring practical co-operation among law enforcement agencies and specific working groups have been established to look at the question of the lawful interception of Internet telecommunications. Work is also being carried out with a view to investigating police and judicial co-operation and the P8 Senior Level group on transnational organized crime is investigating mechanisms to locate, identify and prosecute computer-related crime. In April 1997 a European Commission and Europol communication to European police forces requested that they monitor illegal content on the Internet, seek out 'reporting' points, investigate cross border links, exchange information, reconcile national laws and co-operate on investigations.[15]

In Britain the government's views have been put forcefully in recent years. In responding to a parliamentary question in October 1996, on behalf of the President of the Board of Trade, Ian Taylor MP, stated that 'the basis for the government's approach is that the Internet is not a legal vacuum: the law applies on-line as it does off it'.[16]

Later, the Junior Home Office Minister, Timothy Kirkhope MP, stated that the Internet was being monitored for incidents of minority groups being threatened. He stated that 'the activities of neo-Nazi groups are an increasing worry ... the use of the Internet is a particular concern, because it means that links can be made between these groups and information can be exchanged'.[17]

The police view was given by Sir Paul Condon, Commissioner of the Metropolitan Police in an address to the Inter-Parliamentary Council Against Anti-semitism in February 1997 when he stated that the Telecommunications Act 1984 was among a battery of laws which would provide a basis for prosecuting anti-semitism which incited race hatred on the Internet.

Government spokespeople have continued to make authoritative statements on the UK approach. In January 1998, Home Office Minister, Mike O'Brien stated, in response to a parliamentary question, that 'the Government deplore the distribution – via the Internet or any other medium – of anti-semitism or racially inflammatory material … Material passing over the Internet is subject to the same laws, provided that it falls within our jurisdiction, as material being distributed by other means. The Public Order Act 1986 makes provision to deal with material which is threatening, abusive or insulting and intended or likely to stir up racial hatred.'[18]

In March 1998, he stated, again in response to a parliamentary question about the use of the Internet to spread racist and anti-semitic propaganda, that the National Criminal Intelligence Service (NCIS) had been in close liaison with other countries to combat Internet abuse, and that the G7 Action Plan on High-Tech Crime committed the UK to developing closer links to combat Internet crime more effectively. He added, in response to a further question, that the Home Secretary had recently discussed these matters with G8 colleagues and that it was their belief that the way forward was for the issue to be tackled via international co-operation.[19]

A few months later, in September 1998, the Home Secretary himself stated that the UK was cracking down on racist material published on the Internet and that the Government had asked governments across the world to work together to remove illegal websites and prosecute those responsible. He added that NCIS would be acting against threatening abusive and racist material.[20] A few days later an NCIS spokesman said that NCIS would be combating racism on the Internet, and that it could identify the jurisdiction that illegal material originated from, and would pass such information on to the relevant national authorities.[21]

Police action so far has tended to reflect national judicial attitudes towards hate crime. In Germany and Austria, where Holocaust denial and public manifestations of Nazism are illegal, the governments have acted with a severity that other countries might find unacceptable. In

December 1995, the Munich Public Prosecutor's Office closed down CompuServe as a result of its alleged dissemination of illegal (neo-Nazi) material, and in 1997 forced it to cut worldwide access to offensive sites, although it now appears that no criminal prosecution action will be taken. In January 1996, Deutsche Telekom the largest provider of Internet services in Germany, cut off access to Web Communications, which rents space to the neo-Nazi propagandist Ernst Zundel. However this also resulted in subscribers losing access to another 1,500 websites. In March 1997 the Viennese police raided the offices of the service provider Burgerform, and at least twenty private homes, seizing computers for evidence that they had been used to download and distribute Nazi material originating in America.

In Canada a different approach has been adopted. Canadian law proscribes so-called hate or bias crimes but the courts have yet to adjudicate on such crimes committed on the Internet. However the view generally held is that the medium by which such messages are transmitted is immaterial. In May 1997, the Human Rights Commission began proceedings to indict Ernst Zundel and his web page, the Zundelsite, under the Canadian Human Rights Act. Zundel has argued that his site does not come under Canadian jurisdiction as it is uploaded from California by his colleague Ingrid Rimland, but it has been the contention of those who brought the complaint that Rimland merely acts as his agent and that she receives regular instructions from him as to what is posted. The trial hearing is now into its second year as a consequence of varying objections brought by Zundel and his lawyers.

In British Columbia, Fairview Technology Centre Ltd, run by Bernard Klatt had been hosting American and European neo-Nazi sites, but was forced to close down following complaints to BC Tel, his service provider, that the site hosted customers who promoted race hatred, and that it was in breach of its service contract. Among the sites it hosted were the US Nazi Party, the (British) National Socialist Movement, the European Nationalist Party, the Euro-Christian Defence League and the (French) Charlemagne Hammer-skins. BC Tel refused to renew Klatt's contract and his case is now the subject of a police and judicial investigation, but Klatt himself has moved his operation across the border into the US and continues to post material that would be illegal according to Canadian and European norms.

Any police action that is considered must now inevitably focus on the fact that much offensive and illegal material originates in America, where the First Amendment to the Constitution protects all free expression of opinion except that which directly incites violence. The draft Communications Decency Act, with potentially stringent penalties for improper use of cyberspace, has been challenged by free speech activists, and has been struck down by the Supreme Court but individual states have begun to take legal action bypassing the First Amendment issue. In California legislation was passed that treats electronic words in the same way as written or spoken ones, and speech that 'seriously threatens' is a crime. Maryland has been considering draft legislation to make it illegal to send annoying or embarrassing e-mail. In Pennsylvania, state attorneys brought a successful civil action, requesting injunctive and other equitable relief, against Stormfront and Alpha HQ, its service provider. To lessen the possibility that Stormfront might argue that they were being made martyrs of, the action was bought against everybody along the chain, back to the service provider. On their site Stormfront had identified, by name and photographs, a local human relations council (the Reading-Berks Human Relations Council) and one of its staff members, stating that she was a race traitor and should beware.

The French authorities met less success in November 1998 when a criminal prosecution was brought against Robert Faurisson, a former academic who has been convicted by the French courts on several occasions for promoting Holocaust denial. In this action, which was joined by a number of civil parties representing former members of the French Resistance, deportees and the French League for the Defence of Human Rights, the courts found that it was unable to prove a link between the defendant and the offending texts on the Internet, despite the fact that his name was on the document. The absence of any initiative on the part of the defendant to remove his name from the heading of the offending document was immaterial, and the case was dismissed.[22]

In Britain, the Crown Prosecution Service has also encountered some difficulties, at the time of writing, in a possible case against David Myatt of the National Socialist Movement, who had published a neo-Nazi terrorism manual but had sought to evade British legal jurisdiction by having it uploaded from Bernard Klatt's Fairview Technology site in British Columbia, Canada. This would have been the first UK prosecution.

It is now generally acknowledged by the police and prosecution service that a successful prosecution could now be brought provided the jurisdictional and evidential hurdles have been overcome. The purveyors of hate material however are also quick to spot legal developments and are now registering their sites abroad. This parallels the trend of the early 1990s to print and publish offensive literature and leaflets from the US.

The future for policing the Net

Whilst the two problems mentioned above, that of balancing free speech with the protection of human rights, and the necessity of establishing jurisdiction, are acknowledged, states do now appear to be moving towards policing the most offensive postings, albeit at different paces and in slightly different ways.

It is clear however that there is now a realization that cyberspace provides a new and dangerous arena in which far right extremists can operate and that they are using it to spread their messages of hate, which are designed to offend and to incite violence. Law enforcement agencies appear to be keen to prosecute in most countries, but recognize the dangers and therefore have so far adopted a cautious approach. Pressure on educationalists, service providers, and others who are involved in examining the use of technical options and voluntary codes of conduct to regulate the Internet, will also prove effective in due course. What is important however is to bar access to the promoters of hate without stifling free comment and the expression of ideas and speech. Many extremist groups see the Internet as the last forum free from government interference. Some see the introduction of regulation as part of an external campaign by central governments to destroy 'free' thought. They are likely therefore to resist regulation vigorously and imaginatively. Some of the counter-measures being suggested such as PICS and the use of filters may bar pornographic sites effectively but they are ineffective against hate sites. Greater success is more likely to be achieved through a combination of a complaint-driven regime, by which service providers react to referrals from the public, criminal prosecution of those who post such messages, and an educational process which outlaws race hate through whichever medium it is disseminated.

Notes

1 'Hate Crime on the Internet', *International Police Review*, January/February: 1998: 28.
2 Beam, L. 'Leaderless Resistance', *The Seditionist*, 1992: Issue 12.
3 'Neo-Nazis Go Hi-Tech with Electronic Mailboxes', *The Guardian*, 19 November 1993.
4 Fuhrer, A., 'Rechtsextreme erobern das Internet', *Die Welt*, 23 July 1998; Blohm, D., Mobilmachung via Internet, *DPA*, August 1998.

5 Griffin, N., 'BNP internal communication', March 1999.

6 'The Revolution enters Cyberspace', *Catalyst – The Official Bulletin Of The NR Faction*, London, October 1998.

7 WIN Mission Statement, *Western Imperative Network*, http//www.usaor.net/users/ipn, 24 February 1999.

8 *Resistance Records Raided*, mlemireinterlog.com, 9 April 1999.

9 nswppearthlink.net, 10 March 1997.

10 Final Conflict News E-mail, Issue 759, 9 March 1999.

11 Kleim, M. J. Jr, *On Tactics and Strategy for USENET* 1995, bb748FreeNet. Carlton. CA

12 Ashcroft 1998: 5.

13 Beam, L.R., *The Conspiracy to Erect an Electronic Curtain*, nswppearthlink.net, 6 December 1996.

14 Kleim (see note 11).

15 European Commission (Europol Communication on Criminal Use of the Internet), 9 April 1997.

16 *Hansard*, 17 October 1996.

17 McIlroy, A.J., 'New Moves To Curb Racists On The Internet', *The Daily Telegraph*, 20 February 1997.

18 *Hansard*, vol. 305, no. 105, 26 January 1998.

19 *Hansard*, vol. 307, no. 129, 2 March 1998.

20 'UK Crackdown on Internet Racism', *BBC Online Network*, 15 September 1998.

21 'NCIS to help tackle Internet racism', *The Oxford Times*, 11 September 1998.

22 *The Public Prosecution v. Faurisson*, Paris Regional Court, 17th Chamber, Case No. 9727603115, Judgment of 13 November 1998.

13 Information warfare and the future of the spy

Philip H.J. Davies

Is information warfare a completely new form of conflict that exists because of the burgeoning global information infrastructure or is it merely a new dimension of an old form, like spying, whose origins lie in the 'grayware' of the human brain?

(Schoben 1995)

There were cowboys ever since there were computers. They built the first computers to crack German ice, right? Codebreakers. So there was ice before computers, you wanna look at it that way.

William Gibson *Count Zero* (1987)

Introduction

Information warfare represents one aspect of what has come to be known as the 'revolution in military affairs'. While this somewhat millennial view of how the scope and nature of conflict has changed since the end of the Cold War and the Second Gulf War is more generally accepted in North America than the UK, there can be no doubt that recent information technology, from computers through to satellites, represents a new arena of threats and opportunities, and if military affairs must change to keep pace, so must virtually all other aspects of the national security infrastructure. Amongst the elements of national government facing the burgeoning new 'infosphere', intelligence more than almost any other is *about* information. However, apart from Winn Schwartau's offhand rhetorical arabesque that 'spies are the original information warriors' (1996: 68), the role of *secret* intelligence in this emerging strategic environment is something which has received too little attention, and the thought that has been given the matter requires careful reappraisal and reassessment.

What has emerged in the literature has been two competing views of intelligence. One view stresses the high-tech opportunities of

252 Philip H.J. Davies

cybernetic penetration and disruption, and is concerned with digital espionage and sabotage by Gibsonesque 'console cowboys' who 'hack into' information systems in a globally networked cyberspace. Since the Second World War the primary sources of intelligence 'take' have been technical methods, or TECHINT, traditionally composed mainly of signals intelligence (SIGINT) and imagery intelligence (IMINT). To these the information warfare enthusiast would add cybernetic operations, what might be called, for lack of a better term (although a worse one is hard to imagine), HACKINT.[1] The other approach, however, points to the distributed, easily concealed and pervasively low-intensity conflict world of terrorism, proliferation and transnational organized crime, and anticipates a new age of human intelligence, or HUMINT. Thus intelligence policy-makers, seeking to redesign the world's intelligence communities for the near future and trying to allocate increasingly scarce intelligence resources, are confronted with two competing views of the coming decades: that the future holds either a fast-paced, high-bandwidth TECHINT world, or that it holds instead a dimly-lit Machiavellian HUMINT world. However, neither of these two views adequately represents the situation. In the first place, the technophile view which is put forward underestimates the limitations of technical methods while in the second place the HUMINT view proceeds with a weak understanding of how terrorism, proliferation and serious crime are increasingly using the global infosphere as their operating medium. That intelligence policy-makers must somehow optimize their commitments to human and technical methods may be a truism, but how that balance is to be evaluated is far from a trivial calculation, and what both views of the future underestimate is the *interdependency* between human and technical methods.

HUMINT vs TECHINT I: Woolseyan snakes on the information superhighway

The world of information warfare is, for the most part, a high-bandwidth, high transmission rate universe, and references to espionage and covert action in the literature have, for the most part, reflected that. Martin Libicki of the National Defence University has proposed a sub-class of information warfare that he has termed 'Intelligence-Based Warfare', or IBW. According to Libicki, IBW

> occurs when intelligence is fed directly into operations (notably, targeting and battle damage assessment) rather than used as an

input for overall command and control ... As sensors grow more acute and reliable, as they proliferate in type and number, and as they become capable of feeding fire control systems in real time and near-real-time, the task of developing, maintaining and exploiting systems that sense the battlespace, assess its composition, and send the results to shooters assumes increasing importance for tomorrow's militaries.

(1995)

However, Libicki's concept is very much confined to military *operational* intelligence, to the fast-paced high-bandwidth battlefield of the late twentieth and imagined twenty-first centuries, in which the humble foot soldier holds the grandiose title 'war fighter' and Pentagon press releases assure us that high-tech enhances not only lethality and survivability but also 'operations tempo' (Der Derian 1994: 118). *Secret* intelligence is a very different matter, in which operations are planned and undertaken in terms of months or years rather than minutes and seconds, and the content and sensitivity thereof tend to confine its product to strategic rather than tactical concerns. None the less, a great deal has been made of the potential for cybernetic penetrations to access and disrupt sensitive information systems, with the dangers of 'hacker war' not to be underestimated in an increasingly computer-dependent world. There has also been an accumulating body of evidence that this concern is well founded.

Since Clifford Stoll published *The Cuckoo's Egg* (1990) the world has become well acquainted with the methods employed by Marcus Hess, the 'Hannover Hacker', and his colleagues on behalf of the KGB. However, it might well be argued that the approach of 'hacking into' computer systems is a great deal more limited than might appear in the popular media and some of the more optimistic literature on information warfare. Computer systems can be made secure by physical isolation ('stand alone' systems), or placing them behind hardware defences such as one-way gates and software defences or 'firewalls'. Although Marcus Hess's ring gained access to, according to one estimate, 'fifty military computers at the Pentagon, various defence contractors, the Los Alamos Nuclear Weapons Laboratory, Argonne National Laboratory, the Air Force Space Systems Division' and various US military bases around the world (Madsen 1993: 418), perhaps the most distinctive feature of this effort was the very low grade of information acquired. Stoll, the astronomer-turned-sysop who pursued Hess down the telephone lines to Germany, found US Federal Agencies deeply uninterested in pursuing Hess on the grounds that none of the systems attacked held classified or secret information (Stoll 1990: 233 and *passim*). Indeed, a 1996 report by the US General Accounting Office recently estimated that Pentagon systems had been attacked roughly 250,000 times during 1995, with some 160,000 successful penetrations resulting. The General Accounting Office investigation was brought about by a penetration by a British 16-year old hacker calling himself the 'Datastream Cowboy', acting under the supervision of a figure using the e-mail handle 'Kuji' whom US authorities suspected of being a foreign intelligence officer. Just as with the case of the Hannover Hacker, however, the Pentagon has taken the reports calmly noting that no systems handling classified or secret information has been compromised (Walker 1996). In the event, Kuji and the Datastream Cowboy turned out to be far less sinister than US defence officials expected – two British adolescents determined to find evidence of X-files-reminiscent conspiracies and aliens (Campbell 1997). Curious in all of this, however, is the peculiar combination of one group of US defence information security specialists pursuing a perceived threat to the bitter end while another group write such penetrations off as non-threatening because no 'sensitive compart-mented information' (SCI) has been compromised.

Unfortunately, it is either naive or disingenuous to suggest that non-classified information has no intelligence value. Much of the information compromised in the US defence computers has been logistical, and this alone can be highly revealing about a nation's defence capabilities and intentions.[2] Operationally, cybernetic pene-trations achieved by those such as Marcus Hess and the Datastream Cowboy occupy a grey zone between open sources and covert collection. Much as train watching may be a legitimate, if esoteric, pastime during peace, it has also traditionally been a major field of HUMINT collection monitoring the movements of troops and stores in enemy territory during war (see, for example, Landau 1934 *passim* or Verrier 1983: 188–189). The acquisition of logistical intelligence *becomes* the subject of covert collection as soon as it is locked in office cabinets or placed behind usernames and passwords. Moreover, in many systems, once one is past the front line defences, the data stored there and electronic correspondence traffic is *en claire*. E-mail, especially, represents a potentially rich vein of raw information, in the same league with telephone and postal interception. If nothing else, such non-classified, so-called 'low grade' intelligence can provide an analytical background in the context of which higher grade intelli-gence sources may be interpreted and assessed. Regardless of how one might debate the real intelligence payoff of HACKINT to date, the ability to slip past security protocols and snatch passwords used within a system with sniffer programmes has made the development of 'firewalls', overlaid upon a TCP/IP architecture developed originally to promote wider access rather than constrain it, a growth industry.

With all the discussion of the technical collection methods arising out of the new information technology, it comes, therefore, as something of a surprise that in their book *War and Antiwar*, with its emphasis on high-tech, computer-intensive 'brain force' forms of conflict, Alvin and Heidi Toffler should wheel about and conclude that the prevalent form of intelligence gathering for the 'Third Wave' would be HUMINT. 'The shift to a third wave intelligence system', they propose 'paradoxically, means a stronger emphasis on human spies, the only kind available in the First Wave world. Only now, First Wave spies come armed with sophisticated Third Wave technologies' (Toffler and Toffler 1995: 186). They do not indicate what 'Third Wave' technologies will arm these HUMINT sources, one can only infer that they are referring to improved clandestine communications, since they rule out TECHINT methods. Their reasons are that 'the best satellites can't peer into a terrorist's mind', nor into that of Saddam Hussein. In this sense, the Tofflers are repeating an argument for the virtues of HUMINT which has been in play throughout the increasingly TECHINT-intensive Cold War, which is that satellites can show where an adversary's armies are located, but they cannot tell you what he or she intends to do with them. The Tofflers are also falling in line with a view of the changing priorities of HUMINT and TECHINT which has been propagated by intelligence policy pundits since the end of the Cold War. Briefly put, the small number of large-scale threats presented by the Cold War nuclear stand-off have been replaced by a large number of small-scale threats such as terrorism, local wars and serious crime which while less amenable to imagery and signals intelligence none the less present a very real need for timely and reliable intelligence. As former DCI James Woolsey has observed, the Soviet dragon may have been slain but the global forest is filled with snakes. A number of authors have therefore suggested that intelligence is headed for a new era dependent upon HUMINT to pursue the snakes of the 1980s (Adams 1994: 311–315; Boren 1992: 55–56).

The shift from TECHINT to HUMINT certainly appears compelling if the proliferation of small-scale, distributed intelligence threats after the Cold War is taken out of the context of the growing global infosphere. In February 1996, during a briefing to British academics under the Chatham House rule, a senior UK intelligence officer was asked whether SIGINT had indeed waned in importance as expected. Surprisingly, he responded with a firm denial. 'If anything', he said, 'it is even more important. More terrorists and drug barons are using cellular phones and satellites to talk to each other than ever before.' The lesson here appears to be that the increasing opportunities for technical methods presented by the rapidly expanding, worldwide information infrastructure have more than offset the difficulties of locating and targeting the new threats. Perhaps IMINT may fade in importance, but in its place hacking and communications intelligence are rapidly expanding. During the last decade of the Cold War, the French human source FAREWELL provided documents to the French security service, the *Direction Sécurité Territoriale* (DST) indicating that up to 2.4 per cent of the entire Soviet intelligence effort was taken up by cybernetic penetrations alone (Madsen 1993: 419) – and this in a society with a far lower per capita availability of the necessary hardware and, indeed, skilled operators, than the West, and during a period when cyberspace was a far more radically circumscribed place than it is now. Technical methods produce intelligence *sui generis*; human sources cannot and should not be expected to produce on the same quantitative scale as technical ones. Thus it seems likely that technical methods will remain the large-scale producers, generating the lion's share of the national raw intelligence 'take' for the foreseeable future.

However information technology may be said to 'giveth with one hand, and taketh away with the other', because the same technologies which promise so much to collection may just as easily deny intelligence collectors that wealth. For there is a sting in the tail of the general availability of inexpensive, personal information technology; and that is the general availability of inexpensive, personal information security.

HUMINT vs TECHINT II: of strong encryption and the two-legged spy

It is commonly accepted that HUMINT operations all too often depend upon leads from SIGINT. The wartime double cross depended enormously on the ISOS breaks against German *Abwehr* Enigma traffic, while the VENONA decrypts proved valuable tools in detecting the Soviet atom bomb spies during the opening years of the Cold War. However, what is all too often underestimated is the frequent dependency of TECHINT on initial breaks provided by conventional espionage. Perhaps the most famous, and possibly in global historical terms the most consequential SIGINT breaks ever, were the Allied successes against German, Italian and Japanese Enigma machine codes during the Second World War. While most of the decrypts produced in the Allied cryptanalytical efforts may have relied on mechanical innovations such as multiple, parallel Enigma engines, the so-called 'bombes', and the first generation of computers such as Colossus, the ability to develop these techniques depended initially on a human intelligence coup by the French *Deuxième Bureau* in the form of the clandestine acquisition of detailed drawings of the German Army Enigma provided by walk-in Hans-Thilo Schmidt (Stengers 1984: 127–128). In 1948 Vienna, it was the reports of a human source in the Austrian postal and telecommunications service that alerted the SIS Head of Station to the fact that telephone lines used by Russian forces in the Soviet sector passed under the British sector, leading to the tunnelling operations there and in Berlin during the 1950s (Blake 1990: 8–9). Similarly, Soviet COMINT benefited enormously in the 1970s and early 1980s from the KGB's Walker spy ring providing them with current US Navy keys and other cryptomaterials, while much of their most important information about US satellites came from Andrew Daulton Lee and Christopher Boyce (Andrew and Gordievsky 1990: 437–439, 440–442). In the same fashion, it was Soviet rocketry manuals, provided to the SIS and CIA by Oleg Penkovsky in Soviet Military Intelligence, that helped photo-interpreters identify Soviet missiles in Cuba as well as in the Asian heartland. Because of this interdependency, Britain's SIS has, since the Second World War, maintained a liaison or 'Requirements' Section representing GCHQ, the UK's SIGINT service, at its headquarters circulating intercepts required for SIS operations on the one hand while issuing GCHQ requirements for SIS acquisition of cryptomaterials on the other (Davies 1995). Similarly, the Cold War KGB's foreign operations First Chief Directorate established a separate Sixteenth Department to task *rezidentura* abroad in support of Sixteenth Directorate SIGINT operations (the Sixteenth Department was responsible for sources like the Walker ring and Britain's Geoffrey Prime) (Andrew and Gordievsky, 1990: 440). SIGINT, indeed TECHINT in general, is not a stand-alone collection method, and there are good reasons to believe that HACKINT is likely to be no different from IMINT and SIGINT.

Despite recent successes against DES encryption (Levy 1996: 105–108; Ward 1997b: 19), INFOSEC remains a very real potential limiter in the use of COMINT and HACKINT. The days of negligent sysops leaving factory-issue usernames and passwords in place are fast passing, while at the same time firewall development is a fast-growing industry. Libicki has identified the necessarily *operational* implication of all of this off-handedly, almost by accident.

> Even though many computer systems run with insufficient regard for network security, computer systems can nevertheless be made secure. They can be (*not counting traitors on the inside*), in ways that, say, neither a building nor a tank can be.
>
> (1995)

Although Libicki is undoubtedly overestimating the robustness of INFOSEC techniques, and underestimating the volume of resources which may be directed at a target system by a determined assailant, there can be little doubt that the potential of technical methods against modern information security measures such as 'hacking', intercepting satellite uplink/downlinks and detecting hardware emanations[3] have been likewise exaggerated. Apart from the likelihood that it is far easier to design a computationally intractable encryption algorithm than it is to find a way around that algorithm, there are also very good historical reasons to argue that COMSEC and INFOSEC techniques tend to run ahead of TECHINT, and that technical penetrations tend to require a kick start from less sophisticated intelligence methods. Even with the resources of a national SIGINT service to attack an encrypted system success may prove entirely elusive. Consider the fact that during the Cold War, for ambitious careerist officers within the NSA it was the developing world rather than Soviet bloc divisions that were considered where the real action was. This was because the Soviet machine-based ciphers were almost unassailably strong, and it was more cost-efficient to search the inferior cryptosystems of Soviet bloc satellites in the Third World for Soviet-originated information echoed in their own traffic (Bamford 1983: xx–xxi; Laqueur 1985: 30–31). Similarly, despite the successes of the various Enigma breaks, certain wartime Axis machine codes were *never* broken. Thus although once a system has been penetrated technical methods may produce vast quantities of raw intelligence *sui generis*, the initial break is always a delicate matter, all too often resulting from a human operation. What is said about human sources regarding distributed threats is indeed true: human sources very often can go where technical ones may not – but they are most useful when they make it possible for technical methods to follow.

Information technology makes the kind of information security which drives Libicki's doubts about cybernetic penetrations cheap and readily available. A mathematician-programmer acquaintance of the author once developed a relatively strong eight-digit prime public-key encryption system for his own uses in the mid-1980s, and promptly made that system available in the public domain via a bulletin board system (BBS). Just as it is joked that there is no such thing as a penniless chemistry graduate in Northern Ireland, there is an enormous potential demand for skilled cryptographers in cyberspace, and not always for legitimate national or corporate purposes. There may be various attempts to control strong encryption – it is banned in France, and legally a 'munition' in the United States – such constraints are as likely to be effective in cyberspace as similar attempted blocks on the Internet against the *Big Book of Mischief* or pornography. Indeed, one determined Scandinavian user recently successfully acquired the full *paper* (rather than the actual software) specifications of the non-export version of the Pretty Good Privacy (PGP) encryption software under the constitutional umbrella of freedom of speech (Ward 1997c). Few things are easier to smuggle than information and where export controls may be vigorously enforced, the development of proprietary strong encryption systems, like the early days of programming in general, has all of the possibilities to develop into a fast-growing computer cottage industry in the early twenty-first century. What intelligence and law enforcement policy-makers must accept is that the proliferation of information security technology, like that of nuclear, biological and chemical warfare technologies, is a matter of *when* not *if* (Scallingi 1995).

The upshot of all of this is that just as information technology may indeed have provided a myriad of new opportunities for SIGINT, as well as the emerging field of HACKINT, it has also provided the stuff of countermeasures against SIGINT and HACKINT in the form of readily available and relatively inexpensive encryption. The most readily accessible back door to any secure information network is not some quirk in the code or buried programmer's secret entrance, but the people operating it. Human agents can provide their own passwords to their controllers, upload sniffer programmes to provide their controllers with passwords used by others, or simply access systems themselves, download the data and then pass it on to those controllers. Human sysops can be turned, suborned, influenced or bought outright to provide the keys to their forbidden cybernetic city. Coupled with technical operations such as intercepting satellite streams, tapping the landlines and 'hacking in' from outside – with agent-acquired legitimate protocols to guarantee entry – HUMINT in fact provides precisely the cutting edge

HACKINT and SIGINT are likely to need to continue to be the bulk producer of raw intelligence in a world of 'cheap and cheery' information security.

It is precisely a fear of widespread relatively strong cryptosystems for the masses, criminal or otherwise, which has driven the debate over key-escrow encryption, first in the United States over the ill-fated Clipper Chip, and more recently in Europe, with the UK only recently developing its own programme under the auspices of both GCHQ and the Department of Trade and Industry (Communications Electronics Security Group 1997). The debate in America essentially devolved into two schools of thought based on different articles of faith meeting at loggerheads. On the one hand, libertarians feared increasing encroachment into private communications by government, while on the other side, law enforcement agencies were facing the loss of much of the intelligence and prosecutable evidence that communications intercepts have always provided.[4] By defeating key-escrow legislation, its opponents have in fact created a new problem, and failed to address a no less pernicious problem of civil liberties: denied access to encrypted communications through a law enforcement access field, or keys held by a Trusted Third Party, law enforcement and intelligence agencies will be forced to recruit more and better placed human sources – co-conspirators, accessories, friends, relatives, lovers and spouses. Indeed, as one Canadian national security community official has recently observed, of all the intelligence gathering measures available to domestic intelligence services, the recruitment of human sources is 'one of, if not the, most intrusive means available' (Whitacker 1996: 284–285). A number of Western democracies have had cautionary lessons that they are not immune to overzealous domestic surveillance. The United States, for example, has the legacy of the Hoover years at the FBI and COINTELPRO, while in 1921 the British Secret Service Committee abruptly abolished Basil Thompson's civilian Directorate of Intelligence after only two years of its existence. Their fear was that Thompson's wholesale informant-recruitment in all walks of life was moving towards a 'Continental system of domestic espionage' (Hinsley and Simkins 1991: 6). The recruitment of human sources, moreover, typically does not require the stringent legal controls of judicial or political warrants[5] which are required for communications intercepts or the release of coding keys held in escrow. Thus it is far from clear that in defeating Clipper in America, civil libertarians have, in the long run, struck a blow for or against the civil liberties they strive to protect.

HUMINT vs TECHINT III: special operations and (dis)information warfare

Special operations, or covert action, cover an extremely wide range of tasks. The major covert action functions include: sabotage, in which facilities are destroyed or incapacitated; disinformation, in which false or misleading information is disseminated with an eye to deceiving a target; influence operations, in which propaganda may be disseminated (deceptive or not) or clandestine support may be provided to individuals or groups in a political arena with the intention of skewing the results of a decision or an election in a particular direction; disruptive action, in which 'you set people very discretely against one another'; and special political actions on the scale of engineered coups in which combinations of influence, deception and intelligence are used to overthrow one government and replace it with another.[6] All of these tasks rely on good, comprehensive intelligence from all possible sources, overt as well as covert, to be executed effectively.

The potential of information warfare for special operations has probably been the most major single concern in the literature on the subject. Much has been written and said about the threats from logic bombs and computer viruses which disrupt, corrupt or even physically disable information systems (Arquilla 1998; Arquilla and Ronfeld 1996; Devost *et al.* 1997; Haeni and Hoffman 1996; Johnson 1997; Libicki 1995; Molander *et al.* 1996; Schwartau 1996).[7] A great deal has been made of the *potential* of so-called 'cyberwar', but there is very little evidence that viruses can live up to the hype wrapped around them. To be sure, there have been embarrassing incidents where particularly destructive viruses have been distributed accidentally with brand new 'shrink-wrapped' commercial software, the expensive consequences of the so-called 'Internet worm', and in Israel in 1988 a virus was discovered designed to prompt infected programmes to erase all of their files on May 13 of that year, that is, the fortieth anniversary of the 'demise of Palestine' (Kupperman 1991: 92). As pointed out by Kupperman, this latter device was, however, little more than a 'weapon of political protest', and the potential impact of individual viruses appears to amount to little more than the cybernetic equivalent of blowing trains up in the Resistance.

The analogy between destructive information technologies and wartime sabotage goes considerably further than just individual actions behind enemy lines. During the Second World War, the sabotage measures undertaken by the European Resistance movements in conjunction with the Allied secret services, in particular the British Special Operations Executive (SOE) and the American Office of Strategic Services (OSS) were closely coordinated to act in support of overt, strategic actions. This was most strikingly so in the case of French groups mobilized in conjunction with the D Day landings in June 1944, attacking German lines of communication and logistical support (see, for example, Stafford 1983: 128). Likewise, it would seem most effective to combine cyber-sabotage with other political action methods at a theatre or campaign level. There is a general sentiment that this has yet to happen, and much of the literature deals in 'scenarios' and 'simulations'. However, there is good reason to believe that such an information campaign *has already occurred* in the context of a larger disinformation offensive – during the Cold War.

One fact which the literature on the USSR's disinformation and disruptive actions has not taken into account is that by the end of the Cold War the USSR and its Soviet bloc were the world's largest single source of computer viruses. Of the viruses of known origin (371 types, not including variants; of unknown origin 344), 124 originated in the Soviet bloc (USSR/Russia and Eastern Europe). That is, of the viruses of known origin in circulation, 33.4 per cent of them originated from the Soviet Union and Eastern Europe. Within the Soviet bloc, the USSR was the largest single source, followed closely by Bulgaria and then Poland.[8] This is despite the fact that the USSR had a considerably lower per capita availability of computer facilities than Bulgaria, let alone the Western states (Bontchev 1995). Although there is no conclusive evidence tying the KGB or GRU to the computer-virus explosion at the end of the Cold War, these figures are none the less highly suggestive. Even if the heavy percentage of Soviet bloc originated viruses does indeed represent a coordinated effort rather than being, as Vasselin Bontchev has suggested of the Bulgarian viruses, simply the result of a small number of mischievous or vindictive individual programmers (Bontchev 1995), the fact remains that the presence and wide distribution of viruses throughout the second half of the 1980s amounted to little more than a background noise of nuisance value. The disruptive possibilities of cyber-sabotage may be a genuine cause for some concern, but like the efforts of SOE and the OSS and the various European Resistance movements in 1944, they are unlikely to be an unambiguous war winner, and like the viruses and bacterial munitions of biological warfare there is a very real risk of blow-back.[9]

Another potential of modern information technology for deceptive, disruptive and political actions lies in the Internet as a means of disseminating information – or rather, disinformation. As noted above, much of the data and communications traffic travelling behind the world's firewalls and passwords is *en claire*, and politically useful information is not always Top Secret with a codeword. That background hum of electronic correspondence which can all too easily reveal the jealousies and coalitions that drive the organizational politics of a target group or community can be at least as useful in acting against them as the details of their latest and most secret operational plans. As former SIS officer Baroness Daphne Park observed in 1993 about disruptive action

> Once you get really good inside intelligence about any group you are able to learn where the levers of power are, and what one man fears of another ... you set people discretely against one another ... They destroy each other, we don't destroy them.
>
> (BBC 1993)

This is done, she suggests by way of example, by circulating deceptive information about members or groups within the target group which exploit and exacerbate pre-existing divisions. The same strategy was pursued by the Soviet Union in its 'active measures' disinformation and propaganda campaign during the Cold War by making US and NATO strategy appear threatening to the lives and welfare of Western citizens. This ranged from using various shades of propaganda to suggest that policies such as the Strategic Defence Initiative ('Star Wars') was a direct threat to the survival of Western civilians by increasing the risks of a nuclear conflict (Heather 1987) to fraudulent claims and evidence that US bio-warfare research had led to the creation and release of the Human Immunodeficiency Virus (Andrew and Gordievsky, 1990: 529–530). The rich stream of e-mail and newsgroup traffic within organizations and communities is an ideal medium from which to glean those divisions and hostilities which disruptive action might exploit. The next problem is to generate plausible deceptive materials and then to disseminate them, and in both cases the 'information superhighway' provides a highly promising medium.

There are two main problems to be overcome in circulating disinformation, either as part of a specific disruptive action or as part of a pervasive 'active measures' style campaign: first, getting the disinformation to the people you want to influence, and second, ensuring that information's credibility will be sufficient to convince them. The Internet has vast potential for the first of these problems, but presents real problems in terms of the second. To be sure, it is a communications system with global coverage, and the costs of distributing information over the Internet are negligible compared with the breadth of resulting distribution, especially when compared to alternative means. On top of this, digital information production and storage also opens up previously unmatched opportunities for the falsification of information. As has already been noted in the RAND report:

> Political action groups and other nongovernmental organisations can utilise the Internet to galvanise political support ... Further, the possibility arises that the very 'facts' can be manipulated by multimedia techniques and widely disseminated.
>
> (Schoben 1995)

There have been recent, and telling examples of this kind of action, of which perhaps the most significant were the Malaysian riots that never happened. In this case, a handful of individuals circulated false reports of riots by Indonesian guest workers in the Chow Kit district of Kuala Lumpur by e-mail, reports which circulated faster than they could be countered (*New Straits Times* 1998), and led to a very real heightening of tensions in a country already shaken by the shooting of illegal Acinese immigrants a few months before.

The very opportunities offered by the Internet are, however, its weaknesses. The very ease of dissemination by any group or interest, however ill-informed or extremist, and the very ease of multimedia misrepresentation and digital forgery can potentially make information acquired on the Internet a debased currency. Even in the scientific community, the reliability of scientific data available on the Internet has come into doubt, with one survey of Internet-using research professionals noting that such information was often flawed because:

- units are frequently omitted
- transcription errors often encountered
- this leads to a need to find redundant data
- very few sources have quality assurance statements
- few of the web data sites give the source of the data
- if they do, data are likely to be copied from outdated sources

(Wiggins 1996)

Given the limited credibility of materials available on the Internet, disinformation distributed by World Wide Web or by e-mail would have to be supported by firm *non-Internet* sources to be able to achieve and maintain the kind of credibility that an effective deceptive action requires. Thus the use of cyberspace as a medium of disinformation would be most profitably exploited in combination with other, more conventional human and technical methods.

Conclusion: HUMINT, TECHINT and the future of intelligence

It is, therefore, apparent that while technical methods, in particular SIGINT and HACKINT, are likely to be the large-scale providers of national intelligence 'take' for the foreseeable future, this will have to be in the context of a far closer integration with HUMINT. The twin trends of proliferating, small-scale but, as Bruce Hoffman has argued, disproportionately destructive, intelligence targets (e.g. terrorism, proliferation, transnational crime (Hoffman 1996) and a logarithmi-cally expanding global 'infosphere' (information superhighway, cyberspace, call it what you will) mean that no simple, straight-line shift from TECHINT back to HUMINT nor a continuation of TECHINT's Cold War prevalence provides a plausible picture of intelligence gathering in the next century. As argued above, HUMINT's capacity to work around the 'cheap and cheery' INFOSEC systems increasingly available to terrorists, illegal arms dealers and drug barons can provide precisely the window of opportunity for communications intercepts and cybernetic penetrations to continue to act as the main bulk, raw intelligence producers. However, no matter how much one falls back onto HUMINT, analysts and policy-makers have always and will always prefer information from technical sources (Laqueur 1985: 31). Nevertheless, human sources are likely to prove a vital point of entry past the 'cheap and cheery' information security of the 1990s, a HUMINT vanguard finding a path that the more powerful technical sources can follow. What must be kept in mind is that HUMINT operations have very real and often underestimated civil liberties implications in the context of domestic criminal and counter-intelligence.

No one class of source can be a panacea for intelligence needs in the coming decades. As a result, the issue in allocating intelligence resources in the 1990s and the 2000s is not an either/or of technical versus human methods (indeed, it has never really been so) but how to use them in conjunction with a greater degree of unity, of common targeting and coordination, than has previously been the case.

Notes

1   As a general rule in British literature, the assorted '-ints' are considered something of an American affectation, although their convenience (but not, perhaps, their clarity) has led to a more general usage in the field. The term TECHINT derives from *technical intelligence*, and refers to any source of information derived from technical or mechanical means – which virtually amounts to anything not actually constituting a living human source. As noted above, TECHINT can be very loosely be divided into SIGINT, or *signals* intelligence, and IMINT or *imagery* intelligence. Within IMINT lie PHOTINT, or *photographic* intelligence and 'multi-spectral scanning' (MSS) which employs infrared and microwave imagery as well as visual wavelengths. SIGINT in turn sub-divides into COMINT, or *communications* intelligence (e.g. telecommunications intercepts), and ELINT or *electronic* intelligence which studies non-communicative emissions such as aircraft radars or missile telemetry. In the following discussion I have, for lack of a better alternative, employed the term HACKINT for intelligence gathered from *clandestine*, network-based computer access as compared with what is sometimes called 'Network Based Open-Systems' intelligence or NOSINT, as popularized by figures like Robert Steele of Open Systems Solutions, which relies on overt access to Internet information from open sources (some of the limitations of which are addressed in the discussion of disinformation operations). For good, standard discussions of the various 'int' categories see, for example, Michael Herman (1996), Avram Shulsky (1989), Jeffrey T. Richelson (1989), and Laqueur (1985).

2   A number of commentators have noted this. Clifford Stoll (1990) remarks upon this, as have journalists such as Walker (1996). Acknowledgements also to James Norminton who made this point regarding an earlier version of this chapter.

3   Hardware emanations remain one of the least discussed aspects of information security, while at the same time representing one of the most substantial single points of vulnerability in the current information infrastructure. Although the vulnerability of cathode ray tube (CRT) emissions is reasonably well known (hence the fact that one's password is not echoed verbatim on a computer screen as is one's username), the fact is that central processors generate a very considerable electromagnetic field which can be intercepted and interpreted. NATO standards for electromagnetic insulating of information systems is referred to as TEMPESTing, but effective TEMPESTing is expensive and most organizations do not bother with this feature, even if they spend a great deal on encryption and firewall services. A brief discussion of this risk appears in Schwartau (1996: 221–231), and an embarrassing account of ineffective TEMPESTing on CIA-recommended Wang desktop computers recommended to the SIS by the CIA appears in Urban (1996: 256).

4   By comparison, debate in Britain over the TTP Key Escrow proposals issued jointly by GCHQ's Communications Electronics Security Group and the Department of Trade and Industry have tended to focus not on civil liberties but on the feasibility and potential inefficiencies of the plan. See, for example, the CESG homepage (CESG 1997), and the DTI's 'Licensing of Trusted Third Parties for the Provision of Encryption

Services' (DTI: 1997). A survey of the issue has also appeared in (Ward 1997a.)

5 In Britain's 1985 Interception of Communications Act, the 1989 Security Service Act and the 1994 Intelligence Services Act, communications intercepts *all* require warrants 'signed by the Secretary of State', which in British political parlance means whichever Cabinet Minister whose jurisdiction covers the location of the intercept e.g. the Home Secretary within 'the British Islands' and the Foreign Secretary abroad. British warranting procedures were subject to some criticism in the *1995 Annual Report of the Security Commissioner* (1995), in which it was noted that while the Intelligence and Security Services are subject to the legal strictures of the 1985 IOCA, 1989 SSA and the 1994 ISA, police communication intercepts are only covered by the non-statutory 1984 Guidelines. Reg Whitacker also notes that Federal Canadian reviews of intelligence have proven consistently resistant to extending the practice of judicial warrants from communications intercepts to human source recruitment (1996: 286). Human source selection in Canada is handled by an interdepartmental Targeting Approval and Review Committee (TARC), while all MI5 operations, human or otherwise, require clearance by the Security Service Legal Adviser, and SIS operations need clearance from the SIS Foreign Office Adviser.

6 By way of some degree of complication, both sides of the Atlantic tend to use different jargon, as well as making fine distinctions within the field. Most critically, there is a clear distinction between what the SIS calls *special political actions* and the CIA terms *covert action*, both of which are strictly *political*, and *special operations* (employed by both) to denote actions which involve paramilitary action. In the CIA, this involved two distinct Divisions within the Directorate of Operations, Covert Action and International Activities (formerly Special Operations) (Richelson 1989: 16–17). The equivalent sections of the SIS were defunct by the mid-1970s, with such actions being handled at a geographical rather than central level, and in liaison with either the Foreign and Commonwealth Office or the Ministry of Defence (private information).

7 There is a particular fascination throughout this literature with the issue of terrorism, or of smaller powers clandestinely disrupting the United States military machine and 'critical national infrastructure'. Arquilla's recent piece in *Wired* (1998) deals with the danger of what are known in intelligence circles as 'false-flag' operations by extremist groups, with Devost *et al.* (1997) being explicitly and centrally concerned with terrorism. By comparison, Schwartau's (1996) often alarmist style depends heavily on the idiosyncratic and vaguely melodramatic notion of the 'information warrior', a non-specific creature composed in various parts of terrorist, vandal and opportunist. Although Schwartau provides an informative blow-by-blow description of exactly how information security can be compromised and that often on his own practical experience, for the most part much of the literature depends heavily on disturbing, often worst-case 'scenarios' and simulation exercises of the RAND variety. L. Scott Johnson's article is of considerable interest since it appeared in the semi-annual, unclassified version of the CIA's in-house intelligence studies journal *Studies in Intelligence*. However, Johnson's 1997 discussion

is really yet another threat-assessment of information warfare, rather than any analysis of the role of information warfare and ICTs in intelligence policy and infrastructure. Much the same sentiment is developed in DCI John Deutch's briefing to the US Senate, excerpted in Schwartau (1996: 458–459).

8   These data are drawn from the F-Prot virus descriptions database at http://www.datafellows.fi/ in Iceland in August, 1995. As noted, almost half of the total number of viruses in circulation are of unknown origin. It should also be noted that a small number of the viruses in circulation originated after the Cold War, such as 3APA3A which was found on a University system in Moscow in 1994. It should also be noted that the 1995 version of the F-Prot database distinguished between post-Cold War Federal Russia and the USSR.

9   This is not necessarily a universal risk. China, for example, has concentrated on developing its information infrastructure on the basis of a highly isolated 'Intranet' programme, rather than the open access adopted by most of the rest of the world, providing them with a potential national bunker in cyberspace from which to conduct information warfare on their neighbours or an inconvenient West with near impugnity (Davies 1998).

Bibliography

Adams, James (1994) *The New Spies: Exploring the Frontiers of Espionage* London: Hutchinson

Agreement on Trade-Related Aspects of Intellectual Property Rights (TRIPs), a part of the General Agreement on Tariffs and Trade (GATT) (1994) 33 ILM 1,197–1,225

Ahvenainen, A. (1998) 'Views on IW', SMI Information Warfare Conference, London, 26–27 March

Akdeniz, Y. (1999) 'Regulation of Child Pornography on the Internet', http://www.cyber-rights.org/reports/child.htm (May 1999)

Alberts, D. and Czerwinski, T.J. (eds) (1997) *Complexity, Global Politics and National Security* Washington DC: National Defense University

Altschull, T.H. (1995) *Agents of Power* New York: Longman

Anderson, R., Needham, R. and Shamir, A. (1998) 'The Steganographic File System', presented at the Workshop on Information Hiding, Portland, OR, April 14–17

Andrew, Christopher and Gordievsky, Oleg (1990) *KGB: The Inside Story of Its Foreign Operations* London: Hodder and Stoughton

Ang, I. (1996) *Living Room Wars: Rethinking Media Audiences for a Postmodern World* London: Routledge

Anon. (1999) 'Vozmezdie dlya hackera' ('Revenge to a Hacker') *Computerworld Russia* no. 7 (in Russian)

Antisemitism on the Internet: A Legal Analysis And Proposals For Action (Draft) (1998) London: Denton Hall for the Inter-Parliamentary Council Against Antisemitism

Arquilla, John (1998) 'The Great Cyberwar of 2002', *Wired* 6 (2) (February)

Arquilla, John and Ronfeldt, David (1996) 'Cyberwar is Coming', http://stl.nps.navy.mil/~jmorale/cyberwar.html (15 January 1996)

—— (1997a) 'Cyberwar is Coming', in J. Arquilla and D. Ronfeldt (eds) *In Athena's Camp: Preparing for Conflict in the Information Age* Santa Monica: RAND, pp. 23–60

—— (1997b) 'Information, Power, And Grand Strategy', in J. Arquilla and D. Ronfeldt (eds) *In Athena's Camp: Preparing for Conflict in the Information Age* Santa Monica: RAND, pp. 141–171

Ashcroft, A. (1998) 'NF: Marching along the Information Super-Highway', *The Nationalist* October, London 2: 4

Back, L., Keith, M. and Solomos, J. (1996) 'Techology, Race and Neo-Fascism in a Digital Age: The New Modalities of Racist Culture', *Patterns of Prejudice* 30 (2), JPR, London

—— (1998) 'Racism on the Internet: Mapping neo-Fascist Subcultures in Cyberspace', in J. Kaplan and T. Bjorgos (eds) *Nation And Race – The Developing Euro-American Racist Subculture* Northeastern University Press: Boston

Bainbridge, David (1996) *EC Data Protection Directive* London: Butterworth

Bamford, James (1983) *The Puzzle Palace* London: Sidgwick and Jackson

Bangemann, M. (1994) 'Europe and the Global Information Society, Recommendations to the European Council', 26 May 1994, Brussels (*Bangemann Report*) http://www.earn.net/EC/bangemann.html

Bannister, J., Fyffe, N.R. and Kearns, A. (1988) 'Closed Circuit Television and the City', in Clive Norris, Jade Moran and G. Armstrong (eds) *Surveillance, CCTV and Social Control* (in press)

Baturin, Y. (1987) *Pravo i politika v kompiuternom kruge. (Law and Politics: Computer Aspects)* Moscow: Nauka Publ. (in Russian)

BBC (1993) 'On Her Majesty's Secret Service', *Panorama* BBC Television, 22 November

Bennett, C. (1997) 'Convergence Revisited: Toward a Global Policy for Protection of Personal Data?', in P. Agre and M. Rotenberg (eds) *Technology and Privacy: the New Landscape* MIT Press, pp. 99–124

Bennett, Colin (1992) *Regulating Privacy* Ithaca, NY and London: Cornell University Press

Bennett, Trevor (1990) *Evaluating Neighbourhood Watch* Aldershot: Gower Publishing Company Limited

—— (1994) 'Recent Developments in Community Policing', in M. Stephens and S. Becker *Police Force, Police Service: Care and Control in the Community* London: Macmillan

Benyon, John, Turnbull, Lynne, Willis, Andrew, Woodward, Rachel and Beck, Adrian (1993) *Police Co-operation in Europe: An Investigation* University of Leicester: Centre for the Study of Public Order

Berko, L. (1992) 'Surveying the Surveilled: Video, Space and Subjectivity', *Quarterly Review of Film and Video* 14 (1–2): 61–91

Blake, George (1990) *No Other Choice* London: Jonathan Cape

Blank, S. (1997) 'Preparing for the Next War: Reflections on the Revolution in Military Affairs', in J. Arquilla and D. Ronfeldt (eds) *In Athena's Camp: Preparing for Conflict in the Information Age* Santa Monica: RAND, pp. 61–77

Bloombecker, J. (1993) *Computer Crime Laws* New York: Clark Boardman Callaghan

Blume, Peter (1996) *Personregistrering* third edition, Copenhagen: Akademisk Forlag

—— (1997) 'Privacy as a Theoretical and Practical Concept', *International Review of Law Computers and Technology* 11: 193–202

Bontchev, Vasselin (1995) 'The Bulgarian Virus Factories', http: – HYPERLINK http://www.einet.net/galaxy/Engineering-and-Technology/ Computer – http://www.einet.net/galaxy/Engineering-and-Technology/ Computer – Technology/Security/david-hull/bulgfact.html (20 December 1995)

Boodhoo, N. (1999) 'NATO gets Spammed. Yugoslav Users Disrupt Alliance's Web Site', URL: http://www.pcworld.com/pcwtoday/article/ 0,1510,10358,00.html (23 April 1999)

Boren, David L. (1992) 'The Intelligence Community: How Crucial?' in *Foreign Affairs* (Summer)

Boyan, J. (1997) 'The Anonymizer: Protecting User Privacy on the Web', *Computer-Mediated Communication Magazine* http://www.december.com/ cmc/mag/1997/mag/1997/boyan.html

Brandeis, L. and Warren, S. (1890–91) 'The Right to Privacy', *Harvard Law Review* 4: 193–220

Brunnstein, K., Fischer-Hübner, S. and Schaar, P. (1998) 'Verbraucherbefragung und globale Informationsgesellschaft', in *Computer und Recht aktuell* February, Verlag Dr. Otto Schmidt, pp. 125–126

Brunnstein, K. and Schier, K. (1997) 'Global Digital Commerce: Impacts and Risks for Developments of Global Information Societies', in J. Berleur and Diane Whitehouse (eds) 'An Ethical Global Information Society: Culture and Democracy Revisited', *Proceedings of the IFIP WG 9.2 Corfu International Conference* May 8–10, 1997, Chapman and Hall, pp. 75–82

Budapest Draft (1996) 'International Working Group on Data Protection in Telecommunications', *Data Protection on the Internet, Report and Guidance* (Budapest Draft) http://jilt.law.strath.ac.uk/jilt/consult/iwgdp/ default.htm

Bureau for International Narcotics and Law Enforcement Affairs (1998) *International Narcotics Control Strategy Report (1997)* US Department of State, March at http://www.state.gov/www/global/narcotics_law/1997_ narc_report/index.html

Burroughs, W. (1998a) *Bilet, kotoryi lopnul. Nova express (The Ticket that Exploded. Nova Express)* Kiev: Nika-Tsentr Publ. (in Russian)

—— (1998b) *Golyj zavtrak. (The Naked Lunch)* Moscow: Glagol. (in Russian)

—— (1999) *Myagkaya mashina. (The Soft Machine)* St Petersburg: Azbuka Publ. and Amphora Publ. (in Russian)

Campbell, Douglas (1997) 'More Naked Gun than Top Gun', in *The Guardian* (London) 26 November

Campbell, M. (1998) 'Britain Fights US in Cyber Wargame', *Sunday Times* 7 June

Canada (1995) 'Connection Community Content: The Challenge of the Information Highway', *Final Report of the Canadian Information Highway Advisory Council* September 1995

Capitanchik, D. and Whine, M. (1998) 'Harmful Content on the Internet', *Report for the Intergovernmental Committee* Council of Europe, 24 November

Carrabine, Eamonn (1998) 'The Industry of Prison Control: Power,

Governmentality and Discourse', Institute for Social Research and Department of Sociology, University of Salford

Castells, M. (1996) 'The Information Age: Economy, Society and Culture', Vol. I, *The Rise of the Network Society* Oxford: Blackwell

—— (1998) 'The Information Age: Economy, Society and Culture', Vol. III, *End of Millennium* Oxford: Blackwell

CC (Common Criteria Editorial Board) (1999) 'Common Criteria for Information Technology Security Evaluation', Version 2, August 1999

Chaum, D. (1981) 'Untraceable Electronic Mail, Return Addresses, and Digital Pseudonyms', *Communications of the ACM* 24 (2): 84–88

—— (1985) 'Security Without Identification: Transaction Systems to Make Big Brother Obsolete', *Communications of the ACM* 28 (10): 1,030–1,044

—— (1992) 'Achieving Electronic Privacy', *Scientific American* 8: 76–81

Cisco Systems Inc. (1998) 'Thirteen High-Tech Leaders Support Alternative Solution to Network Encryption Stalemate', press release, July 13

Clarke, Paul, B. (1994) *Citizenship* London: Pluto Press

—— (1996) *Deep Citizenship* London: Pluto Press

Clarke, R. (1996) 'Crypto-Confusion: Mutual Non-comprehension Threatens GII', *Privacy Law and Policy Reporter* 3: 30–33

Clinton, W. (1998) 'Clinton Outlines Cyberthreat Plan', *CNET Newscom* May 22

Cohen, S. (1988) *Visions of Social Control* Cambridge: Polity Press

Coleman, A. (1992) *The Legal Protection of Trade Secrets* London: Sweet and Maxwell

Coleman, R. (1998) 'Surveillance: The Proper Objects of Power and the Regenerated Urban Centre', paper presented at Surveillance: An Interdisciplinary Conference, John Moores University, Liverpool, 6 June

Coleman, Roy and Sim, Joe (1996) 'From the Dockyards to the Disney Store: Surveillance, Risk and Security in Liverpool City Centre', paper presented to the Law and Society Association Conference, University of Strathclyde, July 1996

Colligan, Douglas (Oct./Nov. 1982) 'The Intruder – A biography of Cheshire Catalyst', *Technology Illustrated* http://www.dsl.org/m/doc/arc/nws/cheshire.phk

(CESG) Communications Electronics Security Group (1997) http://www.cesg.gov.uk (5 August 1997)

Conley, Verena (ed.) (1993) *Rethinking Technologies* Minneapolis: University of Minnesota Press

Corcoran, E. (1998) 'Breakthrough Possible in Battle over Encryption Technology', *Washington Post* July 12, p. A8

Corley, Paul (1998) 'ITV's Friend in the North', *Televisual* April: 86

Cottrell, L. (1997) 'Mixmaster and Remailer Attacks', http://www.obscura.com/~loki/remailer/remailer-essay.html

Coupland, Douglas. (1995) *Microserfs* London: Flamingo

CSI (1997) 'Can Your Crypto be Turned Against You? An Interview with Eric Thompson of AccessData', *Computer Security Alert* no. 167, February

Czerwinski, T. (1998) *Coping with the Bounds: Speculations on Nonlinearity in Military Affairs* Washington DC: National Defense University

Dahlgren, Peter (1995) *Television and the Public Sphere: Citizenship, Democracy and the Media* London: Sage

Davies, Philip H.J. (1995) 'Organisational Politics and the Development of Britain's Intelligence Producer/Consumer Interface', *Intelligence and National Security* 10 (4) (October)

—— (1998) 'Infowar, Infosec and Asian Security', in *Asian Defence and Diplomacy* 4 (9) (September)

Davies, S. (1996) *Big Brother: Britain's Web of Surveillance and the New Technological Order* London: Pan Books

Demchenko, V. (1998) 'Zhadnost' hackerov sgubila' ('Greediness Ruined Hackers') *Izvestia* 23 September (in Russian) http://www.cyberpolice.ru/press/0923.html (23 September 1998)

Denning, D.E. and Baugh, W.E., Jr (1997) 'Encryption and Evolving Technologies as Tools of Organized Crime and Terrorism', National Strategy Information Center, Washington DC, July

(DTI) Department of Trade and Industry (1997) 'Licencing of Trusted Third Parties for the Provision of Encryption Services', http://dtiinfo1.dti.gov.uk/pubs/ (5 August)

DERA (1998) 'Cyber Terrorist Threats to the UK', *Conference on Britain and the Revolution in Military Affairs* University of Hull, 25–26 June

Der Derian, James (1994) 'Cyber-Deterrence', *Wired* (September)

Derrida, J. (1981) 'Plato's Pharmacy', in *Dissemination* trans. B. Johnson, London: Athlone Press

De Santis, H. (1998) *Combating Hate On The Internet: An International Comparative Review Of Policy Approaches* Quebec: Multiculturalism Program, Department of Canadian Heritage

Devost, Matthew, Houghton, Brian and Pollard, Neal (1997) 'Information Terrorism: Political Violence in an Information Age', in *Terrorism and Political Violence* 9 (1) (Spring)

Diederich, T. (1999) 'NATO Web Site Hit by Yugoslav Hackers', http://www.computerworld.com/home/news:nsf/all/9904014nato (25 April 1999)

Diffie, Whitfield, Landau, Susan (1998) *Privacy on the Line: The Politics of Wiretapping and Encryption* Cambridge, Mass: MIP Press

Dorril, S. (1999) 'No more James Bond?', *The Observer* 16 May 1999

Dougherty, J. (1999) 'Computer Hacking in Russia Cheap and Widespread. Trail of Pentagon Computer Attack Leads to Russia', *CNN* (in collaboration with Reuters) http://cnn.com/WORLD/europe/9903/05/russia.hackers/index.html (28 April 1999)

DPA annual report 1990, 1992, 1993, Copenhagen: Registertilsynet

Dreyfus, Herbert, L. and Rabinow, Paul (1982) *Michel Foucault: Beyond Structuralism and Hermeneutics* Chicago: Harvester Wheatsheaf

DSTI/ICCP/AH(90)21/REV6 (1997a) *Preamble, Recommendation of the Council Concerning Guidelines for Cryptography Policy*

—— (1997b) *News Release: OECD Adopts Guidelines for Cryptography Policy* 27 March

—— (1997c) *Guidelines for Cryptography Policy*

—— (1998a) *Review of the 1992 Guidelines for the Security of Information Systems* DSTI/ICCP/REG(97)2

—— (1998b) *Inventory of Controls on Cryptographic Technologies* DSTI/ICCP/REG(98)4/FINAL

Eatwell, R. (1996) 'Surfing the Great White Wave: The Internet Extremism and the Problem of Control', *Patterns of Prejudice* 30 (1), JPR, London

EEF (1998) ' "EFF DES Cracker" Machine Brings Honesty to Crypto Debate', press announcement from the Electronic Frontier Foundation, July 17.

EFGA 'Electronic Frontiers Georgia, Reliable Remailer List', http://anon. efga.org/anon/remailers

Emmett, P., Corcoran, M., Ferbrache, D. and Macintosh, J. (1997) 'An Analysis of the Military and Policy Context of Information Warfare' *DERA Report* CIS3/58/8/5, June

EPIC Electronic Privacy Information Center (1997) 'Surfer Beware: Personal Privacy and the Internet', June 1997, http://www.epic.org/reports/surfer-beware.html

Ericson, R.V, Baranek, B.M. and Chan, J.B.L. (1989) *Negotiating Control: A Study of News Sources* Milton Keynes: Open University Press

ERRI (1997) 'Columbian Officials Uncover Drug Cartel Communications Center', http://www.emergency.com (31 May 1997)

EU Directive (1995) Directive 95/46/EC of the European Parliament and of the Council of 24 October 1995, 'On the Protection of Individuals with Regard to the Processing of Personal Data and on the Free Movement of such Data', http://www2.echo.lu/legal/en/dataprot/directiv/directiv.html

European Commission (1997) *Towards a European Framework for Digital Signatures and Encryption* Com(97)503

Evers, S. (1997) 'Pentagon wants NSA to build "threat" database', *Jane's Defence Weekly* 29 October: 11

Farrell, T. (1996) 'Figuring Out Fighting Organisations: The New Organisational Analysis in Strategic Studies', *Journal of Strategic Studies* 19 (1): 122–135

FBI Law Enforcement Bulletin (1970) 'Crime and Cryptology', April: 13–14

Federal Economic Espionage Act (1996) *Title 18, Part 1, Chapter 90*

Fine, D. (1995) 'Why is Kevin Lee Poulsen Really in Jail?', http://www.com/user/fine/journalism/jail.html

Fischer, C. (1998) Presentation at Georgetown University Executive Leadership Seminar, 'Strategic Approaches to Transnational Crime and Civil Society', July 22

Fischer-Hübner, S. (1994) 'Towards a Privacy-Friendly Design and Use of IT-Security Mechanisms', *Proceedings of the 17th National Computer Security Conference* Baltimore, October 1994: 142–152

—— (1997) 'Privacy at Risk in the Global Information Society', in J. Berleur and Diane Whitehouse (eds) 'An Ethical Global Information Society: Culture and Democracy Revisited', *Proceedings of the IFIP WG 9.2 Corfu International Conference* May 8–10, 1997: 261–274

Fiske, John (1987) *Television Culture* London: Methuen

Fitzgerald, M. (1997) 'Russian Views on Electronic and Information Warfare', *Proceedings of the 3rd International Command and Control Research and Technology Symposium* Washington DC: National Defense University, pp. 126–163

Flaherty, David H. (1989) *Protecting Privacy in Surveillance Societies* Chapel Hill and London: University of North Carolina Press

FOA (1997) *Swedish-European Workshop on Information Warfare and National and International Security Challenges in the Information Age* organized by FOA, Sweden 4–26 September

Foucault, M. (1978) *The History of Sexuality: Volume I* trans. R. Hurley, New York: Pantheon

—— (1995) *Discipline and Punish: The Birth of the Prison* trans. A. Sheridan, New York: Vintage Books

Franklin, Bob (1997) *Newszak and News Media* London: Edward Arnold

Freedman, L. (1998) *The Revolution in Strategic Affairs* Adelphi Paper 318, London: ISS

Gallagher, N. (1998) 'Cybercrime, Transnational Crime and Intellectual Property', Congressional Statement, FBI, http://www.fbi.gov/pressrm/congress98/gallagher.htm

Gandy, Oscar (1993) *The Panoptic Sort: A Political Economy of Personal Information* San Francisco/Oxford: Westview Press

Garfinkel, S. and Spafford, G. (1997) *Web Security and Commerce* O'Reilly and Associates Inc.

Gass, N. and Romet, T. (1998) 'A Framework for Modelling the Threat of Information Operations and the Infrastructure of a Country', in A. Campen and D. Dearth, *Cyberwar 2* Fairfax, VA: AFCEA, pp. 345–358

Gearty, C. and Ewing, K. (1997) 'History of a Dog's Dinner: The Police Bill', *London Review of Books* 6 February: 7–10

Gibson, W. (1984) *Neuromancer* New York: Ace Books

—— (1985) *Neuromancer* London: HarperCollins.

—— (1986) *Burning Chrome* London: HarperCollins

—— (1987) *Count Zero* New York: Ace

Gilboa, N. (1994) 'Interview with Chris Goggans at Pumpcon, 1993', *Gray Areas* Fall 1994

Gillard, Michael, S and Flynn, Laurie (1998) 'How Millions were Fooled', *The Guardian* 9 June

Global Internet Liberty Campaign (1998) 'Media Release: GILC Releases Crypto Survey', http://www.eff.org/ (9 February 1998)

Golding, Peter (1990) 'Political Communication and Citizenship: The Media and Democracy in an Inegalitarian Social Order', in M. Ferguson (ed.) *Public Communication: The New Imperatives* London: Sage

Goldschlag, D., Reed, M. and Syverson, P. (1999) 'Onion Routing for

Anonymous and Private Internet Connections', *Communications of the ACM* 42 (2): 39–41

Grabosky, P.N. and Smith, R.G. (1998) *Crime in the Digital Age: Controlling Telecommunications and Cyberspace Illegalities* Transaction Publ.

Graham, Stephen (1998) 'Towards the Fifth Utility? On the Extension and Normalisation of Public CCTV', in C. Norris, C. Moran and G. Armstrong *Surveillance, CCTV and Social Control* (in press)

Gray, C. (1986) *Nuclear Strategy and National Style* London: Hamilton Press

Greenfeld, Karl Taro. (1993) 'The Incredibly Strange Mutant Creatures Who Rule the Universe of Alienated Japanese Zombie Computer Nerds (Otaku to You)', http://www.eff.org/pub/Net_culture/Cyberpunk/otaku.article

Greenleaf, G. (1995) 'The 1995 EU Directive on Data Protection – An Overview', *The International Privacy Bulletin* published by Privacy International, 3 (2)

Grusho, A. and Timonina, E. (1996) *Teoreticheskie osnovy zaschity informatsii (Theoretical foundations of information security)* Moscow: Yakhtsmen Publ.

Habermas, Jürgen (1989/1962) *Structural Transformations of the Public Sphere* Cambridge: Polity Press

Haeni, Reto E. and Hoffman, Lance J. (1996) 'An Introduction to Information Warfare', http://www.seas.gwu.edu/student/reto/infowar/info-war.html (15 January)

Hafner, K. and Markoff, J. (1991) *Cyberpunk: Outlaws and Hackers on the Computer Frontier* New York: Simon and Schuster

Hall, S. (1974) 'The Television Discourse – Encoding and Decoding', *Education and Culture* 25, UNESCO

Halligan, M. (1996) 'The Theft of Trade Secrets is Now a Federal Crime', http://www.execpc.com/~mhallign/unfair.html (30 November)

Hardy, Forsyth (1979) *Grierson on Documentary* London: Faber

Hawn, Matthew. (1996) 'Fear of a Hack Planet: The Strange Metamorphosis of the Computer Hacker', http://www.zdtv.com/0796w3/worl/worl54_071596.html

Heather, Randall W. (1987) 'SDI and Soviet Active Measures', *Mackenzie Paper No. 14* Toronto: Mackenzie Insitute

Herman, M. (1996) *Intelligence Power in Peace and War* Cambridge: Cambridge University Press

Hinsley, F.H. and Simkins, C.A.G. (1991) *British Intelligence in the Second World War Vol. IV: Counter-Espionage and Security* London: HMSO

Hoffman, Bruce (1996) 'Intelligence and Terrorism: Emerging Threats and New Security Challenges in the Post Cold-War Era', in *Intelligence and National Security* 11 (2) (April)

Holvast, J. (1993), 'Vulnerability and Privacy: Are We on the Way to a Risk-Free Society?', in J. Berleur *et al.* (eds) *Facing the Challenge of Risk and Vulnerability in an Information Society* Proceedings of the IFIP-WG9.2 Conference, Namur, May 20–22 1993, Elsevier Science Publ. B.V. (North-Holland), pp. 267–279

IINS News Service (1997) 'Hamas Using Internet for Attack Instructions', Israel, September 28

IITF (1995) Information Infrastructure Task Force – Privacy Working Group, *Privacy and the National Information Infrastructure: Principles for Providing and Using Personal Information* final version, June 1995

IITF (1997) Information Infrastructure Taskforce – Information Policy Committee, *Options for Promoting Privacy on the NII* Executive Summary, April 1997

Illegal and Harmful Content on the Internet (1996) *Communication to the European Parliament, the Council, the Economic and Social Committee and the Committee of the Regions* (CDM(96)487 final) 16 October.

—— (1997) *Resolution, European Parliament* 24 April

International Convention on the Elimination of All Forms of Racial Discrimination (CERD) (1995) *United Nations* December 1965

ITSEC (1991) *Information Technology Security Evaluation Criteria* (Provisional Harmonised Criteria) Luxembourg: Office for Official Publications of the European Communities

Jackson, M. (1998) 'The Development of Australian Law to Protect Undisclosed Business Information', Ph.D. Thesis, Law School, University of Melbourne

Japan (1994) Ministry of International Trade and Industry (MITI) *Programme for Advanced Information Infrastructure* May 1994

Johnson, L. Scott (1997) 'Toward a Functional Model of Information Warfare', in *Studies in Intelligence* No. 1 1997 (unclassified edition)

Johnston, L. (1991) 'Privatisation and the Police Function: From "New Police" to "New Policing" ', *Beyond Law and Order: Criminal Justice Policy and Politics into the 1990's* London: Macmillan

Joubert, Chantal and Bevers, Hans (1996) *Schengen Investigated* The Hague: Kluwer Law International

Junas, G. (1995) 'Angry White Guys with Guns: The Rise of the Citizen Militias', *Covert Action Quarterly* 23 April at http://nwcitizen.com/publicgood/reports/angryguy.html

Kabay, Mitch (1997) 'Strong Capital Sues Allege Hacker-Spammers', *Risks-Forum Digest* 19 (27) 1 August

Kane, Pamela. (1989) *V.I.R.U.S. Protection: Vital Information Resources Under Siege* New York: Bantam

Kaplan, D.E. and Marshall, A. (1996) *The Cult at the End of the World* Crown Publ.

Kapor, M. (1993) 'A Little Perspective, Please', *Forbes Magazine* 21 June 1993

Karsanova, E. (1999) 'Hackery za spravedlivost'. ('Hackers Stand for Justice'). *Moscow News* no. 8, 1999 (in Russian) http://www.mn.ru/1999/08/32.html (28 April 1999)

Keays, A. (1991) 'Software Trade Secret Protection', *Software Law Journal* 4: 577–595

Kelly, Kevin (1994) *Out of Control* Fourth Estate

Knight, V. (1978) 'Comments: Unfair Competition: A Comparative Study of Its Role in Common and Civil Law Systems', *Tulane Law Review* 53: 164–189

Koch, F. (1995) 'European Data Protection – Against the Internet?', *Privacy International Conference on Advanced Surveillance Technologies* Copenhagen, September 1995

Koop, B.-J. (1996) 'Encryption Law – II: A Survey of Cryptography Laws and Regulations', *Computer Law and Security Reporter* 12: 349–355

—— (1999) 'Crypto Law Survey', http://cwis/kub.nl/~frw/people/koops/lawsurvy.htm (February 1999)

Kruyer, P. (1997) 'Recent Developments in Organised Crime', *Proceedings of InfoWarCon 1997* 8–9 May, Brussels ERRI (1997) 'Colombian Officials Uncover Drug Cartel Communications Center', 31 May at http://www.emergency.com

Krylov, V. (1997) *Informazionnye kompjuternye prestupleniya. (Informational Computer Crimes)* Moscow: Infra-M Publ. (in Russian)

Kuehl, D. (1997) 'Defining Information Power', *Strategic Forum* no. 115 (June)

Kupperman, Robert (1991) 'Emerging Techno-Terrorism', in John Marks and Igor Belaiev (eds) *Common Grounds on Terrorism* New York: W.W. Norton

Kyl, Jon (1998) 'Military Computer Hackers Eluded Identification for Four Days During February Gulf Tensions', press release, 10 June 1998 at http://www.emergency.com

Landau, Henry (1934) *All's Fair: The Story of British Secret Service behind German Lines* New York: Puttnam

Laqueur, Walter (1985) *A World of Secrets: The Uses and Limits of Intelligence* New York: Basic

Leary, T., Metzner, R. and Alpert, R. (1999) *Psikhodelicheskii opyt. (Psychodelic experience)* Lviv: Nika-Tsentr Publ. (in Russian)

Leibov, R. (1999) 'Bratya nashi khakery'. ('Hackers – our Younger Brothers'), *Gazeta.RU* (electronic paper) issues, no. 028 and no. 033 (dates of publication: 8 April 1999, and 15 April1999), http://www.gazeta.ru/nl/08–04–1999_hackers_Printed.htm, and: http://www.gazeta.ru/nl/15–04–1999_hackers2_Printed.htm (in Russian) (28 April 1999)

Leistensnider, R. (1987) 'Trade Secret Misappropriation: What is the Proper Length of an Injunction After Public Disclosure?', *Albany Law Review* 51: 271–292

Levy, Steven (1984) *Hackers: Heroes of the Computer Revolution* New York: Bantam Doubleday Bell

—— (1996) 'Wisecrackers', *Wired* 2 (3) (March)

Libicki, Martin (1995) 'What Is Information Warfare?', Washington: US Government Printing Office, http://www.ndu.edu/inss/actpubs/ (19 December)

Littman, J. (1997) *The Watchman: The Twisted Life and Crimes of Serial Hacker Kevin Poulson* Little, Brown and Co.

Loader, B.D. (1997) *The Governance of Cyberspace: Politics, Technology and Global Restructuring* London: Routledge

—— (1998) *Cyberspace Divide: Equality, Agency and Policy in the Information Society* London: Routledge

Lundell, Allan (1989) *Virus! The Secret World of Computer Invaders that Breed and Destroy* Chicago: Contemporary Books

Lundheim, R. and Sindre, G. (1994) 'Privacy and Computing: a Cultural Perspective', in R. Sizer *et al.* (eds) *Security and Control of Information Technology in Society* IFIP WG 9.6 Working Conference, St Petersburg, August 1993, Elsevier Science Publ., pp. 25–40

Lyon, D. (1994) *The Electronic Eye: The Rise of the Surveillance Society* Cambridge: Polity Press

—— (1998) 'The World Wide Web of Surveillance: The Internet and Off-World Power-Flows', *Information Communication and Society* 1: 91–105

Madsen, W. (1992) *Handbook of Personal Data Protection* New York: Macmillan

—— (1993) 'Intelligence Threats to Computer Security', in *International Journal of Intelligence and Counterintelligence* 6 (4) (Winter)

—— (1995) 'Securing Access and Privacy on the Internet', in *Proceedings of the COMPSEC-Conference* London, October 1995, Elsevier Science Publ.

Malhotra, Y. (1996) 'Organizational Learning and Learning Organizations: An Overview', http://www.brint.com/papers/orglrng.htm

Manning, W.M. (1997) 'Should You Be on the Net?' *FBI Law Enforcement Bulletin* January, 18–22.

Markley, Robert (1996) *Virtual Reality and Their Discontents* Baltimore: Johns Hopkins

Markoff, J. (1994) 'Cyberspace's Most Wanted: Hacker Eludes FBI Pursuit', *New York Times* 4 July

—— (1998) 'U.S. Data-Scrambling Code Cracked with Homemade Equipment', *New York Times* 17 July

Markoff, J. and Hafner, K. (1996) 'Hackery' ('Hackers') Kiev: Poligraphkniga Publ. (in Russian)

Mathieson, T. (1997) 'The Viewer Society: Michel Foucault's "Panopticon" Revisited', *Theoretical Criminology* 1: 215–234

May, T.C. (1996a) 'Introduction to BlackNet', reprinted in P. Ludlow (ed.) *High Noon on the Electronic Frontier* MIT Press, pp. 241–243

—— (1996b) 'BlackNet Worries', in Peter Ludlow (ed.) *High Noon on the Electronic Frontier* MIT Press, pp. 245–249

Mayer-Schönberger, V. (1997) 'The Internet and Privacy Legislation: Cookies for a Threat?', *West Virginia Journal of Law and Technology*

McCullah, D. (1997) 'IRS Raids a Cypherpunk', *The Netly News* April 4.

McGrath, John E. (1998) 'After Privacy: Surveillance, Sexuality and the Electronic Self', paper presented at Surveillance: An Interdisciplinary Conference, John Moores University, Liverpool, 6 June

McLuhan, M. (1964) *Understanding Media* New York: New American Library

Meyer, Gordon and Thomas, Jim (1990) 'A Post Modernist Interpretation of the Computer Underground', http://www.eff.org./pub/Net_culture...nk

Michael, James (1994) *Privacy and Human Rights* Aldershot: Dartmouth

Miles, R.H. (1996) *Corporate Comeback: The Story Of Renewal And Transformation At National Semiconductor* Jossey-Bass Publ.

Ministry of Justice (1996) 'Rapport om etablering af et DNA register' ('Report on Establishing a DNA Register'), Copenhagen 1996

Minow, M. (1997) 'Swedish Narcotics Police Demand Telephone Card Database', *Risks-Forum Digest* 9 (7) April 14

Molander, R.C., Riddile, A.S. and Wilson, P. (1996) *Strategic Information Warfare: A New Face of War* Washington DC: RAND

Morley, D. (1980) *The 'Nationwide' Audience* London: British Film Institute

National Research Council (1996) *Cryptography's Role in Securing the Information Society* Washington DC: National Academy Press

Netscape (1997) 'The Open Profiling Standard (OPS)', http://developers. netscape.com/ops/ops.html

New Straits Times (1998) 'Third Suspect Held for Spreading Email Rumours', *New Straits Times* August 14

Nietzsche, F. (1997) *On the Genealogy of Morals* trans. M. Clark and A. Swensen, Indianapolis, IN: Hackett Publishing

Noon, Jeff (1993) *Vurt* Manchester: Ringpull Press

—— (1995) *Pollen* Manchester: Ringpull Press

Norris, C. and Armstrong, G. (1997) 'The Unforgiving Eye: CCTV Surveillance in Public Space', Centre for Criminology and Criminal Justice, The University of Missouri-St Louis

Nosik, A. (1999) 'Otvetny udar' ('Counterattack'), *Moscow News* no. 8, 1999 (in Russian) http://www.mn.ru/1999/08/32.html (28 April 1999)

Nutall, C. (1999) 'Virtual Country "Nuked" on Net' *BBC News* (published 26 January 1999) http://news.bbc.co.uk/hi/sci/tech/newsid_263000/263169.stm (26 January 1999)

(OECD) Organisation for Cooperation and Economic Development (1980) *Explanatory Memorandum to the Guidelines on the Protection of Privacy and Transborder Flows of Personal Data*

—— (1988) *Present Situation and Trends in Privacy Protection in the OECD Area*

—— (1992a) *Explanatory Memorandum to Accompany the Guidelines for the Security of Information Systems*

—— (1992b) *Guidelines for the Security of Information Systems*

—— (1997a) *Preamble, Recommendation of the Council Concerning Guidelines for Cryptography Policy*

—— (1997b) 'News Release: OECD Adopts Guidelines for Cryptography Policy', 27 March

—— (1997c) *Guidelines for Cryptography Policy*

—— (1998a) *Review of the 1992 Guidelines for the Security of Information Systems*, DSTI/ICCP/REG(97)2

—— (1998b) *Inventory of Controls on Cryptographic Technologies*, DSTI/ICCP/REG(98)4/FINAL

Office of the Undersecretary of Defense for Acquisition and Technology (1996) *Defense Science Board Task Force on Information Warfare – Defense* Washington DC: Department of Defense, November

O'Malley, Tom (1994) *Closedown* London: Pluto Press

Orlowski, S. (1997) Special Adviser on IT Security Policy, Commonwealth Attorney-General's Department, *Correspondence* 1 July

Palmer, Gareth (1998) 'Surveillance and Documentary Form', paper presented at Surveillance: An Interdisciplinary Conference, John Moores University, Liverpool, 6 June

Pattison, M. (1997) 'Cryptography and Privacy', Data Privacy and Protection IIR Conference, Sydney, 12 May 1997, pp. 3–10

PCCIP (Presidential Commission on Critical Infrastructure Protection) (1997) *Critical Foundations: Protecting America's Infrastructures* Government Printing Office: Washington DC

Petrakov, A.V. (1997) *Zaschita i okhrana lichnosti, sobstvennosti i informatsii* (*Security and Safeness of Personality, Property, and Information*) Moscow: Radio i Sviaz' Publ. (in Russian)

Philo, Greg and Miller, David (1997) *The Culture of Compliance* Glasgow: Glasgow Media Group

Pillsbury, M. (ed.) (1997) *Chinese Views of Future Warfare* Washington DC: National Defense University

Platonov, V., Medvedovsky, I. and Semjanov, P. (1997) 'Ataka cherez Internet' ('Attack via the Internet') St Peterburg: Mir i Semja Publ. (in Russian)

Poster, Mark (1990) *The Mode of Information: Poststructuralism and Social Context* Cambridge: Polity Press

Postman, Neil (1990) 'Informing ourselves to death', German Informatics Society, Stuttgart, http://www.eff.org/pub/Net culture

Poulsen, K. 'Many Happy Returns', on *The Switchroom* at http://www.catalog.com/Kevin

Powell, W.W. and DiMaggio, P.J. (eds) (1991) *The New Institutionalism in Organizational Analysis* Chicago: University of Chicago Press

Power, R. (1997) 'CSI Special Report: Salgado Case Reveals Darkside of Electronic Commerce', *Computer Security Alert* no. 174, September

Price, D. (1978) 'Comment: Misappropriation of Trade Secrets', *Tulane Law Review* 53: 215–253

Price, Monroe E. (1995) *Television, The Public Sphere and National Identity* Oxford: Clarendon Press

Quittner, J. (1994) 'Technology: Kevin Mitnick's Digital Obsession', *Time* 27 February 1994

Ramo, J.C. (1996) 'Crime Online', *Time Digital* 23 September: 28–32

Rastorguev, S.P. (1998) *Informazionnaya vojna.* (*Informational Warfare*) Moscow: Radio i Sviaz' Publ. (in Russian)

Rathmell, A. (1997a) 'Netwar in the Gulf', *Jane's Intelligence Review* 9 (1): 29–32

—— (1997b) 'Cyberterrorism: The Shape of Future Conflict?' *RUSI Journal* October: 40–45

—— (1998) 'Assessing the IW Capability of Sub-state Groups', in A. Campen and D. Dearth, *Cyberwar 2* Fairfax, VA: AFCEA, pp. 295–312

Rawlings, Philip (1991) 'Creeping Privatisation? The Police, the Conservative Government and Policing in the Late 1980s', in Robert Reiner and

Malcolm Cross (eds) *Beyond Law and Order: Criminal Justice Policy and Politics in the 1990s* London: Macmillan, pp. 41–58

Raymond, E.S. (1996) *Novy slovar' hackera (The New Hacker's Dictionary)* Moscow: TsentrKom Publ. (in Russian)

Regan, Priscilla M. (1995) *Legislating Privacy* Chapel Hill and London: University of North Carolina Press

Registratiekamer (1995) *Privacy-Enhancing Technologies: The Path to Anonymity* Volume II, Achtergrondstudies en Verkenningen 5B, Rijswijk

Registratiekamer/IPC (1995) Registratiekamer, the Netherlands and Information and Privacy Commissioner, Ontario, Canada *Privacy-Enhancing Technologies: The Path to Anonymity* Volume I, Achtergrondstudies en Verkenningen 5A

Reitinger, P.R. (1996) 'Compelled Production of Plaintext and Keys', in *The Law of Cyberspace* The University of Chicago Legal Forum, 1996

Report of the Commission on Illegal and Harmful Content on the Internet (1997) *Committee on Civil Liberties and Internal Affairs* Rapporteur – M. Pierre Pradier, European Parliament, 20 March

Restatement of the Law (1995) (Third) *Unfair Competition* American Law Institute

Restatement of Torts (First) (1939) American Law Institute

Reuters (1998) *Rebel Wars Spread to Cyberspace* 30 March

Richelson, Jeffery (1989) *The US Intelligence Community* New York: Ballinger (second edition)

Ricketson, S. (1984) *The Law of Intellectual Property* Sydney: Law Book Co., reprinted 1991

Rodota, Stefano (1992) 'Protecting Informational Privacy: Trends and Problems', in F. Willem, Altes Korthals, J. Egbert J. Dommering, P. Bernt Hugenholtz, Jan J.C. Kabel (eds) *Information Law Towards the 21st Century* Deventer-Boston, MA: Kluwer Law and Taxation Publisher

Ronfeldt, D. (1996) *Tribes, Institutions, Markets, Networks: A Framework About Societal Evolution* Santa Monica: RAND, P-7967

Rose, N. (1989) *Governing the Soul: The Shaping of the Private Self* London: Routledge

Rosenberg, R. (1992) *The Social Impact of Computers* Academic Press

Ross, Andrew (1991) *Strange Weather: Culture, Science and Technology in the Age of Limits* London: Verso

Sardar, Ziauddin and Ravetz, Jerome (1996) *Cyberfutures: Culture and Politics on the Information Superhighway* London: Pluto Press

Savage, M. (1998) 'Discipline, Surveillance and the "Career": Employment on the Great Western Railway 1833–1914', in A. McKinlay and K. Starkey (eds) *Foucault. Management and Organizational Theory* London: Sage

Scallingi, Paula (1995) 'Proliferation and Arms Control', *Intelligence and National Security* 10 (4) (October)

Scannel, P. (1989) 'Public Service Broadcasting and modern public life', *Media, Culture and Society* 11: 135–166

Schlesinger, Philip and Tumber, David (1994) *Reporting Crime: The Media Politics of Criminal Justice* Oxford University Press: Oxford

Schoben, Ann (ed.) (1995) 'Information Warfare: A Two Edged Sword', in Rand Research Review: *Information Warfare and Cyberspace Security* http://rand.org/RRR/RRR.fall95.cyber, (19 December)

Schwartau, W. (1996) *Information Warfare* New York: Thunder's Mouth Press (second edition)

Security Service Commissioner (1995) *1995 Annual Report of the Security Commissioner* London: HMSO, CMD 2827

Shipilov, A. (1999) 'Hackeram nadajut po mozgam' ('Hackers will be Beaten') *Computerra Online, no. 14* 1999, http://www.computerra.ru.hot/hackers.html?inside (in Russian) (28 April 1999)

Shulsky, Avram (1989) *Silent Warfare: Understanding the World of Intelligence* London: Brasseys

Simon, J. and Freely, M. (1995) 'True Crime: The New Penology and Public Discourse on Crime', in T. Bloomberg and S. Cohen (eds) *Punishment and Social Control* New York: Walter de Gruyter

Simons, John (1995) *Foucault and the Political* London: Routledge

Singapore (1991) National Computer Board (NCB)/ Singapore, *IT2000 – A Vision of an Intelligent Island* August 1991

Soo Hoo, K., Goodman, S. and Greenberg, L. (1997) 'Information Technology and the Terrorist Threat', *Survival* 39 (3): 135–155

Stafford, David (1983) *Britain and European Resistance 1940–1945* Toronto: University of Toronto Press

Starr, B. (1999) 'Pentagon Cyber-War. Attack Mounted Through Russia', *ABC News* http://www.abcnews.go.com/sections/world/DailyNews/pentagonrussia990304.html (21 April 1999)

Stengers, Jean (1984,) 'The French, the British, the Poles and Enigma', in Christopher Andrew and David Dilks (eds) *The Missing Dimension: Governments and Intelligence Communities in the Twentieth Century* Chicago: University of Chicago Press

Stephenson, Neal (1992) *Snow Crash* New York: Bantam Spectra

Sterling, B. (1992) *The Hacker Crackdown: Law and Disorder on the Electronic Frontier* NY: Bantam Books; and http://www.farcaster.com/sterling/contents.html

—— (ed.) (1986) *Mirrorshades: The Cyberpunk Anthology* London: Paladin

Stern, K. (1998) *A Force Upon The Plain – The American Militia Movement and The Politics of Hate* Norman and London, University of Oklahoma Press

Stoll, Clifford (1989) *The Cuckoo's Egg: Tracking a Spy through the Maze of Computer Espionage* New York: Pocket Books

—— (1990) *The Cuckoo's Egg* London: Pan

—— (1996) *Yaitso kukushki (The Cuckoo's Egg)* Moscow: ITS-Garant Publ. (in Russian)

Swinburne, P. (1998) 'Countering Computer Crime', lecture to ICSA seminar series Intelligence and International Security, 3 February

Taylor, Paul (1993) 'Hackers: A Case Study of the Social Shaping of

Computing', Ph.D. dissertation, Research Centre for Social Sciences, University of Edinburgh

—— (1997) 'Them and Us', *Computer Underground Digest* 9 (59), 27 July at http://www-swiss.ai.mit.edu/6805/articles/taylor-them-and-us.txt

TCSEC (1985) *DoD Trusted Computer Systems Evaluation Criteria* DoD 5200.28-STD, Washington DC: Department of Defence

Thompson, J.P. (1990) *Ideology and Modern Culture* Cambridge: Polity Press

Toffler, Alvin and Toffler, Heidi (1995) *War and Antiwar* New York: Warner

Turkle, S. (1984) *The Second Self: Computers and the Human Spirit* NY: Simon and Schuster

Tyrrell, P. (1997) 'The Business of Integrity', *Proceedings of Infowarcon 97* Brussels, 8–9 May 1997

Uniform Trade Secret Act (1985) *Amendments* United States

Urban, M. (1996) *UK Eyes Alpha: The Inside Story of British Intelligence* London: Faber & Faber

US Congress (1997a) Statement of Louis J. Freeh, Director FBI, before the Senate Committee on Commerce, Science, and Transportation, regarding the Impact of Encryption on Law Enforcement and Public Safety, March 19

US Congress (1997b) Jeffrey A. Herig, Special Agent, Florida Department of Law Enforcement, 'The Encryption Debate: Criminals, Terrorists, and the Security Needs of Business and Industry', testimony before the Senate Judiciary Subcommittee on Technology, Terrorism, and Government Information, September 3

US Department of Commerce (1997) *Privacy and Self-Regulation in the Information Age* Washington DC: June 1997, http://www.ntia.doc.gov/reports/privacy/

US Government (1993) *The National Information Infrastructure (NII) Program – Agenda for Action*

Vakka, J. (1997) *Sekrety bezopasnosti v Internet* (*Secrets of the Internet Security*) Kiev: Dialektika Publ (in Russian)

Vallee, Jacques (1984) *The Network Revolution: Confessions of a Network Scientist* London: Penguin Books

Verfassungsschutzbericht (1996) *Bundesministerium des Innern* Bonn

Verfassungsschutzbericht (1997) *Bundesministerium des Innern* Bonn

Verbitskaya, O. (1999) 'Hacker dolzhen sidet' v tiur'me?!' ('A Hacker Should be Imprisoned?!') *Mir Internet* 2: 18––19 (in Russian) http://www.piter-press.ru (22 April 1999)

Verrier, Anthony (1983) *Through the Looking Glass* London: Jonathan Cape

Verstraeten, Hans (1996) 'A Contribution for a Critical Political Economy of the Public Sphere' *European Journal of Communication* 11 (3) 347–370

Virilio, Paul (1980) 'The Work of Art in the Age of Electronic Reproduction', interview in *Block* 14: 4–7

Walker, Martin (1996) 'Datastream Cowboy Fixes Pentagon in his Sights', in *The Guardian* 24 May

Walklate, Sandra (1991) 'Victims, Crime and Social Control', in Robert

Reiner and Malcolm Cross *Beyond Law and Order: Criminal Justice Policy and Politics in the 1990s* London: Macmillan, pp. 204–222

Ward, Mark (1997a) 'Coded Message Plan "Too Complex" ', *New Scientist* 26 April.

—— (1997b) 'Net Surfers Set Cracking Pace', *New Scientist* 28 June

—— (1997c) 'The Secret's Out', in *New Scientist* 6 September

Wark, McKenzie (1992) 'Cyberpunk: from subculture to mainstream', http://www.eff.org./pub/Net_culture...unk_subculture_to_mainstream.paper

Wassenaar Arrangement on Export Controls for Conventional Arms and Dual-Use Goods and Technologies July 1996

Weizenbaum, J. (1976) *Computer Power and Human Reason: From Judgement to Calculation* New York: W.H. Freeman

—— (1982) *Vozmozhnosti vychslitel'nykh mashin i chelovecheskii razum Ot suzhdenii k vychisleniyam. (Computer Power and Human Reason. From Judgement to Calculation)* Moscow: Radio i Svyz' Publ. (in Russian)

Westin, A. (1967) *Privacy and Freedom* New York

Whitacker, Reg (1996) 'The "Bristow Affair": A Crisis of Accountability in Canadian Security Intelligence', in *Intelligence and National Security* 11 (2) April

White House (1995) Remarks by the President to Staff of the CIA and Intelligence Community, Central Intelligence Agency, McLean, VA, July 14

—— (1998a) 'Administration Updates Encryption Policy', statement by the Press Secretary and fact sheet, September

—— (1998b) *White Paper: The Clinton Administration's Policy on Critical Infrastructure Protection: Presidential Decision Directive 63* 22 May

Wiggins, Gary (1996) 'Data Needs of Academic Research on the Internet', http://www.indiana.edu/~cheminfo/gw/nist_csanewsl.html (24 January 1997)

Williams, P. (1994) 'Transnational Criminal Organisations and International Security', *Survival* 36 (1): 96–113

Wise, A. (1981) *Trade Secrets and Know-How Throughout the World* New York: Clark Boardman Company Ltd

Woolgar, Steve and Russell, Geoff (1990) 'The Social Basis of Computer Viruses', *CRICT Discussion Paper* Brunel University

(WIPO) World Intellectual Property Organization (1994) *Protection Against Unfair Competition*

(WTO) World Trade Organisation (1996) 'Intellectual Property Rights – Providing Protection and Enforcement', http://www.wto.org

Worrall, Arme (1997) *Punishment in the Community: The Future of Criminal Justice* New York: Addison Wesley Longman

Zegzhda, D.P. and Ivashko A.M. (1998) 'Kak postroit' zaschischonnuyu informazionnuyu sistemu' ('How to Build a Secure Information System'), St Petersburg: Mir i Semja Publ. (in Russian)

Index